George G. Howard Jr.

Update in Childhood and Adolescent Obesity

Guest Editors

MIRIAM VOS, MD, MSPH
SARAH E. BARLOW, MD, MPH

PEDIATRIC CLINICS
OF NORTH AMERICA

www.pediatric.theclinics.com

December 2011 • Volume 58 • Number 6

SAUNDERS an imprint of ELSEVIER, Inc.

W.B. SAUNDERS COMPANY
A Division of Elsevier Inc.

1600 John F. Kennedy Boulevard • Suite 1800 • Philadelphia, Pennsylvania 19103-2899

http://www.theclinics.com

THE PEDIATRIC CLINICS OF NORTH AMERICA Volume 58, Number 6
December 2011 ISSN 0031-3955, ISBN-13: 978-1-4557-1230-4

Editor: Kerry Holland
Developmental Editor: Donald Mumford

The Pediatric Clinics of North America (ISSN 0031-3955) is published bimonthly by Elsevier Inc., 360 Park Avenue South, New York, NY 10010-1710. Months of issue are February, April, June, August, October, and December. Periodicals postage paid at New York, NY and additional mailing offices. Subscription prices are $191.00 per year (US individuals), $444.00 per year (US institutions), $259.00 per year (Canadian individuals), $591.00 per year (Canadian institutions), $308.00 per year (international individuals), $591.00 per year (international institutions), $93.00 per year (US students and residents), and $159.00 per year (international and Canadian residents and students). To receive students/resident rare, orders must be accompanied by name of affiliated institution, date of term, and the signature of program/residency coordinator on institution letterhead. Orders will be billed at individual rate until proof of status is received. Foreign air speed delivery is included in all *Clinics* subscription prices. All prices are subject to change without notice. **POSTMASTER:** Send address changes to *The Pediatric Clinics of North America*, Elsevier Health Sciences Division, Subscription Customer Service, 3251 Riverport Lane, Maryland Heights, MO 63043. **Customer Service: 1-800-654-2452 (US and Canada). From outside of the US and Canada: 1-314-447-8871. Fax: 1-314-447-8029. For print support, E-mail: JournalsCustomerService-usa@elsevier.com. For online support, E-mail: JournalsOnlineSupport-usa@elsevier.com.**

Reprints. For copies of 100 or more, of articles in this publication, please contact the Commercial Reprints Department, Elsevier Inc., 360 Park Avenue South, New York, NY 10010-1710. Tel.: 212-633-3812; Fax: 212-462-1935; E-mail: reprints@elsevier.com.

The Pediatric Clinics of North America is also published in Spanish by McGraw-Hill Inter-americana Editores S.A., Mexico City, Mexico; in Portuguese by Riechmann and Affonso Editores, Rua Comandante Coelho 1085, CEP 21250, Rio de Janeiro, Brazil; and in Greek by Althayia SA, Athens, Greece.

The Pediatric Clinics of North America is covered in *MEDLINE/PubMed (Index Medicus), Excerpta Medica, Current Contents, Current Contents/Clinical Medicine, Science Citation Index, ASCA, ISI/BIOMED,* and *BIOSIS.*

Printed in the United States of America.

Contributors

GUEST EDITORS

MIRIAM VOS, MD, MSPH
Assistant Professor of Pediatrics, Emory University, and Research Program Director, Children's Healthcare of Atlanta, Atlanta, Georgia

SARAH E. BARLOW, MD, MPH
Associate Professor of Pediatrics, Baylor College of Medicine, and Director of the Center for Childhood Obesity, Texas Children's Hospital, Houston, Texas

AUTHORS

REBECCA BROWN, MD, MHSc
Senior Fellow in Clinical Research, Diabetes, Endocrinology and Obesity Branch, National Institute of Diabetes, Digestive and Kidney Diseases, Bethesda, Maryland

SONIA CAPRIO, MD
Department of Pediatrics, Yale University School of Medicine, New Haven, Connecticut

STEPHEN COOK, MD, MPH, FAAP, FTOS
Department of Pediatrics, Golisano Children's Hospital, University of Rochester Medical Center, Rochester, New York

SOLVEIG A. CUNNINGHAM, PhD
Assistant Professor, Hubert Department of Global Health, Rollins Schools of Public Health, Emory University, Atlanta, Georgia

LAURENCE M. DENIS, MD, MPH
Michael & Susan Dell Center for Healthy Living, University of Texas School of Public Health, Austin, Texas

JOSEPH E. DONNELLY, EdD
Department of Internal Medicine, University of Kansas Medical Center, Kansas City, Kansas

JENNIFER L. FOLTZ, MD, MPH
Division of Nutrition, Physical Activity, and Obesity, National Center for Chronic Disease Prevention and Health Promotion, Centers for Disease Control and Prevention, Atlanta, Georgia

K. GORMAN, MS, RD, LDN
Nutrition and Fitness for Life Program (Pediatric Obesity), Department of Pediatrics, Boston Medical Center, Boston, Massachusetts

KIRSTEN A. GRIMM, MPH
Division of Nutrition, Physical Activity, and Obesity, National Center for Chronic Disease Prevention and Health Promotion, Centers for Disease Control and Prevention, Atlanta, Georgia

JOSEPH G. GRZYWACZ, PhD
Department of Family and Community Medicine, Wake Forest University School of Medicine, Winston-Salem, North Carolina

DIANE M. HARRIS, PhD, MPH
Division of Nutrition, Physical Activity, and Obesity, National Center for Chronic Disease Prevention and Health Promotion, Centers for Disease Control and Prevention, Atlanta, Georgia

CHARLES J. HOMER, MD, MPH
National Initiative for Children's Healthcare Quality; Department of Pediatrics, Harvard Medical School and Children's Hospital, Boston, Massachusetts

MEGAN B. IRBY, MS
Department of Pediatrics, Wake Forest University School of Medicine; Brenner FIT Program, Brenner Children's Hospital, Winston-Salem, North Carolina

ANDREA E. KASS, MA
Department of Psychiatry, Washington University School of Medicine, St Louis, Missouri

RAE ELLEN W. KAVEY, MD, MPH, FAAP, FAHA
Department of Pediatrics, Golisano Children's Hospital, University of Rochester Medical Center, Rochester, New York

GRACE KIM, MD
Department of Pediatrics, Yale University School of Medicine, New Haven, Connecticut

SONIA A. KIM, PhD
Division of Nutrition, Physical Activity, and Obesity, National Center for Chronic Disease Prevention and Health Promotion, Centers for Disease Control and Prevention, Atlanta, Georgia

JOEL KIMMONS, PhD
Division of Nutrition, Physical Activity, and Obesity, National Center for Chronic Disease Prevention and Health Promotion, Centers for Disease Control and Prevention, Atlanta, Georgia

RACHEL P. KOLKO, MA
Department of Psychiatry, Washington University School of Medicine, St Louis, Missouri

KATE LAMBOURNE, PhD
Department of Internal Medicine, University of Kansas Medical Center, Kansas City, Kansas

JOEL E. LAVINE, MD, PhD
Professor of Pediatrics, Division of Pediatric Gastroenterology, Hepatology and Nutrition, Columbia University, New York, New York

C.M. LENDERS, MD, MS, ScD
Associate Professor of Pediatrics, Nutrition and Fitness for Life Program (Pediatric Obesity), Department of Pediatrics, Boston University School of Medicine, Boston Medical Center; Harvard Medical School, Boston, Massachusetts

A. LIM-MILLER, MSW, LICSW
Nutrition and Fitness for Life Program (Pediatric Obesity), Department of Pediatrics, Boston Medical Center, Boston, Massachusetts

ASHLEIGH L. MAY, PhD
Division of Nutrition, Physical Activity, and Obesity, National Center for Chronic Disease Prevention and Health Promotion, Centers for Disease Control and Prevention, Atlanta, Georgia

SARAH MCKETTA, A.B
SM Candidate, Harvard School of Public Health, Boston, Massachusetts

MARIANNE E. MCPHERSON, MS, PhD
National Initiative for Children's Healthcare Quality, Boston, Massachusetts

ALI A. MENCIN, MD
Assistant Professor of Pediatrics, Division of Pediatric Gastroenterology, Hepatology and Nutrition, Columbia University, New York, New York

GARY MILLER, PhD
Department of Health and Exercise Science, Wake Forest University, Winston-Salem, North Carolina

ELISHA R. MITCHELL, MS
Doctoral Candidate, Department of Psychology, Saint Louis University, St Louis, Missouri

J. PRATT, MD
Weight Loss Surgery Program, Department of Surgery, Massachusetts General Hospital, and Harvard Medical School, Boston, Massachusetts

S. PUKLIN, BS
Boston University School of Medicine, Boston Medical Center, Boston, Massachusetts

MICHAEL RICH, MD, MPH
Director, Center on Media and Child Health, Children's Hospital Boston, Boston, Massachusetts

KRISTINA I. ROTHER, MD, MHSc
Senior Staff Clinical Investigator, Diabetes, Endocrinology and Obesity Branch, National Institute of Diabetes, Digestive and Kidney Diseases, Bethesda, Maryland

JOSEPH A. SKELTON, MD, MS
Departments of Pediatrics and Epidemiology and Prevention, Wake Forest University School of Medicine; Brenner FIT Program, Brenner Children's Hospital, Winston-Salem, North Carolina

ALLISON SYLVETSKY, BA
Graduate Division of Biological and Biomedical Sciences, Emory University, Atlanta, Georgia

JILLON S. VANDER WAL, PhD
Associate Professor, Department of Psychology, Saint Louis University, St Louis, Missouri

ELIZABETH A. VANDEWATER, PhD
Associate Professor of Health Promotion and Behavioral Sciences, Michael & Susan Dell Center for Healthy Living, University of Texas School of Public Health, Austin, Texas

JEAN A. WELSH, PhD, MPH, RN
Postdoctoral Fellow, Department of Pediatrics, Emory University School of Medicine, Atlanta, Georgia

DENISE E. WILFLEY, PhD
Department of Psychiatry, Washington University School of Medicine, St Louis, Missouri

Contents

Context

> Childhood obesity is a profoundly complex problem and serves as an example of a biospsychosocial issue. Scientific inquiry has provided incredible insight into the complex etiology of weight gain but must be viewed as an interaction between a human's propensity to conserve calories for survival in a world with an abundance of it. This article provides a brief overview divided between biological (nature) and psychosocial and behavioral (nurture) factors.

Comorbidities

> Over the past 2 decades, the prevalence of obesity and type 2 diabetes mellitus (T2DM) in children and adolescents has risen to epidemic proportions and disproportionately affects racial and ethnic minorities, who are at greater risk. The pathophysiology of T2DM is complex and involves insulin resistance, pancreatic β-cell dysfunction, and visceral adiposity. Current treatments of T2DM are limited to lifestyle intervention, metformin, and insulin therapy; use of these strategies in combination is often most effective. The role of research is to uncover simple biomarkers for insulin sensitivity and optimal and innovative treatment of insulin resistance and T2DM.

> Cardiovascular disease is the leading cause of death in the United States despite a reduction in mortality over the past 4 decades. Much of this success is attributed to public health efforts and more aggressive treatment of clinical disease. The rising rates of obesity and diabetes, especially among adolescents and young adults, raise concern for increases in mortality. National vital statistics have shown a leveling of cardiovascular disease death rates in the fifth decade of life. Public health efforts have begun to address childhood obesity. This article reviews the dyslipidemia associated with obesity in childhood and outlines a proposed approach to management.

5 years of obesity diagnosis is particularly concerning. Because health risk increases with degree of obesity, adolescents who may be eligible for more aggressive obesity treatment should be identified and counseled.

FORTHCOMING ISSUES

RECENT ISSUES

THE CLINICS ARE NOW AVAILABLE ONLINE!

Access your subscription at:
www.theclinics.com

Preface

Update in Childhood and Adolescent Obesity

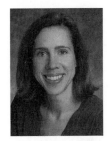 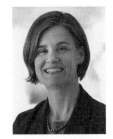

Miriam Vos, MD, MSPH   Sarah E. Barlow, MD, MPH
Guest Editors

It has been just over 10 years since the last time the *Pediatric Clinics of North America* has had an issue focused on Childhood and Adolescent Obesity. Over this time, the epidemic has worsened and then plateaued. The most recent NHANES data available from 2007/2008 show mixed results: prevalence of obesity has not increased significantly since 1999, except among more severely obese boys (**Fig 1**). In women over 20 years of age, a group that strongly influences children, the increase in obesity rates has slowed but not yet decreased. Interpretation of these data is subjective to some extent. The optimist perceives that slowing or stabilization is a response to the valiant efforts extended over the past 10 years and is the first step toward reduction. After all, we applaud weight maintenance in patients as a step toward weight loss. The pessimist observes that not a single state met the US *Healthy People 2010* goal to lower obesity to 15%. In fact, between 2000 and 2010, 12 states crossed the threshold of having ≥30% obese adults. Clearly much work remains to be done. We hope current levels represent the crest and that future surveys will reveal an ebbing of the high numbers of overweight and obese children.

There is certainly evidence that the tide has turned in the *approach* to the problem. In 2001, Guest Editor Dr Dennis Styne wrote about treatment and prevention of childhood obesity and advocated for changes, stating, "it is clear that the medical model of therapy cannot be the answer." Today, prevention of childhood obesity is the focus of a major campaign by the First Lady, Michelle Obama, and is the object of state and city campaigns across the United States as efforts to address the problem expand beyond the health care setting. Over the past 10 years, approaches to childhood obesity have continued to evolve, from individual to comprehensive.

This evolution has occurred perhaps as a result of the failure of the medical model but more importantly because of acknowledgment that community, culture, and society play important roles in the causes of the current epidemic. "Treatment" needs

Pediatr Clin N Am 58 (2011) xv–xvii
doi:10.1016/j.pcl.2011.09.016
0031-3955/11/$ – see front matter © 2011 Elsevier Inc. All rights reserved.

pediatric.theclinics.com

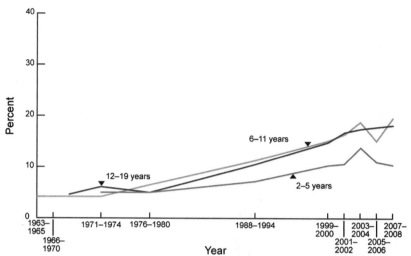

Fig. 1. Trends in obesity among children and adolescents: United States, 1963-2008. Health E-Stat Prevalence of Obesity Among Children and Adolescents: United States, Trends 1963-1965 Through 2007-2008. National Center for Health Statistics. Health, United States, 2000. Hyattsville, MD: Public Health Service; 2010.

to address cause, and, when the cause is the many changes in how we live, a pharmaceutical response is meager at best. We need to modify those lifestyle patterns.

Many aspects of society unintentionally support obesity-promoting behaviors. Although most businesses do not explicitly concern themselves with health, a byproduct of a successful business model may be the promotion of nutrient-poor food. The "individual choice" of a parent at the grocery store is often influenced by a spiderweb of packaging, branding, and marketing, not only in the grocery store but also in media that target parents or children. Health care providers and health-conscious organizations and individuals can ask parents to serve more vegetables, but we need to recognize and moderate the diverse influences shaping parent and child choice. Social policies should evaluate business subsidies and incentives from a perspective of promoting good health.

Schools have focused on test scores because of pressure to improve academic performance. However, schools oversee up to 2 meals per day and half the waking hours of a typical child. Can we really give these institutions a pass on taking care of children's health? Schools are not alone. Comprehensive change means collaboration and participation from churches, daycares, community centers, sport programs, businesses, health care facilities, employers, and government at all levels. All of these entities can have a positive influence on long-term health.

Health care facilities including hospitals and physician offices need to continue to be leaders. For example, Nationwide Children's has removed sugar-sweetened beverages from its campus. Children's Healthcare of Atlanta has initiated a comprehensive employee wellness program including walking paths around the hospital and aerobics classes in the hallways. Physicians have traditionally lacked training in effective counseling techniques, but the tide has changed on this as well with motivational interviewing classes and improved counseling workshops at many conferences and institutions. Setting a good example and effectively educating parents early are two of the top responsibilities of pediatricians and the institutions with which we work.

This issue contains articles from experts in many contributing fields with exciting new information. The authors have summarized the tremendous advancement in the last decade in research on obesity-related medical conditions, including fatty liver disease, in genetic and metabolic contributors to obesity, and in the still-difficult approaches to treatment. In addition, a number of articles summarize topics and directions new to the field of childhood obesity in the last decade: artificial sweeteners, the challenges and potential of social media, and an overview of policies that support obesity prevention. Although the readers of this journal in general are grounded in health care practice, we know pediatric health care providers appreciate the importance of the home and community context of their patients. Historically, pediatric providers strive not only to treat illness but also to promote each child's life trajectory of good health and wellness, appreciating the influences of family, community, and society as a whole.

The medical model is reshaping, and physicians continue to hold a vital leadership role in the integrated model of childhood obesity prevention and in the lives of our individual patients and their families. Pediatricians are using the unique relationship they have with the families of young children to support early introduction of healthy habits that will synergize with the changes in policy, media, behavioral health, and schools.

Much remains to be done, but we seem to have set sail in the right direction.

ACKNOWLEDGMENTS

Dr Vos is supported in part by the National Institutes of Health (NIH)/National Institute of Diabetes and Digestive and Kidney Diseases Grant K23DK080953.

Miriam Vos, MD, MSPH
Emory University and
Children's Healthcare of Atlanta
2015 Uppergate Drive, NE, Atlanta, GA 30322, USA

Sarah E. Barlow, MD, MPH
Baylor College of Medicine
Texas Children's Hospital
6701 Fannin Suite 1010
Houston, TX 77030, USA

E-mail addresses:
mvos@emory.edu (M. Vos)
sbarlow@bcm.edu (S.E. Barlow)

Etiologies of Obesity in Children: Nature and Nurture

Joseph A. Skelton, MD, MS[a,b,c,]*, Megan B. Irby, MS[a,b],
Joseph G. Grzywacz, PhD[d], Gary Miller, PhD[e]

KEYWORDS

- Etiology • Obesity • Pediatrics • Genetics

Scientific inquiry has provided incredible insight into the causes of and contributors to childhood obesity, a profoundly complex biopsychosocial issue. An ecological approach to understanding obesity best captures the overlapping factors involved (**Fig. 1**).[1] In this article, the authors provide a brief overview divided between biological (nature) and psychosocial and behavioral (nurture) factors. However, as with any complex condition, the line between the two can often be blurred.

NATURE

The genetic and biological determinants of weight and obesity are intertwined. With the discovery of leptin in 1994,[2] the understanding of energy regulation, appetite, and adiposity has exploded, and the field has become increasingly complex as a result. Continued discoveries implicate other contributors, from intestinal microbes to stress.

Support: Supported in part by a grant from The Kate B. Reynolds Charitable Foundation (MBI) and NICHD/NIH Mentored Patient-Oriented Research Career Development Award K23 HD061597 (JAS).
[a] Department of Pediatrics, Wake Forest University School of Medicine, Medical Center Boulevard, Winston-Salem, NC 27157, USA
[b] Brenner FIT Program, Brenner Children's Hospital, Medical Center Boulevard, Winston-Salem, NC 27157, USA
[c] Department of Epidemiology and Prevention, Wake Forest University School of Medicine, Medical Center Boulevard, Winston-Salem, NC 27157, USA
[d] Department of Family and Community Medicine, Wake Forest University School of Medicine, Medical Center Boulevard, Winston-Salem, NC 27157, USA
[e] Department of Health and Exercise Science, Wake Forest University, 1834 Wake Forest Road, Winston-Salem, NC 27109, USA
* Corresponding author. Department of Pediatrics, Wake Forest University School of Medicine, Medical Center Boulevard, Winston-Salem, NC 27157.
E-mail address: jskelton@wakehealth.edu

Pediatr Clin N Am 58 (2011) 1333–1354
doi:10.1016/j.pcl.2011.09.006
0031-3955/11/$ – see front matter

pediatric.theclinics.com

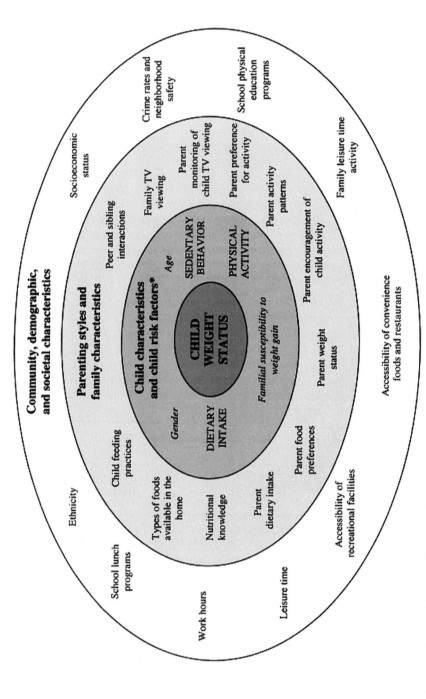

Fig. 1. Ecological model of predictors of childhood obesity.

Neuroendocrine Control of Body Weight

In simplest terms, neuroendocrine control of weight is a balance between short- and long-term control of weight, overall energy intake, and energy expenditure. This balance can also be better understood when divided between the central nervous system (primarily the brain) and the body (primarily the gastrointestinal [GI] tract and adipose tissue).[3–5]

Short-term control

Short-term control of body weight largely concerns control of energy intake.[3,5] Meal initiation is primarily influenced by environmental stimuli such as food, emotions, time of the day, and peers.[6] However, once the meal begins, neuroendocrine factors exert significant influence, thereby affecting the size of the meal, the amount of energy ingested, and when the meal is terminated (**Table 1**).[3,5] Some signals released in response to ingested or circulating nutrients coordinate the digestion and absorption of nutrients and feelings of satiety.[7] Opposing signals, such as those initiated by ghrelin, act to stimulate appetite by increasing before a meal and decreasing after a meal is finished. In obese individuals, serum ghrelin levels are decreased and, alone, are unlikely to be a significant contributor to individual obesity status. However, ghrelin tends to increase during diet-induced weight loss and may explain increased levels of hunger with dieting.[8] Most of the short-term GI signals have local effects, such as slowing gastric emptying and overall proximal GI motility,[7] and also act centrally, either directly or via vagal actions.[3–5,7]

Long-term control

Long-term control is divided between the brain and body through levels of adiposity. These adiposity signals from the body act to communicate energy storage levels centrally, which then act to adjust energy intake and expenditure (**Table 2**).

The primary signals from the body are leptin and insulin, both of which exhibit long-term control of food intake and metabolism.[5] Leptin is secreted in proportion to fat content of adipocytes and downregulates neurons that control food intake in the arcuate nucleus.[3–5] Obese individuals may have relative leptin resistance, similar to

Table 1
Signals involved in the short-term control of body weight

Name	Origin	Action and Effect
Amylin	Pancreas (β-cells); cosecreted with insulin	Reduces meal size via brainstem mechanisms
Cholecystokinin	Intestine (I-cells)	Controls meal size by slowing gastric emptying, stimulates gallbladder contractions, likely activates vagal receptors to terminate meal
Ghrelin	Stomach	Potent appetite stimulation, likely via central nervous system mechanism
Glucagonlike peptide 1	Intestines (L-cells)	Stimulates insulin release, reduces appetite
Oxyntomodulin	Colon	Reduces appetite
Pancreatic polypeptide	Pancreas	Reduces appetite, likely by inhibiting pancreatic, gallbladder, and GI tract activity
Peptide YY (PYY$_{3-36}$)	Intestines (ileum/colon), cosecreted with glucagonlike peptide 1	Reduces appetite, slows gastric emptying

Table 2
Signals involved in the long-term control of body weight

Name	Origin	Action and Effect
Adiponectin	Adipose tissue	Enhances insulin sensitivity, decreases inflammation
Agouti-related peptide	Arcuate nucleus (hypothalamus)	Increases appetite, decreases metabolism
Arcuate nucleus	Hypothalamus	Area of energy regulation; location of CART, POMC, AgRP, NPY
Cocaine-amphetamine– regulated transcript neurons	Arcuate nucleus (hypothalamus)	Reduces energy intake
Insulin	Pancreas	Reduces energy intake
Leptin	Adipose tissue	Reduces energy intake
α-Melanocyte–stimulating hormone	POMC (ARC, hypothalamus)	Reduces energy intake
Neuropeptide Y	Arcuate nucleus	Increases appetite; decreases metabolism
Orexin	Hypothalamus	Increases appetite
Oxyntomodulin	Colon	Reduces appetite
Pro-opiomelanocortin	Arcuate nucleus (hypothalamus)	Releases α-melanocyte–stimulating hormone, reduces energy intake
Periventricular nucleus	Hypothalamus	Appetite and autonomic regulation

insulin resistance, contributing to obesity.[9,10] As with leptin, serum insulin levels increase in proportion to body fat and act centrally to relay energy stores.

An important discovery in the understanding of weight control is the endocrine function of adipose tissue.[11] Leptin has an important role in the long-term control of body weight,[12] whereas other hormones and cytokines released from adipose tissue affect overall health. Adiponectin has an important antiinflammatory function in the body and is generally viewed as a protective countermechanism to inflammatory processes originating in adipose tissues.[13] Visceral adiposity, long known to be linked to the metabolic syndrome and cardiovascular disease, is detrimental to health through inflammatory mechanisms, primarily through adipokines.[11] Interleukin 6, tumor necrosis factor α, plasminogen activator inhibitor 1, and visfatin are adipose-derived signals involved in atherosclerosis, insulin resistance, and inflammation.[3–5]

The brain's principal region for energy balance is the arcuate nucleus, located in the hypothalamus, which controls energy intake (eating) and expenditure (metabolism).[3–5] In addition to direct influence by circulating nutrients indicating satiation (eg, glucose, fatty acids, and some amino acids), the arcuate nucleus receives signals from leptin and insulin, expressing receptors for most adiposity signals regulating long-term control of weight. Neurons controlling these processes are agouti-related peptide/ neuropeptide Y (AgRP/NPY) and pro-opiomelanocortin/cocaine-regulated and amphetamine-regulated transcript (POMC/CART). AgRP/NPY neurons are anabolic in nature, stimulating appetite and reducing metabolism, whereas POMC/CART neurons are catabolic, inhibiting food intake via release of α-melanocyte–stimulating hormone. Neurons of the arcuate nucleus project to many other areas of the brain, particularly the hypothalamic paraventricular nucleus and the lateral hypothalamus.[5] The paraventricular nucleus is a major determinant of energy expenditure, synthesizing anorexigenic factors corticotropin-releasing hormone and oxytocin, thereby regulating the body's response to stress. The lateral hypothalamus is responsible for orexigenic peptides, melanin-concentrating hormone, and orexin. Other areas of the brain key to control of body weight are also influenced by hypothalamic projections. The mesolimbic-dopamine system influences the body's hedonic and reward responses to food. The autonomic centers of the brainstem exert influence on the GI tract. **Fig. 2** illustrates how short- and long-term control of weight across the body and brain are integrated.

The endocannabinoid system, involved in the control of appetite, is found in the central and peripheral nervous system, liver, muscle, GI tract, and adipose tissue.[14] On exposure to palatable food, the system releases endocannabinoids that act on the cannabinoid-1 receptor, which affects satiety.[15] This action overrides satiation, resulting in continued eating. There is some evidence that endocannabinoids play a role in peripheral tissues, linked to ghrelin release and adipose tissue regulation.[16]

Genes and Other Contributors to Obesity

Although many genetic contributors to obesity have been identified in the past few decades, only 176 known cases of obesity have been linked to single-gene mutations in humans.[17] However, an increasing number of mutated genes can be traced to obesity phenotypes. The 2005 Human Obesity Gene Map indicates that 253 quantitative trait loci are related to obesity phenotypes, with 127 candidate genes. Possible candidate genes have been identified on every chromosome except Y. A few genetic

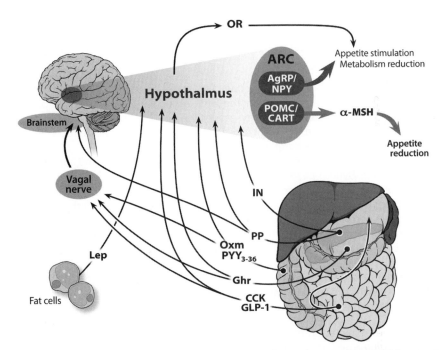

Fig. 2. Signals involved in the control of energy intake and expenditure. ARC, arcuate nucleus; CART, cocaine-amphetamine–regulated transcript neurons; CCK, cholecystokinin; Ghr, ghrelin; GLP-1, glucagonlike peptide 1; In, insulin; Lep, leptin; α-MSH, α-melanocyte–stimulating hormone; NPY, neuropeptide Y; OR, orexin; Oxm, oxyntomodulin; PP, pancreatic polypeptide; PVC, periventricular nucleus; PYY3–36, peptide YY. Skelton J, Cohen G. Obesity, from Pediatric Gastrointestinal and liver disease. Wyllie R, Hyams JS, Kay M, editors. Fourth edition. Philadelphia (PA): Elsevier; p. 157; with permission.

abnormalities have been identified, with only 1 having a treatment avenue presently (see **Fig. 2**).[12,18]

- Leptin deficiency has been described in a few small series of families of Pakistani origin, characterized by severe obesity, hyperphagia, and other abnormalities.[12,18] These rare cases are responsive to leptin therapy. Mutations in the leptin pathway, particularly the receptor gene, may account for up to 3% to 4% of cases of severe early-onset obesity.[4,12] However, these genetic abnormalities are unlikely to respond to leptin therapy.
- Mutations in POMC have been described, resulting in a lack of central appetite signaling and therefore hyperphagia. Affected patients have red hair and adrenal insufficiency as well.[19] Mutations in an enzyme that cleaves POMC have also been identified; these individuals are characterized by hypoglycemia, hypogonadotropic hypogonadism, and intestinal malabsorption.
- The melanocortin 3 (MC3R) and melanocortin 4 (MC4R) receptors are key in feeding behaviors. MC3R abnormalities may have a role in body weight regulation in African American children. MC4R mutations are found in more than 3% of early-onset severe obesity in children.[4,12,19] Heterozygous and homozygous mutations seem to cause obesity, hyperphagia, and hyperinsulinism, as well as tall stature.
- Brain-derived neurotrophic factor is thought to play a role downstream in the leptin pathway and may be linked to early onset-obesity in patients with WAGR syndrome.[4]
- Albright hereditary osteodystrophy (AHO) is associated with pseudohypoparathyroidism, and also involves the leptin pathway.[4] Individuals with AHO also have short stature, developmental delays and mental retardation, brachydactyly, and ectopic ossifications.

Although the connection between a particular single nucleotide polymorphism and obesity is not always clear, large genome-wide association studies hint at possible links, such as the fat mass– and obesity-associated gene and reduced satiety or perilipin A gene and resistance to weight loss.[4] Advances in genomics are rapidly identifying important areas of exploration.

There are numerous genetic syndromes associated with obesity, and, for many, the link is not clear. Syndromes may result in behavioral and health issues that lead to increased energy intake or decreased activity or may have disruptions in the central control of appetite that result in hyperphagia. Typically, obesity is not the presenting sign of the syndrome but is important in the clinical care of the child. For instance, Prader-Willi syndrome (short stature, hypotonia, developmental delay) involves significant hyperphagia, as do Bardet-Biedl (short stature, developmental delay, retinitis pigmentosum, polydactyly) and Alström (blindness or vision loss, hearing loss, hyperinsulinemia) syndromes.[4] Many other syndromes are associated with obesity, including Cohen syndrome, fragile X, Sotos syndrome, Turner syndrome, and Beckwith-Wiedemann syndrome.

Infectious etiologies

Infectious causes include a form of adenovirus (AD36) that results in increased adipose tissue in animal models.[20–22] Laboratory studies using human adipose tissue demonstrates increased adipocyte formation,[23] and individuals with higher obesity levels are more likely to have antibodies to AD36.[24,25] Although it is unlikely the obesity epidemic is a result of widespread adenovirus infection, there seems to be some link between the two.

Gut microbiota

Similar to adenovirus, the predominance of particular strains of colonic bacteria have been associated with higher levels of obesity in animal models, with increasing evidence of an association in humans.[26,27] Theories linking obesity and gut microbes revolve around the bowel flora's use of energy from ingested food, bacterial fermentation of food into readily absorbable fatty acids, and influences on metabolism in peripheral organs.

Stress

Chronic stress affects weight status through dysregulation of the hypothalamic-pituitary-adrenal axis, resulting in altered cortisol metabolism.[28] Stress can result from multiple causes, for example, sleep deprivation, malnutrition, depression, and environmental stressors such as poverty. These factors may be related to obesity risk, even in the prenatal period.[29,30]

Medications

Many medications, particularly antipsychotics, cause weight gain.[31] High-dose inhaled glucocorticoids, oral glucocorticoids, antipsychotics (risperidone, olanzapine, clozapine), mood stabilizers (lithium), antidepressants (tricyclics), anticonvulsants (valproate, carbamazepine), oral contraceptives, and insulin and insulin secretagogues are the more commonly reported ones, but there is a lack of studies in children.[32] Some antihypertensives, such as propranolol, nifedipine, and clonidine, can also lead to weight gain, as do many chemotherapy agents.[4] It is unclear what mechanisms are involved. With antipsychotics, for example, a complex interplay of hunger disruption, metabolic effects, and unknown mechanisms have been reported.[33]

Endocrinologic Conditions

Of children referred for evaluation of obesity, endocrinologic causes are only found in 2% to 3% of cases.[34] **Table 3** lists the most common disorders seen. Cushing syndrome has a prevalence of approximately 1 in a million, whereas insulinomas are even more rare.[4,35] Hypothalamic obesity usually results from damage to the hypothalamus; these cases tend to occur in pediatric patients associated with surgery or radiation therapy. An example is children treated for craniopharyngiomas, which has high rates of obesity development posttreatment.[36,37]

Although pure genetic contributors to obesity, such as the mythical fat gene, are quite rare, there are many genetically linked causes that can increase a child's risk

Table 3
Endocrinologic causes of childhood obesity

Condition	Significant Signs and Symptoms
Hypothyroidism	Short stature and obesity but weight below 95th percentile for age
Growth hormone deficiency	Decreased linear growth velocity with increasing weight gain, increased central adiposity
Cushing syndrome	Decreased linear growth velocity, increased central adiposity, abdominal striae, insulin resistance
Insulinoma	Increased food intake to counteract low blood sugars
Hypothalamic obesity	Hyperphagia, other endocrine disorders;
Pseudohypoparathyroidism type 1A	Multiple other endocrine deficiencies

of obesity. There is evidence for the existence of a thrifty genotype and phenotype.[38,39] The protection of energy stores through famine and hunting/gathering societies has produced a human with a fine-tuned system of weight control described earlier. However, these factors are largely absent for most humans in industrialized nations today.

NURTURE

Although there have been great discoveries in the biological determinants of obesity in children, the rapid increase in obesity prevalence almost certainly points to environmental changes having the greater impact. External influences on obesity vary by life stage, circumstance, and genetic predisposition. Changes in the nutritional and activity environments of children and families over the past several decades have likely had the greatest impact on the present epidemic.

Obesity and the Life Cycle

Prenatal

Antenatal and in utero environment The antenatal environment influences fetal development. Fetal growth may be determined by cell counts, maternal brain centers that control satiety and appetite, and endocrine function even before conception.[40] Antenatal stress or placental insufficiency may also influence altered pancreatic function and insulin sensitivity. These effects can persist into adulthood, increasing the risk for obesity-related conditions, such as metabolic syndrome.[41]

Maternal malnutrition and famine Nutrient restriction from maternal malnutrition in the first 2 trimesters of pregnancy is strongly linked to birth weight and an increased risk of obesity in young children.[41] In a historical cohort study of boys with intrauterine exposure to famine within the first 2 trimesters of development (the "Dutch Hunger Winter" during World War II), an increase of 94% in the risk of developing childhood obesity was found.[42] This may be attributable to structural and functional abnormalities of the endocrine system caused by nutrient restriction and disturbance in insulin and glucose homeostasis.[43,44]

Maternal diabetes Many studies have investigated prenatal exposure to diabetes in utero, indicating an increased prevalence of childhood overweight or obesity if the mother was diabetic during pregnancy.[45] Mechanisms potentially responsible for this increased prevalence include fetal hyperglycemia and hyperinsulinemia caused by the diabetic mother's poor glycemic control.[46,47] Insulin levels in the third-trimester amniotic fluid have also been linked to childhood obesity and the development of insulin resistance and systolic hypertension.[48]

Maternal smoking during pregnancy Children exposed to prenatal cigarette smoke are more likely to exceed the 90th percentile for body mass index (BMI, calculated as weight in kilograms divided by height in meters squared) during adolescence.[49] In one longitudinal study, 14% of 6-year-old children exposed to maternal smoking in the womb were obese, compared with 8% of those who were unexposed.[50] Additional studies confirm these findings,[51] even after adjusting for multiple maternal confounders.[52] Proposed mechanisms for this association include nicotinic effects on leptin[53] and maternal appetite and impaired fetal oxidative metabolism due to carbon monoxide and cyanide compounds found in cigarette smoke.[52]

Maternal weight and pregnancy Maternal weight both before and during pregnancy, and the magnitude of weight gain during pregnancy, are linked to increased risk of overweight or obesity in the offspring.[48] Maternal obesity, especially in the first trimester, markedly increases the risk that a child will be obese by age 4 years.[52,54] Maternal weight gain during pregnancy is also associated with a higher likelihood of childhood obesity,[55,56] and the odds of having a child with a BMI above the 95th percentile at age 7 years increases by 3% for every kilogram of weight gained during pregnancy.[57]

Postnatal

Breastfeeding Breastfeeding versus formula feeding is an important nutritional decision that may affect childhood obesity risk. In some studies, breastfeeding was protective against child[50,58–61] and adolescent[62–64] obesity, whereas others have found little effect.[65–67] The evidence suggests that breastfeeding reduces risk for pediatric weight gain; formula-fed children have an obesity prevalence of 4.5% compared with 2.8% in breast-fed children.[68] More recent investigations indicate that breastfeeding for 6 months or more has a modest protective effect against adolescent obesity but not overweight.[69] In one report, breastfeeding more than 6 months was associated with the lowest risk of overweight and obesity in 5-year-old children.[8]

Early postnatal years As with breastfeeding, overnutrition and early childhood feeding practices are major contributors to childhood obesity, influencing leptin concentrations and adiposity later in life.[70] The rate at which infants gain weight during their first few months, and the type of infant feeding (formula or breast milk), is linked to weight status in later childhood as well as adult cardiovascular disease risk.[61] Independent of birth weight and weight at age 1 year, rapid weight gain even within the first 4 months of life is associated with an increased risk of overweight at age 7 years.[71]

Early childhood feeding and parenting Home and social environments, parenting styles, and family feeding practices are the primary influences on early childhood nutrition behaviors.[72–76] Nearly two-thirds of all meals consumed by children come from home, despite the prevalence of fast-food restaurants and convenient dining establishments.[77] Thus, the home environment and family feeding behaviors are crucial components in the development of childhood nutritional habits and have an undeniable influence on childhood weight status.[78,79]

Authoritarian parenting styles, characterized by restriction, pressures to eat certain food items, and overmonitoring, are most consistently linked to pediatric weight gain.[80,81] However, children raised by authoritative parents who promote responsibility, monitoring, and modeling[80] are more likely to have healthier nutrition and lower BMIs.[82] Child-centered feeding practices,[74] positive nutrition encouragement, and parents' intake of fruits and vegetables are also positively associated with fruit and vegetable consumption in their children.[75] These data support the notion that family factors are crucial components in the prevention and treatment of pediatric obesity.

Early introduction of solid food may have a contribution to the development of obesity. There is some evidence that rapid weight gain in infancy can predict later obesity,[83] with infants already being exposed to unhealthy dietary patterns.[84] Most studies tracking obesity development to infancy have not accounted for age of first solid food introduction.[85] An Australian study found that delayed introduction of solids did significantly reduce the odds of overweight and obesity at age 10 years,[86] and a prevention study seemed to lower risk of obesity development by delaying introduction of solids as part of a multicomponent intervention.[87] One review of the literature did not find an association between age of solid food introduction and obesity development,[88] but available evidence has not answered this question sufficiently.

Adiposity rebound Adiposity rebound, when a child reaches a BMI nadir before body fat increases, typically occurs between ages 5 and 6 years. Normal-weight children with at least 1 overweight parent at the time of adiposity rebound are nearly 5 times as likely to be obese as an adult. If both parents are obese, children before the adiposity rebound have a 13-fold risk of being obese adults.[89] Risk for adult obesity increases with earlier onset of childhood obesity. Children who reach adiposity rebound earlier are 5 times more likely to develop adult obesity, and those who are already overweight at the time of adiposity rebound have 6 times the risk for adult obesity.[89]

Changes in the Family

It is intuitive that changes in family structure affect nutrition and physical activity habits of families. Family meals, fast food, early childhood feeding practices, sleep routines, parenting style, media use, family-based physical activity, adult obesity levels, socio-economic status, and interaction with health services are key factors associated with childhood obesity and are most likely moderated by changes in the family. Families in the United States have experienced substantial changes as the child obesity epidemic has developed. In 1970, approximately 85% of children lived with 2 married parents; by 2010 this estimate decreased to 66%,[90] and most of the change occurred between 1970 and 1990 (**Table 4**). During the same period, children living in a mother-only household increased from 11% to 23%, with significant differences across racial groups.[90] This is important because children from mother-only households are at substantially increased risk for living in poverty,[91] a major risk factor for childhood obesity and poor health outcomes.[92,93] During this same period, there was a substantial growth in women's labor force participation, increasing from 43% in 1970 to 66% by 2009.[94] However, there is little direct evidence linking these changes in the family to obesity risk in children.

Lifestyle and Environment

Diet
Among dietary factors linked to obesity, high-fat and sugar-containing food have been the most studied. Although overconsumption of some food items leads to excessive weight gain and obesity, other patterns (eg, consuming a diet high in fruits and vege-tables) are thought to protect against obesity. Fruits and vegetables have high water

Table 4
Percentage of children living in major family structures by decade between 1970 and 2010

	Living with 2 Married Parents	Living with Mother Only	Living with Father Only	Living with No Parent
1970	85.0	10.9	1.1	3.0
1980	76.6	18.0	1.7	3.7
1990	72.5	21.6	3.1	2.8
2000	69.1	22.4	4.2	4.1
2010	65.7	23.1	3.4	4.1
Decade change				
1970–1980	−10.4	+65.1	+54.5	+23.3
1980–1990	−5.4	+20.0	+82.4	−24.3
1990–2000	−4.7	+3.7	+35.5	+46.4
2000–2010	−4.9	+3.1	+19.0	0.0

Data from Family structure. Child Trends. Available at: http://www.childtrendsdatabank.org/?q=node/231. Accessed July 14, 2011.

and dietary fiber contents, making them low in energy density. Although the mechanisms for their action remain unclear, eating a diet high in fruits and vegetables may help reduce body weight and fat by displacing energy-dense food from the diet.[95,96] Fiber in fruits and vegetables helps reduce total energy intake by initiating satiety[97,98] and altering postprandial hormones through a reduction in glycemic load.[99,100] Yet in a recent review of studies about fruit and vegetable intake and adiposity levels in children,[101] only 1 of 5 observed the expected inverse relationship between fruit and vegetable intake and adiposity.[102] In a cross-sectional analysis, the lifestyle behavioral pattern of eating dinner, cooked meals, and vegetables was inversely related with obesity in children.[103] There are limitations to these studies, with others drawing different conclusions on the link between fruits, vegetables, and obesity.[104] However, no studies show a worsening of weight status with increased vegetable and fruit consumption.

American eating patterns have changed drastically in the past 3 decades. In children aged 2 to 18 years, energy density and portion sizes of key food items, including salty snacks, fruit drinks, french fries, hamburgers, cheeseburgers, pizzas, and Mexican fast food, increased from 1977 to 2006.[105] McConahy and colleagues[106] showed that nearly 20% of variance in daily energy intake can be attributed to portion size. Similarly, portion size, but not energy density, of snacks was the primary determinant of energy intake.[107] At the same time, portion sizes of food items in the American diet have increased in the last several decades.[108,109]

In one study, doubling the portion size of food items offered to preschool-aged children during a 24-hour period increased energy intake by 12%[96] but only in certain food items. However, there was no compensatory reduction in other food items, leading to a higher daily energy intake. In contrast, an earlier study suggested young children can self-regulate energy intake up to 30 hours after a meal.[110] In general, increasing portion sizes and energy density of food items and meals raises meal consumption from approximately 10% to 40% and daily energy intake by 12%.[96,111–114] However, there is a dearth of well-designed studies on how portion size and energy density affect energy intake in children.

Rising rates of obesity coincide with the increased consumption of added sugars.[115] For children and adolescents aged 2 to 18 years, nearly 20% of total energy intake is from added sugars in food items and beverages.[116] Recent systematic reviews ranged from finding no evidence to strong evidence that sugar-sweetened beverages make a significant contribution to BMI in children.[117,118] Cross-sectional studies in children showed positive associations (at least in subgroup analyses) between the use of sugar-sweetened beverages and measures of obesity (weight, BMI, body fat),[119–125] although others showed either weak or no association between these variables.[126–130] In a study of more than 10,000 children and adolescents, overweight people consumed a higher proportion of their total intake from soft drinks than did normal-weight individuals.[131] Observational follow-up studies reported positive associations between intake of sugar-sweetened beverages and overweight/obesity.[120,132–134]

Activity

Arguments that the obesity epidemic is caused largely by reduced physical activity and not energy intake are based on national survey data indicating that daily energy intake is unchanged or reduced in the last several decades. Not only is daily energy expenditure decreasing but also sedentary activities are increasing.[135–137] In one report, children who watched more than 4 hours of television daily had the highest BMIs, and those who watched less than 1 hour daily had the lowest BMIs.[135] In a separate study in Mexico City, the odds ratio of obesity was 1.12 for each hour of television watched per day and 0.90 for each hour of moderate to vigorous physical activity per day.[136] The investigators found no such effect for time playing videogames.

In an early meta-analysis looking at the relationships between sedentary behaviors and obesity in children and youth, a statistically significant association was observed between television viewing and body fatness in children.[138] However, in one study, television viewing only explained approximately 1% of the variance in body fatness, whereas video and computer game use showed no effect with body fatness. Studies have also failed to find correlations between television viewing and BMI.[139] Although there is biological plausibility linking television viewing to body fatness, most of the evidence is from cross-sectional studies, which many demonstrate fairly small responses. In a randomized controlled trial, an intervention specifically geared to reduce television viewing and video game use in children aged 8 to 9 years produced an improvement in body fatness over a 6-month follow-up.[140] Other intervention studies that did not specifically intervene on these sedentary behaviors reported decreases in television viewing and body fatness but were not necessarily causal.[141,142] Currently there is a lack of empirical data to support claims that television viewing, playing video games, or using computers leads to obesity or interferes with physical activity. A possible confounder to these analyses is consumption of energy-dense snacks while participating in sedentary behaviors. As Proctor and colleagues[143] found, children who watched the most television and had a fat intake of more than 34% of their daily kilocalorie consumption gained the most body fat from ages 4 to 11 years.

Overall, low levels of physical activity, defined by not meeting recommended levels, are problematic and mirror increased sedentary activity.[144,145] This disruption in energy balance can explain much of the increase in pediatric obesity.

Sleep

The link between pediatric obesity, higher body fat, and sleep duration has been widely demonstrated in the literature and was recently reviewed in this journal.[146] Although trials are ongoing, no interventions have reported on the manipulation of sleep patterns and the influence on weight gain in children. In adults, however, studies have shown that chronic sleep deprivation may lead to weight gain, which can be attributed to the influence of sleep on hormonal secretions.[147] Restricted sleep is associated with increased food intake, including both meals and snacks,[148,149] thereby increasing obesity risk. Lack of sleep can also lead to reduced physical activity and increased sedentary behaviors.[150,151]

Although causation cannot be established, epidemiologic studies in children have indicated a definitive association between reduced sleep duration at night and increased weight status. Several reviews and meta-analyses agree that children who sleep less have an increased risk for obesity between 56% and 89%.[152,153] Increased BMI in children is associated with reduced sleep duration, which is most likely because of an increase in adipose tissue deposits.[154]

Industrialization and Obesity

Obesity and associated health issues are a worldwide health concern. Increased consumption of a more Western diet means that eating sugar and fat-laden, highly processed, energy-dense food items occurs globally. Popkin[155] describes nutrition transition as existing in several stages, with urbanization, economic growth, and technological changes for work, leisure, and food processing leading the changes in stages. Obesity is evident in stage 4, or the degenerative disease period, characterized by increased intake of fat, sugar, and processed food items and a more prominent presence of technology in work and leisure.

Although urbanization, a demographic factor, improves growth patterns in children, it also increases the proportion of children above the 95th percentile for weight-for-age. Major social and economic changes in communities, such as transitioning from physical to mechanized transportation, introduction of processed food items and supermarkets, and television access, also change obesity and overweight prevalence in children. For example, the proportion of children (5–12 year age group) above the 85th percentile for BMI increased from less than 15% to nearly 50% in less over 20 years in the White Mountain Apache reservation.[156]

The Built Environment

The built environment is a likely explanation for disparities in several health indicators, including the prevalence of obesity. There is substantial evidence showing that alterations in built environments regarding physical activity and eating are a factor in childhood obesity.[157] For example, neighborhood differences in food access influence levels of obesity.[158–161] In adolescents and adults, better availability to healthful food products leads to healthier food intake, including more fruits and vegetables, less dietary fat, and improved diet quality.[162–166] Consequently, lower risks for obesity in children and adolescents are associated with better access to a supermarket.[158,159,161,167]

Schools play a prominent role in a child's nutrition because most children eat at least 1 meal per day at school and spend approximately 6 hours per day in this setting. The presence of fast-food establishments within 0.1 mile from a school was associated with a 5% increase in obesity rates, whereas further distances had no effect on obesity rates in the school.[168]

Urban sprawl is also associated with adult obesity, whereas walkable neighborhoods and communities with sidewalks, safe intersections, accessible destinations, appealing green spaces, and public transit have improved activity levels and health.[169] For each additional hour spent in a car per day, there is a 6% increase in the likelihood of obesity; for each additional kilometer walked, a nearly 5% decrease in obesity is present.[170] A policy statement from the American Academy of Pediatrics has called for a multidisciplinary approach to building communities that promote active lifestyles in children.[171]

SUMMARY

Childhood obesity is a complex medical issue, representing the interplay of physical and environmental factors. The neuroendocrine control of weight contains multiple situations in which genetic variation can influence a person's weight status. However, the unhealthy evolution of food and activity environments has placed children at a higher risk for obesity and associated weight problems than they ever have been before.

ACKNOWLEDGMENTS

The authors would like to thank Karen Klein (Research Support Core, Office of Research, Wake Forest University Health Sciences) for her assistance in editing this manuscript.

REFERENCES

1. Davison KK, Birch LL. Childhood overweight: a contextual model and recommendations for future research. Obes Rev 2001;2(3):159–71.
2. Zhang Y, Proenca R, Maffei M, et al. Positional cloning of the mouse obese gene and its human homologue. Nature 1994;372(6505):425–32.

3. de Kloet AD, Woods SC. Molecular neuroendocrine targets for obesity therapy. Curr Opin Endocrinol Diabetes Obes 2010;17(5):441–5.

4. Crocker MK, Yanovski JA. Pediatric obesity: etiology and treatment. Endocrinol Metab Clin North Am 2009;38(3):525–48.

5. Korner J, Woods SC, Woodworth KA. Regulation of energy homeostasis and health consequences in obesity. Am J Med 2009;122(4 Suppl 1):S12–8.

6. Woods SC. The control of food intake: behavioral versus molecular perspectives. Cell Metab 2009;9(6):489–98.

7. Cummings DE, Overduin J. Gastrointestinal regulation of food intake. J Clin Invest 2007;117(1):13–23.

8. Korner J, Aronne LJ. Pharmacological approaches to weight reduction: therapeutic targets. J Clin Endocrinol Metab 2004;89(6):2616–21.

9. Considine RV, Sinha MK, Heiman ML, et al. Serum immunoreactive-leptin concentrations in normal-weight and obese humans. N Engl J Med 1996; 334(5):292–5.

10. Marx J. Cellular warriors at the battle of the bulge. Science 2003;299(5608):846–9.

11. Sell H, Eckel J. Adipose tissue inflammation: novel insight into the role of macrophages and lymphocytes. Curr Opin Clin Nutr Metab Care 2010;13(4):366–70.

12. Farooqi IS. Genetic, molecular and physiological insights into human obesity. Eur J Clin Invest 2011;41(4):451–5.

13. Phillips SA, Kung JT. Mechanisms of adiponectin regulation and use as a pharmacological target. Curr Opin Pharmacol 2010;10(6):676–83.

14. Andre A, Gonthier MP. The endocannabinoid system: its roles in energy balance and potential as a target for obesity treatment. Int J Biochem Cell Biol 2010; 42(11):1788–801.

15. Di Marzo V, Goparaju SK, Wang L, et al. Leptin-regulated endocannabinoids are involved in maintaining food intake. Nature 2001;410(6830):822–5.

16. Cani PD, Montoya ML, Neyrinck AM, et al. Potential modulation of plasma ghrelin and glucagon-like peptide-1 by anorexigenic cannabinoid compounds, SR141716A (rimonabant) and oleoylethanolamide. Br J Nutr 2004;92(5):757–61.

17. Rankinen T, Zuberi A, Chagnon YC, et al. The human obesity gene map: the 2005 update. Obesity (Silver Spring) 2006;14(4):529–644.

18. Farooqi IS, Wangensteen T, Collins S, et al. Clinical and molecular genetic spectrum of congenital deficiency of the leptin receptor. N Engl J Med 2007;356(3):237–47.

19. Farooqi S. Insights from the genetics of severe childhood obesity. Horm Res 2007;68(Suppl 5):5–7.

20. Dhurandhar NV, Kulkarni P, Ajinkya SM, et al. Effect of adenovirus infection on adiposity in chicken. Vet Microbiol 1992;31(2–3):101–7.

21. Dhurandhar NV, Israel BA, Kolesar JM, et al. Increased adiposity in animals due to a human virus. Int J Obes Relat Metab Disord 2000;24(8):989–96.

22. Dhurandhar NV, Whigham LD, Abbott DH, et al. Human adenovirus Ad-36 promotes weight gain in male rhesus and marmoset monkeys. J Nutr 2002; 132(10):3155–60.

23. Pasarica M, Mashtalir N, McAllister EJ, et al. Adipogenic human adenovirus Ad-36 induces commitment, differentiation, and lipid accumulation in human adipose-derived stem cells. Stem Cells 2008;26(4):969–78.

24. Dhurandhar NV, Kulkarni PR, Ajinkya SM, et al. Association of adenovirus infection with human obesity. Obes Res 1997;5(5):464–9.

25. Atkinson RL, Dhurandhar NV, Allison DB, et al. Human adenovirus-36 is associated with increased body weight and paradoxical reduction of serum lipids. Int J Obes (Lond) 2005;29(3):281–6.

26. Backhed F. Changes in intestinal microflora in obesity: cause or consequence? J Pediatr Gastroenterol Nutr 2009;48(Suppl 2):S56–7.

27. Reinhardt C, Reigstad CS, Backhed F. Intestinal microbiota during infancy and its implications for obesity. J Pediatr Gastroenterol Nutr 2009;48(3):249–56.

28. Bose M, Olivan B, Laferrere B. Stress and obesity: the role of the hypothalamic-pituitary-adrenal axis in metabolic disease. Curr Opin Endocrinol Diabetes Obes 2009;16(5):340–6.

29. Barker DJ. Maternal nutrition, fetal nutrition, and disease in later life. Nutrition 1997;13(9):807–13.

30. Barker DJ. Fetal nutrition and cardiovascular disease in later life. Br Med Bull 1997;53(1):96–108.

31. Correll CU, Lencz T, Malhotra AK. Antipsychotic drugs and obesity. Trends Mol Med 2011;17(2):97–107.

32. Clinical practice guidelines for the management of overweight and obesity in children and adolescents. National Health and Medical Research Council Australia; 2003. Available at: http://www.health.gov.au/internet/main/publishing.nsf/Content/893169B10DD846FCCA256F190003BADA/$File/children.pdf. Accessed September 6, 2011.

33. Coccurello R, Moles A. Potential mechanisms of atypical antipsychotic-induced metabolic derangement: clues for understanding obesity and novel drug design. Pharmacol Ther 2010;127(3):210–51.

34. Crino A, Greggio NA, Beccaria L, et al. Diagnosis and differential diagnosis of obesity in childhood. Minerva Pediatr 2003;55(5):461–70 [in Italian].

35. Ning C, Yanovski JA. Endocrine disorders associated with pediatric obesity. In: Goran MI, Sothern MS, editors. Handbook of pediatric obesity: etiology, pathophysiology, and prevention. Boca Raton (FL): CRC Press, Taylor & Francis Group; 2006. p. 135–55.

36. Hoffman HJ, De Silva M, Humphreys RP, et al. Aggressive surgical management of craniopharyngiomas in children. J Neurosurg 1992;76(1):47–52.

37. Muller HL, Bueb K, Bartels U, et al. Obesity after childhood craniopharyngioma—German multicenter study on pre-operative risk factors and quality of life. Klin Padiatr 2001;213(4):244–9.

38. Prentice AM. Early influences on human energy regulation: thrifty genotypes and thrifty phenotypes. Physiol Behav 2005;86(5):640–5.

39. Prentice AM, Rayco-Solon P, Moore SE. Insights from the developing world: thrifty genotypes and thrifty phenotypes. Proc Nutr Soc 2005;64(2):153–61.

40. Dietz WH. Overweight in childhood and adolescence. N Engl J Med 2004;350(9):855–7.

41. Barker DJ, Eriksson JG, Forsen T, et al. Fetal origins of adult disease: strength of effects and biological basis. Int J Epidemiol 2002;31(6):1235–9.

42. Ravelli GP, Stein ZA, Susser MW. Obesity in young men after famine exposure in utero and early infancy. N Engl J Med 1976;295(7):349–53.

43. Armitage JA, Khan IY, Taylor PD, et al. Developmental programming of the metabolic syndrome by maternal nutritional imbalance: how strong is the evidence from experimental models in mammals? J Physiol 2004;561(Pt 2):355–77.

44. Terroni PL, Anthony FW, Hanson MA, et al. Expression of agouti-related peptide, neuropeptide Y, pro-opiomelanocortin and the leptin receptor isoforms in fetal mouse brain from pregnant dams on a protein-restricted diet. Brain Res Mol Brain Res 2005;140(1–2):111–5.

45. Huang JS, Lee TA, Lu MC. Prenatal programming of childhood overweight and obesity. Matern Child Health J 2007;11(5):461–73.

46. Plagemann A, Harder T, Rake A, et al. Hypothalamic insulin and neuropeptide Y in the offspring of gestational diabetic mother rats. Neuroreport 1998;9(18): 4069–73.

47. Weiss PA, Hofmann HM, Kainer F, et al. Fetal outcome in gestational diabetes with elevated amniotic fluid insulin levels. Dietary versus insulin treatment. Diabetes Res Clin Pract 1988;5(1):1–7.

48. Cho NH, Silverman BL, Rizzo TA, et al. Correlations between the intrauterine metabolic environment and blood pressure in adolescent offspring of diabetic mothers. J Pediatr 2000;136(5):587–92.

49. Power C, Jefferis BJ. Fetal environment and subsequent obesity: a study of maternal smoking. Int J Epidemiol 2002;31(2):413–9.

50. Bergmann KE, Bergmann RL, Von Kries R, et al. Early determinants of childhood overweight and adiposity in a birth cohort study: role of breast-feeding. Int J Obes Relat Metab Disord 2003;27(2):162–72.

51. Wideroe M, Vik T, Jacobsen G, et al. Does maternal smoking during pregnancy cause childhood overweight? Paediatr Perinat Epidemiol 2003;17(2):171–9.

52. Salsberry PJ, Reagan PB. Dynamics of early childhood overweight. Pediatrics 2005;116(6):1329–38.

53. Li MD, Kane JK. Effect of nicotine on the expression of leptin and forebrain leptin receptors in the rat. Brain Res 2003;991(1–2):222–31.

54. Whitaker RC. Predicting preschooler obesity at birth: the role of maternal obesity in early pregnancy. Pediatrics 2004;114(1):e29–36.

55. Olson CM, Demment MM, Carling SJ, et al. Associations between mothers' and their children's weights at 4 years of age. Child Obes 2010;6(4):201–7.

56. Oken E, Taveras EM, Kleinman KP, et al. Gestational weight gain and child adiposity at age 3 years. Am J Obstet Gynecol 2007;196(4):322 e321–8.

57. Wrotniak BH, Shults J, Butts S, et al. Gestational weight gain and risk of overweight in the offspring at age 7 y in a multicenter, multiethnic cohort study. Am J Clin Nutr 2008;87(6):1818–24.

58. Liese AD, Hirsch T, von Mutius E, et al. Inverse association of overweight and breast feeding in 9 to 10-y-old children in Germany. Int J Obes Relat Metab Disord 2001;25(11):1644–50.

59. Toschke AM, Vignerova J, Lhotska L, et al. Overweight and obesity in 6- to 14-year-old Czech children in 1991: protective effect of breast-feeding. J Pediatr 2002;141(6):764–9.

60. Armstrong J, Reilly JJ. Breastfeeding and lowering the risk of childhood obesity. Lancet 2002;359(9322):2003–4.

61. von Kries R, Koletzko B, Sauerwald T, et al. Breast feeding and obesity: cross sectional study. BMJ 1999;319(7203):147–50.

62. Elliott KG, Kjolhede CL, Gournis E, et al. Duration of breastfeeding associated with obesity during adolescence. Obes Res 1997;5(6):538–41.

63. Grummer-Strawn LM, Mei Z. Does breastfeeding protect against pediatric overweight? Analysis of longitudinal data from the Centers for Disease Control and Prevention Pediatric Nutrition Surveillance System. Pediatrics 2004;113(2): e81–6.

64. Poulton R, Williams S. Breastfeeding and risk of overweight. JAMA 2001; 286(12):1449–50.

65. Hediger ML, Overpeck MD, Kuczmarski RJ, et al. Association between infant breastfeeding and overweight in young children. JAMA 2001;285(19):2453–60.

66. Parsons TJ, Power C, Manor O. Infant feeding and obesity through the lifecourse. Arch Dis Child 2003;88(9):793–4.

67. Victora CG, Barros F, Lima RC, et al. Anthropometry and body composition of 18 year old men according to duration of breast feeding: birth cohort study from Brazil. BMJ 2003;327(7420):901.
68. Arenz S, Ruckerl R, Koletzko B, et al. Breast-feeding and childhood obesity–a systematic review. Int J Obes Relat Metab Disord 2004;28(10):1247–56.
69. Shields L, O'Callaghan M, Williams GM, et al. Breastfeeding and obesity at 14 years: a cohort study. J Paediatr Child Health 2006;42(5):289–96.
70. Singhal A, Farooqi IS, O'Rahilly S, et al. Early nutrition and leptin concentrations in later life. Am J Clin Nutr 2002;75(6):993–9.
71. Stettler N, Zemel BS, Kumanyika S, et al. Infant weight gain and childhood overweight status in a multicenter, cohort study. Pediatrics 2002;109(2):194–9.
72. Patrick H, Nicklas TA. A review of family and social determinants of children's eating patterns and diet quality. J Am Coll Nutr 2005;24(2):83–92.
73. Polfuss ML, Frenn M. Parenting and feeding behaviors associated with school-aged African American and white children. West J Nurs Res 2011. [Epub ahead of print].
74. Vereecken C, Rovner A, Maes L. Associations of parenting styles, parental feeding practices and child characteristics with young children's fruit and vegetable consumption. Appetite 2010;55(3):589–96.
75. Pearson N, Atkin AJ, Biddle SJ, et al. Parenting styles, family structure and adolescent dietary behaviour. Public Health Nutr 2009;13(8):1245–53.
76. Rhee KE, Lumeng JC, Appugliese DP, et al. Parenting styles and overweight status in first grade. Pediatrics 2006;117(6):2047–54.
77. Adair LS, Popkin BM. Are child eating patterns being transformed globally? Obes Res 2005;13(7):1281–99.
78. Birch LL, Davison KK. Family environmental factors influencing the developing behavioral controls of food intake and childhood overweight. Pediatr Clin North Am 2001;48(4):893–907.
79. Dietz WH, Gortmaker SL. Preventing obesity in children and adolescents. Annu Rev Public Health 2001;22:337–53.
80. Hubbs-Tait L, Kennedy TS, Page MC, et al. Parental feeding practices predict authoritative, authoritarian, and permissive parenting styles. J Am Diet Assoc 2008;108(7):1154–61 [discussion: 1161–2].
81. Clark HR, Goyder E, Bissell P, et al. How do parents' child-feeding behaviours influence child weight? Implications for childhood obesity policy. J Public Health (Oxf) 2007;29(2):132–41.
82. Sleddens EF, Gerards SM, Thijs C, et al. General parenting, childhood overweight and obesity-inducing behaviors: a review. Int J Pediatr Obes 2011; 6(2–2):e12–27.
83. Dennison BA, Edmunds LS, Stratton HH, et al. Rapid infant weight gain predicts childhood overweight. Obesity (Silver Spring) 2006;14(3):491–9.
84. Fox MK, Pac S, Devaney B, et al. Feeding infants and toddlers study: what foods are infants and toddlers eating? J Am Diet Assoc 2004;104(1 Suppl 1):s22–30.
85. Owen CG, Martin RM, Whincup PH, et al. Effect of infant feeding on the risk of obesity across the life course: a quantitative review of published evidence. Pediatrics 2005;115(5):1367–77.
86. Seach KA, Dharmage SC, Lowe AJ, et al. Delayed introduction of solid feeding reduces child overweight and obesity at 10 years. Int J Obes (Lond) 2010; 34(10):1475–9.
87. Paul IM, Savage JS, Anzman SL, et al. Preventing obesity during infancy: a pilot study. Obesity (Silver Spring) 2011;19(2):353–61.

88. Yew KS, Webber B, Hodges J, et al. Clinical inquiries: are there any known health risks to early introduction of solids to an infant's diet? J Fam Pract 2009;58(4):219–20.

89. Whitaker RC, Pepe MS, Wright JA, et al. Early adiposity rebound and the risk of adult obesity. Pediatrics 1998;101(3):E5.

90. Family structure. Child Trends. Available at: http://www.childtrendsdatabank. org/?q=node/231. Accessed July 14, 2011.

91. Chau M. Low income children in the United States: National and state trend data, 1998-2008. Available at: http://www.nccp.org/publications/pdf/text_907. pdf. Accessed July 14, 2011.

92. Drewnowski A, Specter SE. Poverty and obesity: the role of energy density and energy costs. Am J Clin Nutr 2004;79(1):6–16.

93. Phipps SA, Burton PS, Osberg LS, et al. Poverty and the extent of child obesity in Canada, Norway and the United States. Obes Rev 2006;7(1):5–12.

94. U.S. Department of Labor, Bureau of Labor Statistics. Women in the labor force: a databook. US Bureau of Labor Statistics; 2011. Available at: http://www.bls. gov/cps/wlf-databook-2005.pdf. Accessed September 6, 2011.

95. Rolls BJ, Ello-Martin JA, Tohill BC. What can intervention studies tell us about the relationship between fruit and vegetable consumption and weight management? Nutr Rev 2004;62(1):1–17.

96. Fisher JO, Liu Y, Birch LL, et al. Effects of portion size and energy density on young children's intake at a meal. Am J Clin Nutr 2007;86(1):174–9.

97. Ludwig DS, Pereira MA, Kroenke CH, et al. Dietary fiber, weight gain, and cardiovascular disease risk factors in young adults. JAMA 1999;282(16):1539–46.

98. Howarth NC, Saltzman E, Roberts SB. Dietary fiber and weight regulation. Nutr Rev 2001;59(5):129–39.

99. Livesey G, Taylor R, Hulshof T, et al. Glycemic response and health–a systematic review and meta-analysis: relations between dietary glycemic properties and health outcomes. Am J Clin Nutr 2008;87(1):258S–68S.

100. Ebbeling CB, Leidig MM, Sinclair KB, et al. A reduced-glycemic load diet in the treatment of adolescent obesity. Arch Pediatr Adolesc Med 2003;157(8):773–9.

101. Ledoux TA, Hingle MD, Baranowski T. Relationship of fruit and vegetable intake with adiposity: a systematic review. Obes Rev 2011;12(5):e143–50.

102. Wang Y, Ge K, Popkin BM. Why do some overweight children remain overweight, whereas others do not? Public Health Nutr 2003;6(6):549–58.

103. Yannakoulia M, Ntalla I, Papoutsakis C, et al. Consumption of vegetables, cooked meals, and eating dinner is negatively associated with overweight status in children. J Pediatr 2010;157(5):815–20.

104. Newby PK. Plant foods and plant-based diets: protective against childhood obesity? Am J Clin Nutr 2009;89(5):1572S–87S.

105. Piernas C, Popkin BM. Food portion patterns and trends among U.S. children and the relationship to total eating occasion size, 1977-2006. J Nutr 2011;141(6): 1159–64.

106. McConahy KL, Smiciklas-Wright H, Mitchell DC, et al. Portion size of common foods predicts energy intake among preschool-aged children. J Am Diet Assoc 2004;104(6):975–9.

107. Looney SM, Raynor HA. Impact of portion size and energy density on snack intake in preschool-aged children. J Am Diet Assoc 2011;111(3):414–8.

108. Nielsen SJ, Popkin BM. Patterns and trends in food portion sizes, 1977-1998. JAMA 2003;289(4):450–3.

109. Smiciklas-Wright H, Mitchell DC, Mickle SJ, et al. Foods commonly eaten in the United States, 1989-1991 and 1994-1996: are portion sizes changing? J Am Diet Assoc 2003;103(1):41–7.

110. Birch LL, Deysher M. Caloric compensation and sensory specific satiety: evidence for self regulation of food intake by young children. Appetite 1986; 7(4):323–31.

111. Rolls BJ, Engell D, Birch LL. Serving portion size influences 5-year-old but not 3-year-old children's food intakes. J Am Diet Assoc 2000;100(2): 232–4.

112. Birch LL, Fisher JO, Davison KK. Learning to overeat: maternal use of restrictive feeding practices promotes girls' eating in the absence of hunger. Am J Clin Nutr 2003;78(2):215–20.

113. Fisher JO. Effects of age on children's intake of large and self-selected food portions. Obesity (Silver Spring) 2007;15(2):403–12.

114. Fisher JO, Arreola A, Birch LL, et al. Portion size effects on daily energy intake in low-income Hispanic and African American children and their mothers. Am J Clin Nutr 2007;86(6):1709–16.

115. Popkin BM, Nielsen SJ. The sweetening of the world's diet. Obes Res 2003; 11(11):1325–32.

116. Reedy J, Krebs-Smith SM. Dietary sources of energy, solid fats, and added sugars among children and adolescents in the United States. J Am Diet Assoc 2010;110(10):1477–84.

117. Malik VS, Schulze MB, Hu FB. Intake of sugar-sweetened beverages and weight gain: a systematic review. Am J Clin Nutr 2006;84(2):274–88.

118. Gibson S. Sugar-sweetened soft drinks and obesity: a systematic review of the evidence from observational studies and interventions. Nutr Res Rev 2008; 21(2):134–47.

119. Ariza AJ, Chen EH, Binns HJ, et al. Risk factors for overweight in five- to six-year-old Hispanic-American children: a pilot study. J Urban Health 2004;81(1):150–61.

120. Berkey CS, Rockett HR, Field AE, et al. Sugar-added beverages and adolescent weight change. Obes Res 2004;12(5):778–88.

121. French SA, Jeffery RW, Forster JL, et al. Predictors of weight change over two years among a population of working adults: the Healthy Worker Project. Int J Obes Relat Metab Disord 1994;18(3):145–54.

122. Giammattei J, Blix G, Marshak HH, et al. Television watching and soft drink consumption: associations with obesity in 11- to 13-year-old schoolchildren. Arch Pediatr Adolesc Med 2003;157(9):882–6.

123. Gillis LJ, Bar-Or O. Food away from home, sugar-sweetened drink consumption and juvenile obesity. J Am Coll Nutr 2003;22(6):539–45.

124. Liebman M, Pelican S, Moore SA, et al. Dietary intake, eating behavior, and physical activity-related determinants of high body mass index in rural communities in Wyoming, Montana, and Idaho. Int J Obes Relat Metab Disord 2003; 27(6):684–92.

125. Nicklas TA, Yang SJ, Baranowski T, et al. Eating patterns and obesity in children. The Bogalusa Heart Study. Am J Prev Med 2003;25(1):9–16.

126. Andersen LF, Lillegaard IT, Overby N, et al. Overweight and obesity among Norwegian schoolchildren: changes from 1993 to 2000. Scand J Public Health 2005;33(2):99–106.

127. Bandini LG, Vu D, Must A, et al. Comparison of high-calorie, low-nutrient-dense food consumption among obese and non-obese adolescents. Obes Res 1999; 7(5):438–43.

128. Forshee RA, Anderson PA, Storey ML. The role of beverage consumption, physical activity, sedentary behavior, and demographics on body mass index of adolescents. Int J Food Sci Nutr 2004;55(6):463–78.

129. Forshee RA, Storey ML. Total beverage consumption and beverage choices among children and adolescents. Int J Food Sci Nutr 2003;54(4):297–307.

130. Rodriguez-Artalejo F, Garcia EL, Gorgojo L, et al. Consumption of bakery products, sweetened soft drinks and yogurt among children aged 6-7 years: association with nutrient intake and overall diet quality. Br J Nutr 2003;89(3): 419–29.

131. Troiano RP, Briefel RR, Carroll MD, et al. Energy and fat intakes of children and adolescents in the united states: data from the national health and nutrition examination surveys. Am J Clin Nutr 2000;72(Suppl 5):1343S–53S.

132. Ludwig DS, Peterson KE, Gortmaker SL. Relation between consumption of sugar-sweetened drinks and childhood obesity: a prospective, observational analysis. Lancet 2001;357(9255):505–8.

133. Phillips SM, Bandini LG, Naumova EN, et al. Energy-dense snack food intake in adolescence: longitudinal relationship to weight and fatness. Obes Res 2004; 12(3):461–72.

134. Welsh JA, Cogswell ME, Rogers S, et al. Overweight among low-income preschool children associated with the consumption of sweet drinks: Missouri, 1999-2002. Pediatrics 2005;115(2):e223–9.

135. Andersen RE, Crespo CJ, Bartlett SJ, et al. Relationship of physical activity and television watching with body weight and level of fatness among children: results from the Third National Health and Nutrition Examination Survey. JAMA 1998;279(12):938–42.

136. Hernandez B, Gortmaker SL, Colditz GA, et al. Association of obesity with physical activity, television programs and other forms of video viewing among children in Mexico city. Int J Obes Relat Metab Disord 1999;23(8):845–54.

137. Sisson SB, Broyles ST, Baker BL, et al. Screen time, physical activity, and overweight in US youth: national survey of children's health 2003. J Adolesc Health 2010;47(3):309–11.

138. Marshall SJ, Biddle SJ, Gorely T, et al. Relationships between media use, body fatness and physical activity in children and youth: a meta-analysis. Int J Obes Relat Metab Disord 2004;28(10):1238–46.

139. DuRant RH, Baranowski T, Johnson M, et al. The relationship among television watching, physical activity, and body composition of young children. Pediatrics 1994;94(4 Pt 1):449–55.

140. Robinson TN. Reducing children's television viewing to prevent obesity: a randomized controlled trial. JAMA 1999;282(16):1561–7.

141. Gortmaker SL, Peterson K, Wiecha J, et al. Reducing obesity via a school-based interdisciplinary intervention among youth: Planet Health. Arch Pediatr Adolesc Med 1999;153(4):409–18.

142. Epstein LH, Saelens BE, O'Brien JG. Effects of reinforcing increases in active behavior versus decreases in sedentary behavior for obese children. Int J Behav Med 1995;2(1):41–50.

143. Proctor MH, Moore LL, Gao D, et al. Television viewing and change in body fat from preschool to early adolescence: the Framingham Children's Study. Int J Obes Relat Metab Disord 2003;27(7):827–33.

144. Duke J, Huhman M, Heitzler C, Centers for Disease Control and Prevention (CDC). Physical activity levels among children aged 9-13 years: United States, 2002. MMWR Morb Mortal Wkly Rep 2003;52(33):785–8.

145. Grunbaum JA, Kann L, Kinchen S, et al. Youth risk behavior surveillance- United States, 2003. MMWR Surveill Summ 2004;53(2):1–96.
146. Hart CN, Cairns A, Jelalian E. Sleep and obesity in children and adolescents. Pediatr Clin North Am 2011;58(3):715–33.
147. Copinschi G. Metabolic and endocrine effects of sleep deprivation. Essent Psychopharmacol 2005;6(6):341–7.
148. Nedeltcheva AV, Kilkus JM, Imperial J, et al. Sleep curtailment is accompanied by increased intake of calories from snacks. Am J Clin Nutr 2009;89(1):126–33.
149. Brondel L, Romer MA, Nougues PM, et al. Acute partial sleep deprivation increases food intake in healthy men. Am J Clin Nutr 2010;91(6):1550–9.
150. Dru M, Bruge P, Benoit O, et al. Overnight duty impairs behaviour, awake activity and sleep in medical doctors. Eur J Emerg Med 2007;14(4):199–203.
151. Schmid SM, Hallschmid M, Jauch-Chara K, et al. Short-term sleep loss decreases physical activity under free-living conditions but does not increase food intake under time-deprived laboratory conditions in healthy men. Am J Clin Nutr 2009;90(6):1476–82.
152. Cappuccio FP, Taggart FM, Kandala NB, et al. Meta-analysis of short sleep duration and obesity in children and adults. Sleep 2008;31(5):619–26.
153. Chen X, Beydoun MA, Wang Y. Is sleep duration associated with childhood obesity? A systematic review and meta-analysis. Obesity (Silver Spring) 2008; 16(2):265–74.
154. Bayer O, Rosario AS, Wabitsch M, et al. Sleep duration and obesity in children: is the association dependent on age and choice of the outcome parameter? Sleep 2009;32(9):1183–9.
155. Popkin BM. An overview on the nutrition transition and its health implications: the Bellagio meeting. Public Health Nutr 2002;5(1A):93–103.
156. Owen GM, Garry PJ, Seymoure RD, et al. Nutrition studies with White Mountain Apache preschool children in 1976 and 1969. Am J Clin Nutr 1981;34(2): 266–77.
157. Sallis JF, Glanz K. The role of built environments in physical activity, eating, and obesity in childhood. Future Child 2006;16(1):89–108.
158. Morland K, Diez Roux AV, Wing S. Supermarkets, other food stores, and obesity: the atherosclerosis risk in communities study. Am J Prev Med 2006;30(4):333–9.
159. Powell LM, Auld MC, Chaloupka FJ, et al. Associations between access to food stores and adolescent body mass index. Am J Prev Med 2007;33(Suppl 4): S301–7.
160. Powell LM, Chaloupka FJ, Bao Y. The availability of fast-food and full-service restaurants in the United States: associations with neighborhood characteristics. Am J Prev Med 2007;33(Suppl 4):S240–5.
161. Powell LM, Chaloupka FJ, Slater SJ, et al. The availability of local-area commercial physical activity-related facilities and physical activity among adolescents. Am J Prev Med 2007;33(Suppl 4):S292–300.
162. Bodor JN, Rose D, Farley TA, et al. Neighbourhood fruit and vegetable availability and consumption: the role of small food stores in an urban environment. Public Health Nutr 2008;11(4):413–20.
163. Laraia BA, Siega-Riz AM, Kaufman JS, et al. Proximity of supermarkets is positively associated with diet quality index for pregnancy. Prev Med 2004;39(5): 869–75.
164. Rose D, Richards R. Food store access and household fruit and vegetable use among participants in the US Food Stamp Program. Public Health Nutr 2004; 7(8):1081–8.

165. Wang MC, Cubbin C, Ahn D, et al. Changes in neighbourhood food store environment, food behaviour and body mass index, 1981–1990. Public Health Nutr 2008;11(9):963–70.

166. Jago R, Baranowski T, Baranowski JC, et al. Distance to food stores & adolescent male fruit and vegetable consumption: mediation effects. Int J Behav Nutr Phys Act 2007;4:35.

167. Sturm R, Datar A. Body mass index in elementary school children, metropolitan area food prices and food outlet density. Public Health 2005;119(12):1059–68.

168. Currie J, DellaVigna S, Moretti E, et al. The Effect of Fast Food Restaurants on Obesity. Available at: www.econ.berkeley.edu/~sdellavi/wp/fastfoodJan09.pdf. Accessed May 28, 2011.

169. Brownson RC, Hoehner CM, Day K, et al. Measuring the built environment for physical activity: state of the science. Am J Prev Med 2009;36(Suppl 4): S99–123. e112.

170. Frank LD, Andresen MA, Schmid TL. Obesity relationships with community design, physical activity, and time spent in cars. Am J Prev Med 2004;27(2): 87–96.

171. Council on Sports Medicine and Fitness, Council on School Health. Active healthy living: prevention of childhood obesity through increased physical activity. Pediatrics 2006;117(5):1834–42.

Diabetes and Insulin Resistance in Pediatric Obesity

Grace Kim, MD, Sonia Caprio, MD*

KEYWORDS
- Diabetes • Insulin resistance • Pediatric obesity

EPIDEMIOLOGY OF DIABETES AND INSULIN RESISTANCE

Before the 1990s, type 2 diabetes mellitus (T2DM) was rarely diagnosed in children. In 1994, however, T2DM represented nearly 16% of new cases of diabetes in children in urban areas.[1] By 1999, the percent of new cases of diabetes that are T2DM ranged from 8% to 45% and was disproportionately represented in minority populations.[2,3] Most overweight children have metabolic abnormalities associated with insulin resistance without T2DM.[4] Metabolic syndrome represents a cluster of metabolic abnormalities associated with obesity and insulin resistance (ie, increased waist circumference, hypertension, low high-density lipoprotein, hypertriglyceridemia, and abnormal glucose tolerance).[4] These metabolic abnormalities put children an increased risk for premature cardiovascular disease.[4]

Recent population-based data from the SEARCH for Diabetes in Youth study indicate that approximately 3700 children and adolescents are diagnosed with type T2DM annually,[5] with the highest prevalence in the 10-year-old to 19-year-old age group[6] and in minority populations. Population-based studies differ by usage of diagnostic tests and classification scheme for diabetes and often do not account for undiagnosed or asymptomatic cases of T2DM, making comparisons between studies difficult.

AUTOIMMUNITY AND DIAGNOSIS

The classification of diabetes is determined by the clinical presentation and course of the disease.[7] Making the distinction between type 1 diabetes and T2DM is often difficult in overweight children and adolescents.[5] Diabetes-associated autoantibodies are measured to aid in diagnosis (islet cell antibodies [ICAs], antibodies against insulin, glutamic acid decarboxylase [GAD], and insulinoma-associated protein 2 [IA-2] or islet cell antigen 512 [ICA512]). The SEARCH study is the first population-based study to present estimates on the incidence of different forms of diabetes mellitus in youth.

Department of Pediatrics, Yale University School of Medicine, Department of Pediatrics, 333 Cedar Street PO Box 208064, New Haven, CT 06520, USA
* Corresponding author.
E-mail address: sonia.caprio@yale.edu

Pediatr Clin N Am 58 (2011) 1355–1361
doi:10.1016/j.pcl.2011.09.002
0031-3955/11/$ – see front matter © 2011 Published by Elsevier Inc.

pediatric.theclinics.com

This study measured GAD65 and IA2 antibodies. The SEARCH study reported 21% of children with T2DM aged 10 to 19 years had GAD65 positivity,[7] whereas the treatment options for type 2 diabetes in adolescents and youth (TODAY) study reported a rate of 10% islet cell autoimmunity in children clinically diagnosed with T2DM[8]—5.9% of subjects were positive for single antibody and 3.9% of subjects were positive for both antibodies.[9] Diabetes autoimmunity was significantly associated with ethnicity and gender, and the higher rates of antibody positivity may have been due to the large non-Hispanic white population in the SEARCH study.[8] Subjects both with and without diabetes autoimmunity were classified as overweight or obese, but the median body mass index (BMI) and BMI z scores were lower in the antibody-positive group.[8] This is not surprising the antibody-positive group was less likely to have clinical and laboratory findings of T2DM and metabolic syndrome.[8] As described previously, there are clinical characteristics that differ between those with and without diabetes autoimmunity; autoantibodies or phenotype methods cannot be used in isolation to distinguish between type 1 diabetes or T2DM.[8]

PATHOPHYSIOLOGY
Insulin Resistance and Insulin Secretion Defects

Glucose is the most important regulator of insulin release.[9] Normally, there is a nonlinear dose-related effect of glucose on insulin secretion.[9] The relationship between glucose and insulin secretion follows a sigmoidal curve.[9] The threshold to secrete insulin corresponds to nonfasting glucose levels and the steepest portion corresponds to postprandial glucose levels.[9] Data show that chronic exposure to hyperglycemia (glucotoxicity) reduces expression of genes important in β-cell function, specifically insulin gene.[9] T2DM is a progressive disease involving insulin resistance and impaired insulin secretion.[10] Insulin resistance is a state where peripheral tissues are insensitive to insulin action, resulting in increased insulin production by the β cells of the pancreas.[10] Both prediabetes and diabetes develop when the β-cells are unable to compensate for the lack of insulin sensitivity in target tissues, resulting in hyperglycemia.[11]

Because insulin resistance is a major factor in the development of T2DM, various strategies have been developed to identify high-risk children.[10] The gold standard method for measuring insulin resistance is hyperglycemic-euglycemic clamp.[10] This test requires an overnight fast followed by constant infusion of insulin and glucose with periodic sampling of insulin and glucose concentrations.[12] It is cumbersome test, making it difficult to use in the outpatient setting. Another common assessment technique uses the frequently sampled intravenous glucose tolerance test (FSIVGTT).[10] These tests are not recommended for mass population screening due to their labor-intensive nature and high cost.[9] Alternatively, the homeostasis model assessment of insulin resistance (HOMA-IR), which estimates insulin resistance through fasting glucose and insulin levels, has been used in large epidemiologic studies.[10] In studies of nondiabetic children, HOMA-IR was highly correlated with clamp and FSIVGTT, supporting its potential usefulness in diagnosing T2DM in a pediatric population.[10]

The National Health and Nutrition Examination Survey (NHANES) from 1999 to 2002 examined the prevalence of insulin resistance, defined as HOMA-IR greater than 4.39 (upper 2.5 percentile) or greater than 2 SD above mean HOMA-IR, and determined that obesity was a major determinant of insulin resistance independent of age, gender, or ethnicity.[10] Prevalence of insulin resistance in obese adolescents was 52.1%, and girls had higher HOMA-IR than boys.[10] Furthermore, Mexican-American children had higher HOMA-IR than white children, whereas HOMA-IR in black and white children was not statistically different.[10]

Ectopic Fat Deposition

Body fat distribution is an important component effecting the development of insulin resistance.[13] Disruption of insulin signal transduction occurs due to presence of fatty acid derivatives of intramyocellular lipid deposition, which leads to decreased glucose uptake and is associated with insulin resistance.[14] Despite similar adiposity, obese adolescents with impaired glucose tolerance (IGT) were more insulin resistant than those with normal glucose tolerance (NGT).[11] Subjects with IGT had increased intra-myocellular lipid content, increased visceral fat, and decreased subcutaneous fat deposition, which is not surprising because increased visceral fat has been related to increased insulin resistance in obese children.[14]

It has been proposed that fat deposited into visceral fat and other nonadipose tissue is the result of overflow from subcutaneous fat.[15–17] In adult data, increased fat cell size is a sign of impaired adipogenesis and was shown related to the development of T2DM.[15,18] Another study reported that an increased proportion of small adipocytes and an impaired expression of adipogenesis markers were also related to insulin resistance.[16,19] To explore this concept, obese adolescents were divided into two groups: high or low ratio of visceral adipose tissue to visceral plus subcutaneous adipose fat ratio (VAT/[VAT+SAT]).[15] The high ratio group had smaller proportion of large adipocytes and less expression of adipogenesis markers.[15] Large adipocytes down-regulate lipogenic genes to limit triglyceride storage and prevent metabolic dysfunction.[15,20] Meanwhile, decreased gene expression involved in adipose cell differentiation was observed in insulin-resistant offspring of patients with T2DM compared with insulin-sensitive controls in a previous study.[15,20] Thus, it can be concluded that reduced fraction of large subcutaneous adipocytes may play a part in abnormal abdominal fat partitioning and insulin resistance.[15]

Progression to Type 2 Diabetes in Youth

In adults, the progression from NGT to overt T2DM involves an intermediate stage of hyperglycemia, characterized by impaired fasting glucose and/or IGT, now known as prediabetes.[21] Reports have documented a high prevalence of prediabetes among obese children and adolescents.[22] The authors' cross-sectional study measured the prevalence of IGT in a multiethnic clinic-based population of 167 obese children and adolescents; IGT was detected in 25% of the obese children and 21% of the obese adolescents, and diabetes was identified in 4% of the obese adolescents, irrespective of ethnicity.[22] In this study, the risk factors associated with IGT in order of importance were insulin resistance (HOMA-IR), fasting proinsulin, 2-hour insulin level, and fasting insulin.[22] This study was the first to highlight the high prevalence of prediabetes in the midst of the childhood obesity epidemic.[22] Meanwhile, high prevalence of IGT has been also reported in obese children from other parts of the world, including Thailand[23] and the Philippines.[24]

Similarly, Goran and colleagues[25] found that 28% of obese Hispanic children with a positive family history for T2DM had IGT but found no cases of T2DM. Additionally, Weigand and colleagues[26] reported that the prevalence of IGT was 36.3% among an obese multiethnic cohort of children and adolescents with a risk factor for T2DM. Finally, the authors' longitudinal study was conducted in a multiethnic clinic-based population of 117 nondiabetic obese children and adolescents. IGT was initially detected in 25% of the obese youth.[27,28] After almost 2 years' follow-up, 10% of the NGT group converted to IGT and 45% reverted to NGT.[27] In the baseline IGT group, 24% developed diabetes and 30% remained IGT.[27] All subjects who developed diabetes had previously been IGT at baseline.[27] Measures derived from oral glucose tolerance test (ie, disposition index) were helpful to predict changes in glucose metabolism but fasting measures (ie, fasting insulin and glucose) were not. Disposition index is calculated as the product of insulin secretion and insulin sensitivity.[11] This study supports the need for sensitive and reliable diagnostic methods. The identification of children with abnormal glucose metabolism allows clinicians to intervene and prevent the progression to T2DM.

MANAGEMENT

Obesity has been connected to sedentary lifestyle and poor nutrition. Children are consuming more fast food and foods containing high fat and sugar. Physical activity has decreased among children and adolescents. Both lifestyle modification and drug therapies are recommended in the management of T2DM.

Lifestyle modification programs are geared to changing high-risk lifestyle behaviors.[29] A multidisciplinary family-based approach is critical factor to success.[29] These programs focus on dietary change, physical activity, and psychosocial support.[29] Weight loss and improvement in insulin resistance have been observed with lifestyle modification programs.[30] A randomized controlled trial showed the beneficial effects of a weight management program.[30] The intervention group was a family-based program, which included nutrition, exercise, and behavior modification.[30] Savoye and colleagues[30] showed a sustained treatment effect at 24 months for BMI z score, BMI, percent body fat, and HOMA-IR.

Because behavior change is difficult to achieve, most adolescents with T2DM require pharmacologic therapy early in their disease course.[31] There are no current guidelines regarding drug therapy initiation. Metformin is a biguanide and is a Food and Drug Administration (FDA)-approved treatment of T2DM in children 10 years or older[32] and decreases hepatic glucose production while improving peripheral insulin sensitivity.[33] A randomized, double-blind, placebo-controlled study of metformin showed safety and efficacy in pediatric subjects.[34] Subjects were treated with metformin ($\geq$2000mg daily) or placebo for 16 weeks.[34] Significant improvement in hemoglobin A1c was observed (7.5% vs 8.6%, $P<.001$).[34] Larger, prospective studies are needed to elucidate the role of monodrug therapy or combination therapy (lifestyle changes or other drugs).[29]

At this time, there is no FDA-approved medication for isolated insulin resistance.[35] Metformin, however, has been used off-label in obese children with insulin resistance and a meta-analysis, with 5 randomized controlled trials demonstrated positive effects of metformin in adolescents with prediabetes and/or insulin resistance.[36] After 6 months of metformin in children and adolescents, fasting insulin, HOMA-IR, and BMI decreased significantly.[36] Adult studies have shown more benefits from lifestyle intervention in combination with pharmacotherapy than the interventions alone.[36] There is no published study, however, on this relationship in children/adolescent age group.[36]

Metformin with insulin is the first choice in combination therapy.[37–39] There are few data on the efficacy and safety of other antihyperglycemic medications alone or in combination in children with T2DM.[29] Antihyperglycemic medications are divided by mechanism of action: insulin sensitizers (thiazolidinediones) and insulin secretagogues (DPP-IV inhibitors, incretin mimetics, meglitinides, and sulfonylureas).[29] These medications are not FDA approved for the treatment of T2DM in children.[29]

An ongoing clinical trial on treatments of T2DM in children and adolescents, Treatment Options for Type 2 Diabetes in Adolescent and Youth (TODAY), is being conducted.[33] The TODAY trial involves 3 treatment groups: metformin (1000 mg bid), metformin plus rosiglitazone (4 mg bid), and metformin plus intensive lifestyle intervention.[33] TODAY results are currently pending and may shed light on the optimal management for T2DM in children and adolescents.[6]

SUMMARY

Over the past 2 decades, the prevalence of obesity and T2DM in children and adolescents has risen to epidemic proportions and disproportionately affects racial and ethnic minorities, who are at greater risk. The pathophysiology of T2DM is complex and involves insulin resistance and pancreatic β-cell dysfunction as well as visceral adiposity. Children who have impaired fasting glucose or IGT display abnormal insulin secretion, which can lead to T2DM. Current treatments of T2DM are limited to lifestyle intervention, metformin, and insulin therapy, and use of these strategies in combination is often most effective. The role of research is to uncover simple biomarkers for insulin sensitivity and optimal and innovative treatment of insulin resistance and T2DM.

REFERENCES

1. Pinhas-Hamiel O, Dolan LM, Daniels SR, et al. Increased incidence of non-insulin diabetes mellitus among adolescents. J Pediatr 1996;128:608–15.
2. Dabelea D, Pettitt DJ, Jones KL, et al. Type 2 diabetes mellitus in minority children and adolescents: an emerging problem. Endocrinol Metab Clin North Am 1999; 28:709–29.
3. Rosenbloom AL, Young RS, Joe JR, et al. Emerging epidemic of type 2 diabetes in youth. Diabetes Care 1999;22:345–54.
4. Nathan BM, Moran A. Metabolic complications of obesity in childhood and adolescence: more than just diabetes. Curr Opin Endocrinol Diabetes Obes 2008;15:21–9.
5. The Writing Group for the SEARCH for Diabetes in Youth Study Group. Incidence of diabetes in youth in the United States. JAMA 2007;297:2716–24.
6. Amed S, Daneman D, Mahmud FH, et al. Type 2 diabetes in children and adolescents. Expert Rev Cardiovasc Ther 2010;8(3):393–407.
7. Cali AM, Caprio S. Prediabetes and type 2 diabetes in youth: an emerging epidemic disease? Curr Opin Endocrinol Diabetes Obes 2008;15:123–7.
8. Klingensmith GJ, Pyle L, Arslaian S, et al. The presence of GAD and IA-2 antibodies in youth with type 2 diabetes phenotype. Diabetes Care 2010;33:1970–5.
9. Grodsky G. The kinetics of insulin release. In: Hasselblatt A, Bruchhausen F, editors. Handbook of Experimental Pharmacology, vol. 32. Berlin: Springer-Verlag; 1975. p. 1–19.
10. Lee JM, Okumura MJ, Davis MM, et al. Prevalence and determinants of insulin resistance among US adolescents. Diabetes Care 2006;29:2427–32.
11. D'Adamo E, Caprio S. Type 2 diabetes in youth: epidemiology and pathophysiology. Diabetes Care 2011;34:S161–5.
12. Nelson RA, Bremer AA. Insulin resistance and metabolic syndrome in the pediatric population. Metab Syndr Relat Disord 2010;8:1–14.
13. Tfayli H, Arslanian S. Pathophysiology of type 2 diabetes mellitus in youth: the evolving chameleon. Arq Bras Endocrinol Metabol 2009;53:165–74.
14. Weiss R, Kaufman F. Metabolic complications of childhood obesity. Diabetes Care 2008;31:S310–5.

15. Kursawe R, Cali A, D'Adamo E, et al. Cellularity and adipoegnic profile of the abdominal subcuatbeous adipose tissue from obese adolescents: association with insulin resistance and hepatic steatosis. Diabetes 2010;59:288–2296.

16. Danforth E Jr. Failure of adipocyte differentiation causes type II diabetes mellitus? Nat Genet 2000;26:13.

17. Shulman GI. Cellular mechanisms of insulin resistance. J Clin Invest 2000;106: 171–6.

18. Azuma K, Heilbronn LK, Albu JB, et al, Look AHEAD Adipose Research Group. Adipose tissue distribution in relation to insulin resistance in type 2 daibetes mellitus. Am J Physiol Endocrinol Metab 2007;293:E435–42.

19. McLaughlin T, Sherman A, Tsao P, et al. Enhanced proportion of small adipose cells in insulin-resistant obese individuals vs insulin sensitive obese individuals implicates impaired adipogenesis. Diabetologia 2007;50:1707–15.

20. Roberts R, Hodson L, Dennis AL, et al. Markers of de novo lipogenesis in adipose tissue associations with small adipocytes and insulin sensitivity in humans. Diabetologia 2009;52:882–90.

21. Genuth S, Alberti KG, Bennett P, et al. Expert Committee on the Diagnosis and Classification of Diabetes Mellitus. Follow-up report on the diagnosis of diabetes mellitus [review]. Diabetes Care 2003;26(11):3160–7.

22. Sinha R, Fisch G, Teague B, et al. Prevalence of impaired glucose tolerance among children and adolescents with marked obesity. N Engl J Med 2002;346: 802–9.

23. Keamseng C, Likitmaskul S, Kiattisathavee P, et al. Risk of metabolic disturbance and diabetes development in Thai obese children, 29th Annual Meeting of the International Society for Pediatric and Adolescent Diabetes. Saint-Malo (France), September 3–6, 2003.

24. Lee W, Tang J, Karim H, et al. Abnormalities of glucose tolerance in severely obese Singapore children, 29th Annual Meeting of the International Society for Pediatric and Adolescent Diabetes. Saint-Malo (France), September 3–6, 2003.

25. Goran MI, Bergman RN, Avila Q, et al. Impaired glucose tolerance and reduced beta-cell function in overweight Latino children with a positive family history for type 2 diabetes. J Clin Endocrinol Metab 2004;89(1):207–12.

26. Wiegand S, Maikowski U, Blankenstein O, et al. Type 2 diabetes and impaired glucose tolerance in European children and adolescents with obesity—a problem that is no longer restricted to minority groups. Eur J Endocrinol 2004;151(2): 199–206.

27. Weiss R, Taksali SE, Tamborlane WV, et al. Predictors of changes in glucose tolerance status in obese youth. Diabetes Care 2005;28(4):902–9.

28. Cali AM, Caprio S. Primary defects in β-cell Function further exacerbated by worsening of insulin resistance mark the development of impaired glucose tolerance in obese adolescents. Diabetes Care 2009;32:456–69.

29. Fleishmann A, Rhodes ET. Management of obesity, insulin resistance and type2 diabetes in children: consensus and controversy. Diabetes Metab Syndr Obes 2009;2:185–202.

30. Savoye M, Nowicka P, Shaw M, et al. Long-term results of an obesity program in an ethnically diverse pediatric population. Pediatrics 2011;127:402–10.

31. Pinhas-Hamiel O, Zeitler P. Clinical presentation and treatment of type 2 diabetes in children. Pediatr Diabetes 2007;8(Suppl 9):16–27.

32. Nathan DM, Buse JB, Davidson MB, et al. Medical management of hyperglycemia in type 2 diabetes: a consensus algorithm for the initiation and adjustment of therapy. Diabetes Care 2009;32:193–203.

33. Yanovski JA, Krakoff J, Salaita C, et al. Effects of metformin on body weight and body composition in obese insulin-resistant children. Diabetes Care 2011;60: 477–85.
34. Jones KL, Arslanian S, Peterokova VA, et al. Effect of metformin in pediatric patients with type 2 diabetes: a randomized controlled trial. Diabetes Care 2002;25:89–94.
35. Burgert TS, Taksali SE, Dziura J, et al. Alanine aminotransferase levels and fatty liver in childhood obesity: associations with insulin resistance, adiponectin, and visceral fat. J Clin Endocrinol Metab 2006;91:4287–94.
36. Garnett SP, Baur LA, Noakes M, et al. Researching Effective Strategies to Improve insulin Sensitivity in Children and teenagers- RESIST. A randomised control trial investigating the effects of two different diets on insulin sensitivity in young people with insulin resistance and/or pre-diabetes. BMC Public Health 2010;10:1–10.
37. Svoren B, Wolfsdorf JI. Management of diabetes mellitus in children and adolescents. Int Diabetes Monitor 2006;18(5):9–18.
38. Zuhri-Yafi MI, Brosnan PG, Hardin DS. Treatment of type 2 diabetes mellitus in children and adolescents. J Pediatr Endocrinol Metab 2002;15(Suppl 1):541–6.
39. Gemmill JL, Brown RJ, Nandagopal R, et al. Clinical trials in youth with type 2 diabetes. Pediatr Diabetes 2011;12:50–7.

Dyslipidemia and Pediatric Obesity

Stephen Cook, MD, MPH, FTOS*, Rae Ellen W. Kavey, MD, MPH

KEYWORDS

- Obesity • Dyslipidemia • Metabolic syndrome • Epidemiology
- Children • Adolescents • Waist circumference
- Insulin resistance

Cardiovascular disease (CVD) remains the leading cause of death in the United States despite a steady reduction in mortality over the past 4 decades, attributed to public health efforts to reduce cardiovascular risk factors and more aggressive treatment of clinical disease.[1] Concealed in the reduced overall mortality are increasing mortality rates due to obesity and diabetes.[1] When CVD mortality middle age adults, ages 35 to 54 years is considered separately, there is an unsettling plateau in the net rate of CVD deaths that can be traced to the steady rise in childhood obesity and diabetes over the past 4 decades.[2] This is interpreted as the leading edge of a new wave of CVD mortality.[3] Current adolescent overweight is forecast to increase future adult obesity by 5% to 15% by 2035, resulting in more than 100,000 excess prevalent cases of CVD.[4]

Concern about clinical events in middle-aged and older adults has been the primary focus in CVD but research over the past 2 decades has shown that the atherosclerotic process has its beginnings in childhood.[5,6] Management of hypercholesterolemia in pediatrics has traditionally focused on the identification of children and adolescents with severe elevation in total cholesterol (TC) and low-density lipoprotein cholesterol (LDL-C) levels, usually familial hypercholesterolemia (FH).[7,8] This lipid pattern occurs in 1 in 500 individuals and is inherited as autosomal dominant. It is not associated with obesity. Children with FH have severely elevated TC and LDL-C levels from birth and are at established high risk for premature CVD.[7,8] The focused approach on children with severe LDL elevation in the context of FH comes from the desire to identify youth and young adults who are at greatly elevated risk for premature coronary artery disease.[7] The number of children with LDL elevations, however, who meet criteria for drug treatment is small. Ford and colleagues[9,10] reported the rate of hypercholesterolemia from a nationally representative sample of US adolescents from 1999 to 2006, using the defined levels from the last National Heart, Lung, and Blood Institute (NHLBI) guidelines for management of hypercholesterolemia in childhood published in 1992[7] (TC $\geq$200 mg/dL and LDL-C $\geq$130 mg/dL) and found 5.2% with elevated LDL-C and

Department of Pediatrics, Golisano Children's Hospital, University of Rochester Medical Center, 601 Elmwood Avenue, PO Box 777, Rochester, NY 14642, USA
* Corresponding author.
E-mail address: stephen_cook@urmc.rochester.edu

Pediatr Clin N Am 58 (2011) 1363–1373
doi:10.1016/j.pcl.2011.09.003
0031-3955/11/$ – see front matter © 2011 Elsevier Inc. All rights reserved.

10.7% with elevated TC. They next examined the proportion of US adolescents with an elevated LDL-C that would trigger pharmacologic treatment based on recent American Academy of Pediatrics recommendations[9]: (1) LDL-C greater than 190 mg/dL with no other risk factors (likely genetic origin); (2) LDL-C greater than 160 mg/dL with greater than or equal to 2 additional risk factors (obesity, hypertension, smoking, or family history of premature CVD); and (3) LDL-C greater than 130 mg/dL among youth with diabetes mellitus. Only 0.8% of US teens had an LDL-C value elevated enough to consider starting drug treatment, and among these, less than half had LDL-C greater than 190 mg/dL.[9] From these findings, the number of children who meet criteria for drug treatment for hypercholesterolemia is small.

TRENDS AND PREVALENCE IN OBESITY AMONG PEDIATRIC POPULATIONS

Unfortunately, the pediatric obesity epidemic has resulted in a second and much larger population of children with abnormal lipids, those with secondary combined dyslipidemia. Childhood obesity rates have tripled in the past 30 years with as many as 17% of US adolescents and 16% of US children, 2 to 11 years of age, defined as obese.[11] Alarmingly, prevalence rates among black and Hispanic children and adolescents in the United States are even higher.[11] Severe obesity is formally defined by the 2007 Centers for Disease Control (CDC)/American Medical Association/Department of Health and Human Services childhood obesity expert committee recommendations as a body mass index (BMI) greater than the 99th percentile for age. In a recent report from a national sample of US children and adolescents,[12] almost 4%, or nearly 2.7 million of today's youth were severely obese. This study also examined the change in the prevalence of severe obesity from the 1980s to present and found alarming disparities, with Hispanic and African American children and adolescents as well as those in the lowest poverty group showing the greatest increase in rates of severe obesity over the past 3 decades.

Abdominal obesity is a special concern because of its known association with insulin resistance and the metabolic syndrome. In adults, the metabolic syndrome is defined as 3 or more of the following risk factors: elevated waist circumference, triglyceride (TG) levels, blood pressure, fasting glucose, and reduced high-density lipoprotein cholesterol (HDL-C). In the United States, the metabolic syndrome is said to affect between 34% and 39% of adults, including 7% of men and 6% of women in the 20-year-old to 30-year-old age group. As yet, there is no consensus on use of the diagnosis of the metabolic syndrome in children but the cluster of findings seen in adults often occurs with obesity in children.[13] In the first study to define the metabolic syndrome among US adolescents, abdominal obesity (defined as by waist circumference above the 90th percentile for age/gender) was found to be strongly associated with other cardiovascular risk factors defined in the metabolic syndrome, as in adults.[14] Li and colleagues[15,16] examined changes in measures of abdominal obesity from National Health and Nutrition Examination Survey (NHANES) data in 2 national cohorts of US children from 1988 to 1994 and from 1999 to 2004. Waist circumference had increased at a higher rate than BMI during that time period. Mean waist circumference for the population had increased from 2% to 8% depending on age and gender. Comparing these 2 cohorts, the overall relative increase in abdominal obesity for boys was 65.4% (10.5%–17.4%) and for girls 69.4% (10.5%–17.8%). This is important when considering the implications of abdominal obesity for identifying overweight or obese youth who may also have increased visceral fat. Visceral fat is strongly associated with the atherogenic dyslipidemia seen in the metabolic syndrome and insulin resistance. The rate of the metabolic syndrome found among US teens has also increased along with this trend in abdominal obesity.[15]

PATHOPHYSIOLOGY OF DYSLIPIDEMIA AND PEDIATRIC OBESITY

Childhood obesity appears with a powerful array of cardiovascular risk factors, including combined dyslipidemia, insulin resistance, and hypertension,[17] and has been shown to be associated with pathologic evidence of accelerated atherosclerosis in autopsy studies in this age group.[18] The dyslipidemia pattern associated with pediatric obesity consists of a combination of elevated TGs, decreased HDL-C, and top normal to mildly elevated LDL-C.[8] Normal lipid values in childhood have been developed from major epidemiologic studies, including the Bogalusa Heart Study and the Lipid Research Clinics Study, and are shown in **Table 1**.[7,8] Normal TG levels are less than 100 mg/dL in children younger than age 10 years and less than 130 mg/dL at ages 10 to18 years.[7,8] In the dyslipidemia associated with obesity, TG levels are usually between 100 and 400 mg/dL.[8] Recent NHANES data indicate this pattern is highly prevalent, present in 42.9% of children with BMI greater than the 95th percentile.[19] Insulin resistance, another common feature in obese children and adolescents, contributes significantly to development of the combined dyslipidemia of obesity by enhancing hepatic delivery of nonesterified free fatty acids for TG production and sequestration into TG-rich lipoproteins.[20] High TG levels are processed into small, dense LDL and small, less stable HDL; there is both an increase in small, dense LDL and in overall LDL particle number and a reduction in total HDL-C and in large HDL particles with analysis by nuclear magnetic resonance spectroscopy.[21,22] The combined dyslipidemia pattern seen with traditional lipid profile analysis identifies the atherogenic pattern seen with nuclear magnetic resonance spectroscopy analysis.[20]

The root cause of atherogenesis remains subendothelial retention of LDL-containing lipoproteins.[23] The combined dyslipidemia of obesity is particularly atherogenic for multiple reasons: small, dense LDL particles are inefficiently cleared by LDL receptors, elevated total circulating LDL particles heighten the risk of entrapment in the subendothelial matrix, and decreased large HDL particles limit reverse cholesterol transport.[24,25] The atherogenicity of the combined dyslipidemia seen with childhood obesity manifests in structural and functional vascular changes assessed

Table 1
Acceptable, borderline high, and high plasma lipid and lipoprotein concentrations (mg/dL) for children and adolescents[a]

Category	Acceptable	Borderline High	High[b]
Total cholesterol	<170	170–199	≥200
LDL–C	<110	110–129	≥130
Triglyceride			
0–9 years	<75	75–99	≥100
10–19 years	<90	90–129	≥130
Category	Acceptable	Borderline high	Low[b]
HDL-C	>45	40–45	<40

To convert to SI units, divide the results for TC, LDL-C, HDL-C, and non–HDL-C by 38.6; for TGs, divide by 88.6.

[a] Values for plasma lipid and lipoprotein levels are from the National Cholesterol Education Program (NCEP) "Expert Panel on Blood Cholesterol Levels in Children and Adolescents."[7] Non–HDL-C values are from the Bogalusa Heart Study and are equivalent to the NCEP pediatric panel cutpoints for LDL-C.

[b] The cutpoints for high and borderline high represent approximately the 95th and 75th percentiles, respectively. Low cutpoints for HDL-C represent approximately the 10th percentile.

noninvasively as increased carotid intima-media thickness (cIMT) and increased arterial stiffness.[26,27] In adults, combined dyslipidemia is the most prevalent pattern seen in individuals presenting with early clinical cardiovascular events.[21,22,28,29] In children, a recent report from the longitudinal Cardiovascular Risk in Young Finns Study revealed that, at 21-year follow-up, subjects with the combined dyslipidemia pattern beginning in childhood had significantly increased cIMT compared with normolipidemic controls, even after adjustment for other risk factors; cIMT was further increased when the dyslipidemia occurred in the context of the metabolic syndrome.[30] An article from the CDC evaluated multiple CVD risk factors in US children, specifically, systolic blood pressure, fasting glucose, and components of the lipid profile.[31] The mean and median values of TC, LDL-C, and glucose remained unchanged over multiple cohorts of US children and adolescents. Over successive cohorts, however, there was a significant increase in mean and median values of TGs and systolic blood pressure and a decrease in HDL-C, all components of the metabolic syndrome cluster. So, whether or not the metabolic syndrome is considered a separate entity, pediatric lipid profiles are qualitatively worse, even if TC and LDL-C levels have not increased. Thus, the combined dyslipidemia pattern seen with obesity in childhood is increasing in prevalence and predicts vascular dysfunction in young adulthood and early clinical events in adult life.

LIFESTYLE MANAGEMENT OF COMBINED DYSLIPIDEMIA

Treatment of combined dyslipidemia of obesity is primarily lifestyle change and this is often highly effective. Combined dyslipidemia has been shown to be responsive to even small changes in weight status, diet composition, and activity. Most importantly, in obese children, adolescents, and adults, even small amounts of weight loss are associated with significant decreases in TG levels and increases in HDL-C levels.[32–36] Even without weight loss, exercise training is associated with a significant decrease in TG levels and an increase in HDL-C, with reversion to baseline when subjects became less active.[34,37–39] A diet that limits both simple carbohydrate intake and calories addresses both combined dyslipidemia and obesity. In adults with hypertriglyceridemia, diet patterns like this significantly decreased TGs by a mean of 63% and increased HDL-C by 8%.[40,41] In adolescents, a low-carbohydrate diet associated with minimal weight loss significantly reduced TG levels.[42] A 12-month follow-up study of 21-month-old children with elevated TG levels treated with a carbohydrate-restricted diet showed that a decrease in sugar and carbohydrate intake was associated with a significant decrease in TG levels from a mean of 274.1 ± 13.1 mg/dL before treatment to 88.8 ± 13.3 mg/dL, within normal limits.[43] The concept of glycemic load has also been evaluated in the setting of obesity and combined dyslipidemia in adolescents and adults. The glycemic index is a measure of the blood glucose response to a 50-g portion of a selected carbohydrate; the glycemic load is the mathematic product of the glycemic index and the carbohydrate amount. In adolescents and young adults, there is evidence that low glycemic-load diets are at least as effective as low-fat diets in achieving weight loss, with decreased TGs and increased HDL in subjects on the low glycemic-load diet.[44–47] For all dietary change in children and adolescents, family-based training with a registered dietitian has been shown to be the most effective way to both begin and sustain change. A straightforward approach using a diet low in simple carbohydrates and sugar with controlled calories and a regular exercise schedule is shown in **Boxes 1** and **2**, **Table 2**, and **Fig. 1**; the latter was derived from just-released NHLBI guidelines for management of cardiovascular

---

Box 1
Diet composition: healthy lifestyle/combined dyslipidemia diet

These diet recommendations are those recommended for all healthy children over age 2 with specific differences focused on appropriate portion size and limitation of simple carbohydrate intake.

- Teach portions based on estimated energy requirements (EERs) for age/gender/activity level (see **Table 2**).

- Primary beverage: fat-free unflavored milk. No sugar-sweetened beverages; encourage water intake.

- Limit refined carbohydrates (sugars, baked goods, white rice, white bread, and plain pasta), replacing with complex carbohydrates (brown rice, whole grain bread, and whole grain pasta).

- Encourage dietary fish content.[a]

- Fat content:
  - Total fat 25%–30% of daily kcal/EER. Saturated fat ≤8% of daily kcal/EER. Avoid trans fats as much as possible. Monounsaturated and polyunsaturated fat up to 20% of daily kcal/EER; cholesterol <300 mg/d.

- Encourage high dietary fiber intake from naturally fiber-rich foods (fruits, vegetables, and whole grains) with a goal of "age plus 5 g/d."

[a] The Food and Drug Administration (FDA) and the Environmental Protection Agency are advising women of childbearing age who may become pregnant, pregnant women, nursing mothers, and young children to avoid some types of fish and shellfish and eat fish and shellfish that are lower in mercury. For more information, call the FDA's food information line toll free at 1–888–SAFEFOOD or visit http://www.cfsan.fda.gov/~dms/admehg3.html. Accessed August 3, 2011.
Data from Strong WB, Malina RM, Blimkie CJ, et al. Evidence based physical activity for school-age youth. J Pediatr 2005;146(6):732–7; and 2008 Physical Activity Guidelines for Americans. Available at: www.health.gov/paguidelines.

---

risk factors in childhood.[48] This is usually all that is necessary to address combined dyslipidemia in most obese children and adolescents.

DRUG THERAPY FOR COMBINED DYSLIPIDEMIA

In the rare child with combined dyslipidemia and severe hypertriglyceridemia for whom diet and exercise interventions are insufficient, there are nutriceutical and

---

Box 2
Activity recommendations for obese children

- Take activity and screen time history from child and parents at each visit.

- In children over age 6 years, prescribe moderate to vigorous activity[a] 1 h/d, with vigorous intensity physical activity[b] on 3/7 days.

- Combined leisure screen time should not exceed 2 h/d.

- Match physical activity recommendations with energy intake (see **Table 2**).

- No TV in child's bedroom.

[a] Examples of moderate to vigorous physical activities are walking briskly and jogging.
[b] Examples of vigorous physical activities are running, playing singles tennis, and soccer.
Data from Strong WB, Malina RM, Blimkie CJ, et al. Evidence based physical activity for school-age youth. J Pediatr 2005;146(6):732–7; and 2008 Physical Activity Guidelines for Americans. Available at: www.health.gov/paguidelines. Accessed August 3, 2011.

Table 2
EER (in kilocalories) for gender and age groups at three levels of physical activity[a]

Gender	Age (Years)	Sedentary[b]	Moderately Active[c]	Active[d]
			Activity Level[b,c,d]	
Child	2–3	1000	1000–1400[e]	1000–1400[e]
Female	4–8	1200	1400–1600	1400–1800
	9–13	1600	1600–2000	1800–2200
	14–18	1800	2000	2400
	19–30	2000	2000–2200	2400
Male	4–8	1400	1400–1600	1600–2000
	9–13	1800	1800–2200	2000–2600
	14–18	2200	2400–2800	2800–3200
	19–30	2400	2600–2800	3000

Estimates are rounded to nearest 200 calories and were determined using the Institute of Medicine (IOM) equation.

[a] These levels are based on EERs from the IOM *Dietary Reference Intakes* macronutrients report (2005), calculated by gender, age, and activity level for reference-size individuals. "Reference size," as determined by the IOM, is based on median height and weight for ages up to age 18 years and median height and weight for that height to give BMIs of 21.5 for adult women and 22.5 for adult men.

[b] A sedentary activity level in childhood, as in adults, means a lifestyle that includes only the light physical activity associated with typical day-to-day life.

[c] Moderately active in childhood means a lifestyle that includes some physical activity, equivalent to an adult walking approximately 1.5 to 3 miles per day at 3 to 4 miles per hour, in addition to the light physical activity associated with typical day-to-day life.

[d] Active means a lifestyle that includes more physical activity, equivalent to an adult walking more than 3 miles per day at 3 to 4 miles per hour, in addition to the light physical activity associated with typical day-to-day life.

[e] The calorie ranges shown recognize the needs of different ages within the group. For growing children and adolescents, more calories are needed at older ages.

Data from National Academy of Sciences. Institute of Medicine. Food and Nutrition Board. Dietary reference intakes for energy, carbohydrate, fiber, fat, fatty acids, cholesterol, protein, and amino acids (macronutrients). Washington, DC: Institute of Medicine, National Academies Press, 2005; with permission.

medication options that can be considered. The TG level and the timing for consideration of more advanced therapy are outlined in the algorithm (see **Fig. 1**). A recent systematic review demonstrated that omega-3 fish oil capsules are both safe and effective in adults, reducing TGs by 30% to 45%, with significant associated increases in HDL-C.[49] For children, the safety of omega-3 fish oil was observed in their use in children with immunoglobulin A nephropathy and in a small series of children with dyslipidemia.[50] Because fish oil preparations are marketed directly to the public, pediatric care providers can expect to encounter children who are taking these supplements and should be prepared to offer guidance about their use. There are many generic forms of fish oil capsules that are commercially available. The University of Wisconsin maintains a preventive cardiology patient education Web site, http://www.heartdecision.org. The "fish oil" section includes information about the content of various preparations. The Web site is updated every 6 months (https://www.heartdecision.org/chdrisk/v_hd/patient_edu_docs/Fish_Oil_11-2007.pdf). There is one FDA-approved omega-3 fish oil preparation, called Lovaza. Each capsule contains 1 g of fish oil with a recommended dose of 4 g/d, given either all at once or as 2 g twice a day. At the recommended dosage, there are almost no reported side effects for fish oil preparations except a fishy after taste and increased burping. In some studies, there has been a 5% to 10% dose-related increase in LDL-C levels. Allergic reactions can occur in individuals who have allergies to fish. The statin

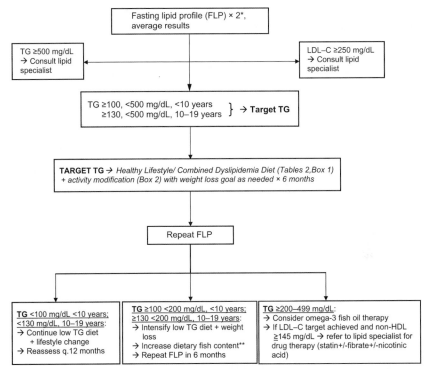

Fig. 1. Algorithm for management of combined dyslipidemia/high TGs. *Obtain fasting lipid profiles (FLPs) at least 2 weeks but no more than 3 months apart. **The FDA and the Environmental Protection Agency are advising women of childbearing age who may become pregnant, pregnant women, nursing mothers, and young children to avoid some types of fish and shellfish and eat fish and shellfish that are lower in mercury. For more information, call the FDA's food information line toll free at 1–888–SAFEFOOD or visit http://www.cfsan.fda. gov/~dms/admehg3.html. (*Data from* National Institutes of Health. National Heart, Lung and Blood Institute. NHLBI Pediatric Guidelines for Cardiovascular Health and Risk Reduction. Available at: http://www.nhlbi.nih.gov/guidelines/cvd_ped. Accessed August 3, 2011.)

medications have been studied in adults with combined dyslipidemia and have been shown to reduce total LDL particle numbers and to selectively decrease small, dense LDL.[51] One trial in children with familial hypercholesterolemia showed similar results with a significant decrease in total LDL particle number and in small, dense LDL concentration.[52] In adults, fibrates have been used to lower TG levels, and a small series in children demonstrated effective reductions in TG levels and an associated increase in HDL-C levels.[53] Finally, niacin has been used extensively in adults, but there is limited experience in children, with a single series demonstrating a high rate of side effects.[54] The use of any medication except omega-3 fish oil in youths with combined dyslipidemia should be undertaken only with the assistance of a lipid specialist.

SUMMARY

The prevalence of obesity has continued to rise over the past 3 decades. The obesity epidemic is already having an impact on the cardiovascular health of today's adults in their 30s and 40s. In children, obesity—especially abdominal obesity—is strongly associated with insulin resistance and with a high prevalence of the atherogenic combined dyslipidemia described in this article. Although these cardiometabolic abnormalities have not resulted in measurable increases in TC or LDL-C, adult and pediatric data have revealed qualitative changes in LDL-C and HDL-C associated with elevated measures of atherosclerosis among adolescents and with clinical disease in adults. A focused, family-based approach to management of these lipid abnormalities is critical and requires randomized trials of enhanced lifestyle approaches that will result in evidence-based treatment strategies.

REFERENCES

1. Ford ES, Ajani UA, Croft JB, et al. Explaining the decrease in U.S. deaths from coronary disease, 1980-2000. N Engl J Med 2007;356:2388–98.
2. Ford ES, Capewell S. Coronary heart disease mortality among young adults in the U.S. from 1980 through 2002: concealed leveling of mortality rates. J Am Coll Cardiol 2007;50:2128–32.
3. Heidenreich PA, Trogdon JG, Khavjou OA, et al. Forecasting the future of cardiovascular disease in the United States: a policy statement from the American Heart Association. Circulation 2011;123(8):933–44.
4. Bibbins-Domingo K, Coxson P, Pletcher MJ, et al. Adolescent overweight and future adult coronary heart disease. N Engl J Med 2007;357:2371–9.
5. McGill HC Jr, McMahan CA, Zieske AW, et al. Associations of coronary heart disease risk factors with the intermediate lesion of atherosclerosis in youth. The Pathobiological Determinants of Atherosclerosis in Youth (PDAY) Research Group. Arterioscler Thromb Vasc Biol 2000;20(8):1998–2004.
6. Berenson GS, Srinivasan SR, Bao W, et al. Association between multiple cardiovascular risk factors and atherosclerosis in children and young adults. The Bogalusa Heart Study. N Engl J Med 1998;338(23):1650–6.
7. NCEP Expert Panel of Blood Cholesterol Levels in Children and Adolescents. National Cholesterol Education Program (NCEP): highlights of the report of the Expert Panel on Blood Cholesterol Levels in Children and Adolescents. Pediatrics 1992;89:495–501.
8. Kwiterovich PO Jr. Recognition and management of dyslipidemia in children and adolescents. J Clin Endocrinol Metab 2008;93(11):4200–9.
9. Ford ES, Li C, Zhao G, et al. Concentrations of low-density lipoprotein cholesterol and total cholesterol among children and adolescents in the United States. Circulation 2009;119:1108–15.
10. Daniels SR, Greer FR, AAP Committee on Nutrition. Lipid screening and cardiovascular health in childhood. Pediatrics 2008;122:198–208.
11. Ogden CL, Carroll MD, Curtin LR, et al. Prevalence of high body mass index in US children and adolescents, 2007–2008. JAMA 2010;303:242–9.
12. Skelton J, Cook S, Auinger P, et al. Prevalence and trends of severe obesity among US children and adolescents. Acad Pediatr 2009;9(5):322–9.
13. Grundy SM, Cleeman JI, Daniels SR, et al. Diagnosis and management of the metabolic syndrome: an American Heart Association/ National Heart, Lung and Blood Institute Scientific Statement. Circulation 2005;112:2735–52.
14. Cook S, Weitzman M, Auinger P, et al. Prevalence of a metabolic syndrome phenotype in adolescents: findings from the third National Health and Nutrition Examination Survey, 1988-1994. Arch Pediatr Adolesc Med 2003;157:821–7.
15. Li C, Ford E, Mokdad A, et al. Recent waist circumference trends and waist-to-height ratio among US children and adolescents. Pediatrics 2006;118(5):e1390–8.

16. Cook S, Auinger P, Li C, et al. Metabolic Syndrome Rates in U.S. Adolescents, from the National Health and Nutrition and Examination Survey 1999-2002. J Pediatr 2008;152(2):165–70.

17. Freedman DS, Mei Z, Srinivasan SR, et al. Cardiovascular risk factors and excess adiposity among overweight children and adolescents: the Bogalusa Heart Study. J Pediatr 2007;150(1):12–7.

18. McGill HC, McMahan CA, Herderick EE, et al. Obesity accelerates the progression of coronary atherosclerosis in young men. Circulation 2002;105:2712–8.

19. Centers for Disease Control and Prevention. Prevalence of abnormal lipid levels among youths—United States, 1999-2006. MMWR Morb Mortal Wkly Rep 2010; 59:29–33.

20. Laakso M, Sarlund H, Mykkanen L. Insulin resistance is associated with lipid and lipoprotein abnormalities in subjects with varying degrees of glucose tolerance. Arteriosclerosis 1990;10:223–31.

21. Blake GJ, Otvos JD, Rifai N, et al. Low-density lipoprotein particle concentration and size as determined by nuclear magnetic resonance spectroscopy as predictors of cardiovascular disease in women. Circulation 2002;106:1930–7.

22. Kuller L, Arnold A, Tracy R, et al. Nuclear magnetic resonance spectroscopy of lipoproteins and risk of coronary heart disease in the cardiovascular health study. Arterioscler Thromb Vasc Biol 2002;22:1175–80.

23. Tabas I, Williams KJ, Boren J. Subendothelial lipoprotein retention as the initiating process in atherosclerosis: update and therapeutic implications. Circulation 2007;116:1832–44.

24. Campos H, Arnold KS, Balestra ME, et al. Differences in receptor binding of LDL subfractions. Arterioscler Thromb Vasc Biol 1996;16:794–801.

25. Barter P, Gotto AM, LaRosa JC, et al. HDL cholesterol, very low levels of LDL cholesterol, and cardiovascular events. N Engl J Med 2007;357:1301–10.

26. Paramsothy P, Knopp RH, Bertoni AG, et al. Association of combinations of lipid parameters with carotid intima-media thickness and coronary artery calcium in the MESA (Multi-Ethnic Study of Atherosclerosis). J Am Coll Cardiol 2010; 56(13):1034–41.

27. Koivistoinen T, Hutri-Kahonen N, Juonala M, et al. Apolipoprotein B is related to arterial pulse wave velocity in young adults: the Cardiovascular Risk in Young Finns Study. Atherosclerosis 2011;214:220–4.

28. Kathiresan S, Otvos JD, Sullivan LM, et al. Increased small low-density lipoprotein particle number: a prominent feature of the metabolic syndrome in the Framingham Heart Study. Circulation 2006;113:20–9.

29. Cromwell WC, Otvos JD, Keyes MJ, et al. LDL Particle Number and Risk of Future Cardiovascular Disease in the Framingham Offspring Study—Implications for LDL Management. J Clin Lipidol 2007;1:583–92.

30. Juonala M, Viikari JS, Ronnemaa T, et al. Associations of dyslipidemias from childhood to adulthood with carotid intima-media thickness, elasticity, and brachial flow-mediated dilatation in adulthood: the Cardiovascular Risk in Young Finns Study. Arterioscler Thromb Vasc Biol 2008;28(5):1012–7.

31. Ford ES, Mokdad AH, Ajani UA. Trends in risk factors for cardiovascular disease among children and adolescents in the United States. Pediatrics 2004;114:1534–44.

32. Epstein LH, Kuller LH, Wing RR, et al. The effect of weight control on lipid changes in obese children. Am J Dis Child 1989;143(4):454–7.

33. Nemet D, Barkan S, Epstein Y, et al. Short- and long-term beneficial effects of a combined dietary-behavioral-physical activity intervention for the treatment of childhood obesity. Pediatrics 2005;115(4):e443–9.

34. Kang HS, Gutin B, Barbeau P, et al. Physical training improves insulin resistance syndrome markers in obese adolescents. Med Sci Sports Exerc 2002;34(12): 1920–7.

35. Becque MD, Katch VL, Rocchini AP, et al. Coronary risk incidence of obese adolescents: reduction by exercise plus diet intervention. Pediatrics 1988; 81(5):605–12.

36. Siri-Tarino PW, Williams PT, Fernstrom HS, et al. Reversal of small, dense LDL subclass phenotype by normalization of adiposity. Obesity (Silver Spring) 2009; 17:1768–75.

37. Ferguson MA, Gutin B, Le NA, et al. Effects of exercise training and its cessation on components of the insulin resistance syndrome in obese children. Int J Obes Relat Metab Disord 1999;23(8):889–95.

38. Watts K, Beye P, Siafarikas A, et al. Effects of exercise training on vascular function in obese children. J Pediatr 2004;144(5):620–5.

39. Woo KS, Chook P, Yu CW, et al. Effects of diet and exercise on obesity-related vascular dysfunction in children. Circulation 2004;109(16):1981–6.

40. Pieke B, von Eckardstein A, Gulbahce E, et al. Treatment of hypertriglyceridemia by two diets rich in unsaturated fatty acids or in carbohydrates: effects on lipoprotein subclasses, lipolytic enzymes, lipid transfer proteins, insulin and leptin. Int J Obes Relat Metab Disord 2000;24:1286–96.

41. Musunuru K. Atherogenic dyslipidemia: cardiovascular risk and dietary intervention. Lipids 2010;45:907–14.

42. Sondike SB, Copperman N, Jacobson MS. Effects of a low-carbohydrate diet on weight loss and cardiovascular risk factors in overweight adolescents. J Pediatr 2003;142(3):253–8.

43. Ohta T, Nakamura R, Ikeda Y, et al. Follow up study on children with dyslipidaemia detected by mass screening at 18 months of age: effect of 12 months dietary treatment. Eur J Pediatr 1993;152(11):939–43.

44. Pereira MA, Swain J, Goldfine AB, et al. Effects of a low-glycemic load diet on resting energy expenditure and heart disease risk factors during weight loss. JAMA 2004;292(20):2482–90.

45. Ebbeling CB, Leidig MM, Sinclair KB, et al. Effects of an ad libitum low-glycemic load diet on cardiovascular disease risk factors in obese young adults. Am J Clin Nutr 2005;81(5):976–82.

46. Ebbeling CB, Leidig MM, Feldman HA, et al. Effects of a low glycemic-load vs low fat diet in obese young adults. JAMA 2007;297:2092–102.

47. Ebbeling CB, Leidig MM, Sinclair KB, et al. A reduced glycemic load diet in the treatment of adolescent obesity. Arch Pediatr Adolesc Med 2003;157: 773–9.

48. NHLBI expert panel on integrated guidelines for cardiovascular health and risk reduction in children and adolescents: Summary report. Pediatrics 2011; (Suppl 128)6.

49. Goldberg RB, Sabharal AK. Fish oil in the treatment of dyslipidemia. Curr Opin Endocrinol Diabetes Obes 2008;15:167–74.

50. Engler MM, Engler MB, Malloy MJ, et al. Effect of docosahexaenoic acid on lipoprotein subclasses in hyperlipidemic children (the EARLY study). Am J Cardiol 2005;95(7):869–71.

51. Guerib M, Egger P, Soudant C, et al. Dose dependent action of atorvastatin in type IIB hyperlipidemia: preferential and progressive reduction of atherogenic apoB-containing lipoprotein subclasses (VLDL-2, IDL, small dense LDL) and stimulation of cellular cholesterol efflux. Atherosclerosis 2002;163:287–96.

52. van der Graaf A, Rodenburg J, Vissers MN, et al. Atherogenic lipoprotein particle size and concentrations and the effect of pravastatin in children with familial hypercholesterolemia. J Pediatr 2008;152(6):873–8.

53. Wheeler KA, West RJ, Lloyd JK, et al. Double blind trial of bezafibrate in familial hypercholesterolaemia. Arch Dis Child 1985;60(1):34–7.

54. Colletti RB, Neufeld EJ, Roff NK, et al. Niacin treatment of hypercholesterolemia in children. Pediatrics 1993;92:78–82.

Advances in Pediatric Nonalcoholic Fatty Liver Disease

Ali A. Mencin, MD, Joel E. Lavine, MD, PhD*

KEYWORDS

- Nonalcoholic fatty liver disease (NAFLD)
- Nonalcoholic steatohepatitis (NASH) • Pediatric • Obesity
- Metabolic syndrome • PNPLA3

Nonalcoholic fatty liver disease (NAFLD) is the most common cause of liver disease in children and its increase is coincident with the obesity epidemic. NAFLD is defined as the presence of macrovesicular steatosis in greater than 5% of hepatocytes in the absence of significant alcohol consumption, drug use, or other recognized disorders that may result in fatty liver. The disease includes a range of disease severity from simple steatosis, which is thought to have a relatively benign prognosis, to nonalcoholic steatohepatitis (NASH), which can progress to cirrhosis. Among children, it is estimated that 5% of normal or overweight and 38% of children who are obese have evidence of NAFLD.[1] Given that obesity rates in the United States approach 30% in many areas, the prevalence of the disease is staggering.[2] Obesity trends in children are not isolated to the United States and are found worldwide.[3–8] Among those patients with NAFLD, a subset will develop NASH. Current evidence suggests that 1% to 3% of the Western population has NASH, making this disease a significant public health problem.[9]

Clinically, NAFLD is primarily a silent disease that is often suspected incidentally on physical examination or on routine blood testing. On physical examination, most patients will be overweight or obese and will commonly have acanthosis nigricans on the back of the neck, intertrigenous areas, or joints. Hepatomegaly can usually be appreciated, although palpating the liver is often challenging in obese individuals. Alanine aminotransferase (ALT) and aspartate aminotransferases (AST) can be abnormal in NAFLD, usually less than 200 U/L. Patients can also complain of abdominal pain as a presenting symptom, which may relate to stretching of the liver capsule as the liver expands or may be the result of other known obesity-related

Funding Disclosure: Dr Lavine is a consultant for Quark Pharmaceuticals and has received grant support from Raptor Pharmaceuticals.

Division of Pediatric Gastroenterology, Hepatology and Nutrition, Columbia University, 3959 Broadway, CHN 702, New York, NY 10032, USA

* Corresponding author.

E-mail address: jl3553@columbia.edu

Pediatr Clin N Am 58 (2011) 1375–1392
doi:10.1016/j.pcl.2011.09.005
0031-3955/11/$ – see front matter © 2011 Elsevier Inc. All rights reserved.

pediatric.theclinics.com

gastrointestinal comorbidities, such as reflux, constipation, or biliary tract disease. Abdominal pain often prompts the clinician to order an abdominal ultrasound, which sometimes demonstrates echogenicity of the liver that is highly suggestive of fatty infiltration.

Although the diagnosis of NAFLD may be strongly suspected based on clinical parameters, liver function tests and ultrasound, staging and grading of the disease still requires liver biopsy. Liver biopsy not only can confirm NAFLD but can differentiate between simple steatosis and NASH, which is relevant given differences in natural history. Laboratory testing to exclude other forms of liver disease, such as viral hepatitis, alpha-1 antitrypsin deficiency, Wilsons disease, hemochromatosis, and autoimmune hepatitis should be performed before liver biopsy as part of a general hepatitis evaluation in patients with persistently abnormal liver function tests.

This review endeavors to provide a clinically relevant general overview of pediatric NAFLD by using the most up-to-date literature on the topic. Our understanding of this disease has improved significantly in the last several years, and there have been many interesting advancements in the areas of diagnosis, pathophysiology, genetics, and management.

EPIDEMIOLOGY AND NATURAL HISTORY

The true prevalence of pediatric NAFLD is difficult to determine because screening guidelines are not established and the diagnosis can only be made definitively by liver biopsy. ALT is a nonspecific marker of liver injury in NAFLD, which can be easily obtained; unfortunately normal ALT values have not been clearly established in children.[10] Furthermore, it has been shown that up to 23% of children with NAFLD can have a normal ALT with liver fibrosis.[11] Although abnormal ALT is seen in numerous other liver diseases, most abnormal ALT levels in large populations are attributable to NAFLD. Despite limitations in sensitivity and specificity, ALT can be a valuable screening tool and has been used in numerous studies looking at the prevalence of NAFLD.[12] Data collected from the National Health and Nutrition Examination Survey on 5586 adolescents found elevated ALT in 8% of the study population. Elevated ALT correlated with male sex, Mexican American ethnicity, waist circumference, and fasting insulin levels.[13] The metabolic syndrome, which includes overweight or obesity, insulin resistance, elevated blood pressure, and abnormal waist circumference, has been strongly correlated with the development of NAFLD and disease severity.[14,15] In a European cohort of 16,390 overweight children and adolescents, 11% of the study population was found to have abnormal liver function tests that significantly correlated with high insulin levels, older age, increasing obesity, and male gender.[16] NAFLD prevalence in Asia seems to be as high or higher, although pediatric data is limited.[17] No official position statement by the major pediatric professional societies recommend routine screening for NAFLD, but plasma ALT may be an easily obtainable, although nonspecific, screening tool in patients considered high risk.

NAFLD is a clinicopathologic diagnosis and, therefore, liver tissue is required to determine true prevalence data in children. The only practical means to obtain this data has been to obtain autopsy specimens from children who had an accidental death. In a landmark article using 742 autopsy specimens from children in San Diego County, 17.3% of the children were aged from 15 to 19 years, were found to have the disease.[1] NAFLD was also found to be more common in boys and children of Asian (10.2%) and Hispanic (11.8%) background. African Americans had the lowest rates of NAFLD at 1.5%. Of note, most Hispanic subjects in this study were of Mexican background. Multiple studies have confirmed that male gender and Asian and Mexican ethnicity are risk factors for NAFLD, whereas African Americans seem to be protected.[18–21] It is worth noting that although boys are more likely to have NAFLD, boys and girls with NAFLD have an equal chance of developing NASH.[1,22]

The natural history of NAFLD in the pediatric population is not clearly understood because of a lack of prospective studies evaluating children over time. It seems that those patients with simple steatosis have a benign course, whereas those with NASH can progress to severe liver disease. In one study that retrospectively analyzed 66 pediatric patients with NAFLD over a period of 20 years, 4 patients developed type II diabetes and 4 progressed to cirrhosis.[23] Adult data indicate that one-third of patients with early NASH will progress to cirrhosis in 5 to 10 years, and it is a risk factor for hepatocellular carcinoma (HCC).[24–26] A recent study identified 4406 cases of HCC from a health care claims database and found that NASH was the leading etiologic risk factor (53%) followed by diabetes (36%).[27]

In addition to liver disease, NAFLD has been associated with the development of risk factors for cardiovascular disease and impaired quality of life.[28] In adults with NASH, death is more likely to result from cardiovascular disease than from liver disease.[29] NAFLD in children is associated with multiple cardiovascular risk factors, including abnormal waist circumference, dyslipidemia, hypertension, and insulin resistance.[30] Carotid intima media thickness (cIMT) is increased in children with NAFLD.[31–33] In one study, cIMT and flow-mediated dilatation of the brachial artery (FMD) were measured in 150 children with NAFLD and were compared with 100 obese controls. Those children with NAFLD had significantly worse cIMT and FMD, demonstrating that NAFLD is a risk factor independent of obesity in the development of cardiovascular disease.[34]

PATHOLOGY

NAFLD encompasses a range of disease severity spanning simple steatosis to NASH.[35] Simple steatosis refers to the accumulation of liver fat without apparent inflammation. Simple steatosis has a benign prognosis compared with NASH. However, emerging adult data suggest that a significant, albeit diminished, proportion of patients with simple steatosis may progress to NASH.[36] NASH describes a pattern in which there is both hepatic steatosis and inflammation. With prolonged liver inflammation, the liver responds with collagen deposition resulting in fibrosis and eventually cirrhosis. There exists both an adult pattern of NASH (type 1) and a unique pediatric pattern (type 2).[22] Type 1 NASH is characterized by inflammatory changes and fat accumulation around the central hepatic venule (**Fig. 1**). In type 2 NASH, inflammation and fibrosis are found around the portal tract (**Fig. 2**). Type II NASH has been associated more strongly with male sex and Hispanic and Asian background. Many patients have been noted to have overlapping features.[37]

IMAGING

There are 2 primary imaging modalities used in the assessment of NAFLD, including ultrasound and magnetic resonance imaging (MRI). Computerized tomography is not used because of radiation considerations. With ultrasound, a NAFLD liver seems echogenic or bright and is usually enlarged. Although readily available and of comparatively low cost, ultrasound has a few significant limitations. The first limitation is that liver echogenicity is only seen when approximately 30% or more of hepatocytes are steatotic, which results in diminished sensitivity. Other limitations of ultrasound include that it only visualizes part of the liver, provides no information on liver injury,

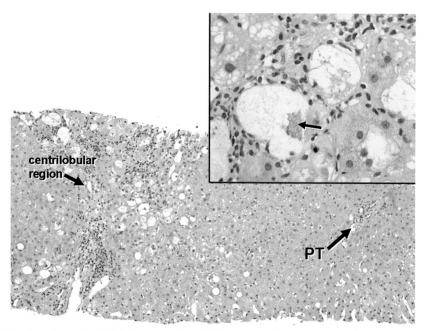

Fig. 1. Type I nonalcoholic steatohepatitis (adult type). At lower power, inflammatory cells are noted within the centrilobular region where indicated, whereas the area around the portal tract (PT) is relatively spared. Lipid droplets are more prominent in the centrilobular region (hematoxylin-eosin, original magnification ×40). The (*arrow*) inset image (hematoxylin-eosin, original magnification ×400) demonstrates a cytoplasmic aggregate known as a Mallory hyaline body. Mallory hyaline bodies and ballooned hepatocytes are more typical of type I NASH (hematoxylin-eosin, original magnification ×400).

and interpretation is operator dependent. Nevertheless, ultrasound is abundantly used both in clinical practice and some research studies because of its low cost and non-invasiveness. MRI shows the most promise as an imaging technique not only to assess liver fat content but to also assess liver fibrosis. MR spectroscopy provides

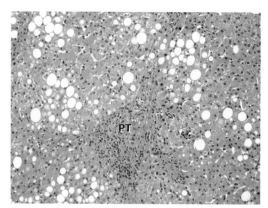

Fig. 2. Type II nonalcoholic steatohepatitis (pediatric type). Lower-power magnification demonstrates prominent steatosis and presence of inflammatory cells around the portal tract (PT) (hematoxylin-eosin, original magnification ×200).

the most accurate assessment of liver fat and a technique called MR elastography can be used to quantify fibrosis. The use of MR in NAFLD is still primarily a research tool.[38–40] Another device that may prove useful in the staging of liver disease involves transient elastography (known as FibroScan, Echosens, Paris, France). This device assesses liver stiffness, which correlates with hepatic fibrosis, using vibration through a topically applied transducer similar to an ultrasound probe. Elastography has been found in adult studies of NAFLD to correlate well with histologic fibrosis scoring.[41,42] In one study of 52 pediatric patients with biopsy proven NAFLD, this technique identified patients without fibrosis and those with significant fibrosis relatively well but was less useful for discriminating intermediate grades of fibrosis.[43] The utility of transient elastography is often limited by the large amount of subcutaneous fat in affected patients.

BIOMARKERS

Considering the high prevalence of NAFLD and that the current diagnosis requires a liver biopsy, which can be associated with significant, although uncommon, complications, the need for noninvasive biomarkers to diagnose and follow liver injury is critical. In the previous section, the authors briefly discussed the use of imaging studies for this purpose, but serum biomarkers offer the potential of diagnosis and monitoring disease activity at a low cost and with a simple blood test. The investigation of biomarkers has revolved around 3 different approaches.[44] The first approach is to use known markers of liver disease in isolation or in combination as an algorithm that can be correlated with NAFLD disease severity. The second is to investigate new markers based on what is known about NAFLD pathophysiology. The third method is to perform nonhypothesis-driven genome-wide association studies (GWAS) or proteomic studies to uncover genes or proteins that can be used clinically as markers of disease or disease activity. Most studies have been conducted in adult cohorts. For a full review of this topic, the authors recommend referral to recently published articles.[44,45]

The enhanced liver fibrosis test (ELF) comprises a panel of serum markers of liver fibrosis, including hyaluronic acid, amino terminal propeptide of collagen type III, and tissue inhibitor of metalloproteinase, combined in an algorithm to predict liver fibrosis.[46] In a study limited by the paucity of patients with moderate or severe fibrosis, the ELF test was used on 112 pediatric patients with biopsy-proven NAFLD.[47] Another pediatric study attempted to improve on the ELF by combining it with the NAFLD fibrosis index (age, waist circumference, and triglycerides) and the results showed promise in predicting the absence or presence of fibrosis.[48] Maffeis and colleagues[49] used a model combining the height-to-waist ratio, Homeostasis Model of Assessment-Insulin Resistance, adiponectin, and ALT in 56 obese 10-year-old children and found this algorithm to be predictive of NAFLD, although the study population was small. In adults, other biomarker profiles have also been used, including the FIB-4 (AST, ALT, platelet count, patient age), which has shown encouraging results.[50]

A potential marker of NAFLD severity is serum cytokeratin-18 (CK18), which is a protein filament cleaved by caspase-3 during apoptosis and released into the circulation. Feldstein and colleagues[51] published data comparing CK18 levels in 139 patients with biopsy-proven NAFLD versus 150 healthy controls. Serum levels of CK18 were found to both predict the presence of NASH and its severity with the area under the receiver operator curve at 0.83 (0.74, 0.91) for the diagnosis of NASH. CK18 may only be useful as a measure of disease activity once the diagnosis of NAFLD has already been confirmed because apoptosis is not unique to NAFLD.

The use of biomarkers in the staging and diagnoses of NAFLD can only be advocated for research purposes, especially in pediatrics, but advancements in the field show great promise and the authors anticipate that biomarkers will be used in the future for staging disease.

PATHOPHYSIOLOGY

Over the last several years, there have been many advances toward understanding the pathophysiology of NAFLD. From a simplistic point of view, the cause of NAFLD can be attributed to overnutrition, which can be defined as excessive caloric intake in the absence of appropriate caloric expenditure. The biologic mechanisms by which overnutrition leads to NAFLD are multifactorial and interrelated.[42,52,53] Although the epidemic of obesity can largely be ascribed to the decreased activity levels and poor food choices (or options) typical of many modern lifestyles, dozens of genes have been implicated in the development of obesity primarily through appetite regulation. The effect of single genes is small but combinations may have additive effects whose end result may promote obesity development.[54] However, given the rapid increase in obesity rates in the developing world, the role of genes in obesity development is likely small compared with the behavioral and environmental components.

Overnutrition is fundamental to the development of NAFLD, but excessive ingestion or deficiency of particular dietary components may play a significant role. One of the most widely discussed dietary factors is fructose, a constituent of both sucrose and high fructose corn syrup. Fructose, unlike glucose, is processed almost exclusively by the liver and is preferentially shunted into the lipogenesis pathway via glyceraldehyde-3-phosphate.[55] Fructose consumption has been associated with increased central obesity, hepatic lipogenesis, dyslipidemia, insulin resistance, and increased uric acid levels.[56,57] This finding is particularly relevant because fructose consumption in the form of sugar-sweetened beverages over the last several decades has increased considerably. As a percentage of total caloric intake in children aged 2 to 19 years, dietary surveys indicate that between 1977 and 2001 soft drink consumption increased from 3.0% to 6.9%, whereas fruit drink consumption increased from 1.8% to 3.4%.[56,58] In adult studies, consumption of soft drinks has been shown to be a risk factor for the development of NAFLD and increased liver fibrosis.[59–61] Although the deleterious effect of fructose consumption on NAFLD in pediatrics has still yet to be proven, one study has demonstrated a correlation between uric acid levels (a surrogate marker for fructose consumption) and NAFLD severity.[62] Mouse models provide further data that fructose intake may be harmful in NAFLD. A recent murine study revealed that a high-fat diet accompanied with high fructose and carbohydrate intake worsened hepatic fibrosis when compared with mice of the same weight on a high-fat diet alone.[63]

Other dietary components that may play a role in the development of NAFLD include saturated fatty acids and *trans* fatty acids. Both have been found to have a role in the development of the metabolic syndrome.[64–66] Rodent models have demonstrated reasonable causality between these two types of fats and NAFLD.[67–69]

Overnutrition eventually leads to the development of obesity and the accumulation of fat stores. Previously it was thought that adipose tissue was merely an inert storage site for lipid but now it is clear that it is metabolically active. Central obesity resulting from the accumulation of visceral adipose tissue (VAT) is strongly linked to the metabolic syndrome and seems to be key in NAFLD development.[70] Interestingly, VAT is the primary source of liver fat in adults with NAFLD, contributing 59% of the triglyceride (main fat component in NAFLD) found in the liver.[71] VAT is also fundamental to the proinflammatory state seen in the metabolic syndrome through the production of inflammatory cytokines (tumor necrosis factor [TNF]-α, interleukin [IL]-6) and free fatty acids (FFA), all of which promote insulin resistance, hepatic fat accumulation, and steatohepatitis (**Fig. 3**).[53,72] The cause of the release of proinflammatory mediators from adipose tissue may relate to adipose tissue hypoxia. There is evidence to suggest that as the adipose bed expands, adipocytes suffer from a microhypoxic environment resulting in cellular injury and death, which can then lead to an upregulation of the inflammatory cascade.[73,74] This finding is particularly interesting because there are data to suggest that hypoxia induced by obstructive sleep apnea in patients who are obese may worsen NAFLD.[75]

In addition to the production of proinflammatory cytokines, VAT produces the adipocytokines leptin and adiponectin. Leptin is a peptide hormone that acts centrally as an appetite suppressant. High levels of leptin are often seen in obese individuals, who commonly develop leptin resistance. In this resistant state, some of the protective effects of leptin are lost, such as the promotion of fatty oxidation and the prevention of hepatic lipogenesis.[76] There is also evidence that leptin directly promotes hepatic fibrogenesis and may play a role in the development of hepatocellular carcinoma.[77–79] Adiponectin has been shown to improve insulin sensitivity as well as have an antiinflammatory effect.[80] Increased VAT results in decreased adiponectin, low levels of which have been associated in the development of NAFLD in both epidemiologic studies and mouse models.[81–84] The effects of adiponectin on glucose homeostasis seem to be at least partially mediated through AMP-activated protein kinase and its upstream regulator liver kinase B1.[85] The antiinflammatory properties of adiponectin

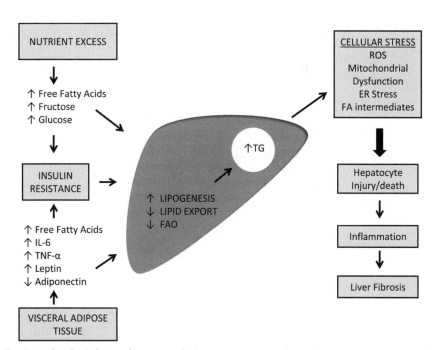

Fig. 3. Pathophysiology of NASH. Caloric excess, VAT, and insulin resistance promote fat deposition in the liver. In a subset of patients with NAFLD, fat deposition progresses from simple steatosis to NASH if cellular injury with concomitant inflammation occurs. Liver fibrosis may result. ER stress, endoplasmic reticulum stress; ROS, reactive oxygen species.

relate to the inhibition of TNF-α, upregulation of the antiinflammatory cytokine IL-10, and suppression of the lipopolysaccharide–induced inflammatory cascade.[83,86] Both increased leptin and decreased adiponectin have been associated with increased steatosis in NAFLD.[87]

One of the primary physiologic results of the proinflammatory cytokines and adipocytokines, which are produced in the obese state, is insulin resistance, which has been closely linked with the development of NAFLD, specifically NASH. Insulin is an anabolic hormone that promotes glucose uptake in liver, skeletal muscle, and adipose tissue as well as increasing hepatic and peripheral glycogenesis and lipogenesis. In obesity-related insulin resistance, glucose uptake is blunted, lipogenesis is increased, and there is increased breakdown and uptake of FFAs resulting in high serum FFAs.[72] Much of these FFAs are taken up by the liver where they are invariably processed into triglyceride (TG).[55,71] The increased fat deposition in the liver caused by insulin is mediated by sterol regulatory binding element (SREBP-1c), which upregulates many lipogenic genes.[88] As insulin resistance develops, elevated serum glucose levels activate the carbohydrate responsive element binding protein, which also promotes lipogenesis.[89] Chronic overnutrition resulting in obesity, therefore, creates an inflammatory cycle that promotes insulin resistance and hepatic lipid deposition.

As triglyceride accumulates within the hepatocyte, large fat vacuoles develop within the cytoplasm. The pathogenicity of this fat accumulation has been debated. Wanless and Shiota[90] postulated that extracellular fat accumulation after hepatocyte necrosis might impair hepatic blood flow through the hepatic veins but this remains unproven. Choi and Diehl[91] suggested that the formation of lipid droplets may actually be protective by sequestering away toxic FFAs in the form of triglyceride. When this sequestering process exceeds capacity, certain FFAs begin to exert their toxic effect.[91] This concept is supported by mouse work done by the same group, which demonstrated that when the final step in triglyceride synthesis (DGAT2) was inhibited with antisense oligonucleotides, hepatic fat accumulation decreased but liver damage worsened as measured by necroinflammation and fibrosis.[92] Conversely, upregulation of DGAT2 resulting in increased hepatic TG creation was associated with no significant increase in liver inflammatory markers.[93] FFAs and their lipotoxic intermediates have been implicated in hepatocellular injury by promoting inflammation, endoplasmic reticulum stress, mitochondrial dysfunction, and oxidant stress.[14,94] As a result of these processes, hepatocytes begin to die and release inflammatory cytokines and reactive oxygen species (ROS), which then further fuel an already upregulated obesity-related inflammatory environment. The role of cell death in the progression of disease has been demonstrated in a mouse model of NASH in which administration of a pan-caspase inhibitor, which mitigates hepatocyte death, resulted in decreased markers of liver fibrosis.[95] Hepatocyte injury and death directly and indirectly activate the hepatic stellate cells, which are the primary collagen-forming cells in the liver. This activation can result in the development of fibrosis and, if activation is chronic, cirrhosis.[96]

GENETICS

Evidence for a genetic contribution to NAFLD is supported by increased prevalence in boys, certain ethnicities and races, and family clustering. In children with biopsy-proven NAFLD, 59% of their siblings and 78% of their parents were found to have evidence of fatty liver on MRI, significantly more than in relatives of age and body mass index (BMI)-matched children without NAFLD.[40] There are many potential genetic contributors to NAFLD but those affecting lipid metabolism, insulin sensitivity, inflammation, oxidative stress, and fibrosis show particular promise as contributers.[97]

One of the most exciting recent developments has been the association between NAFLD and variants of the adiponutrin gene, otherwise known as patatinlike phospholipase 3 (PNPLA3). GWAS conducted by Romeo and colleagues[98] found that the PNPLA3 rs738409 SNP was seen more commonly in Hispanics and was associated with increased liver fat and hepatic inflammation, whereas the rs6006460 was seen more commonly in African Americans and correlated with less fat accumulation. A study of 475 obese and overweight children with a mean age of 10 years noted that homozygosity for the rs738409 variant was associated with a 52% increase in mean ALT levels compared with homozygous controls.[99] Another study of 83 obese children using MRI to quantify hepatic lipid content found that the rs738409 variant was associated with both increased steatosis and Hispanic ethnicity.[100] In a large adult cohort of 894 patients with biopsy-proven NAFLD, rs738409 correlated with worse hepatic inflammation and fibrosis. The same study also had a sizable pediatric cohort of 224 children, and although the investigators could not link the rs738409 SNP with histologic NAFLD severity, they found that this variant was associated with an earlier presentation of disease.[101] A recent meta-analysis that reviewed 11 studies, including 2651 patients with biopsy-proven NAFLD confirmed that PNPLA3 polymorphisms could be correlated with increased fat deposition and worse histologic injury.[102] In addition to its role in NAFLD, rs348409 seems to worsen disease severity in other liver diseases associated with hepatic fat accumulation, such as hepatitis C and alcohol-induced fatty liver disease, adding further proof to the importance of this gene variant.[103,104]

The mechanism by which the PNPLA3 rs738409 SNP affects liver disease is still under investigation. In humans, PNPLA3 is most robustly expressed in liver but it is also found in muscle and adipose tissue.[105] Expression seems to be directly related to nutritional intake, being downregulated in the fasting state and upregulated during feeding.[106] In vitro and mouse work have shown that SREBP-1, which is activated by insulin, induces PNPLA3, which then promotes hepatic lipogenesis and modulates glucose homeostasis.[107,108] Interestingly, the role of PNPLA3 on insulin resistance in humans remains controversial, with 2 studies in children demonstrating no association.[100,109] PNPLA3 is the most widely studied gene affecting the development of NAFLD but the role of many other genes is being investigated.

A recent study by Speliotes and colleagues[110] performed GWAS on subjects pooled from 3 large adult studies (Family Heart Study, Framingham Study, and Amish) to identify candidate genes in patients with evidence on NAFLD on computed tomography scan. Candidate genes were then correlated with histologic and metabolic liver data gathered in patients enrolled in the NASH Clinical research Network. This study demonstrated an association not only between PNPLA3 but also 3 other candidate genes in the development of histologically confirmed NAFLD. PNPLA3 rs738409 conferred the highest odds ratio of developing NAFLD at 3.26, confirming the significant role of PNPLA3. The other candidate genes included neurocan, lysophospholipaselike 1, and glucokinase regulatory protein and were associated with odds ratios of developing NAFLD of 1.6, 1.37, and 1.45, respectively. The function and mechanism of these candidate genes remain to be fully characterized.

Variants of apolipoprotein C3 (APOC3) have also been implicated in the development of NAFLD. Petersen and colleagues[111] conducted a study on 95 healthy Indian Asian men and found that 2 variants in APOC3 (rs2854116 and rs28541) were associated with a 30% increase in the fasting plasma APOC3 concentration and an approximately 60% increase in fasting plasma triglycerides. A total of 30% of those patients possessing one of these variants of APOC3 were found to have fatty liver disease on MR spectroscopy. No patients with wild-type APOC3 had evidence of fatty liver disease, and these findings were reproduced in a cohort of 163 non–Indian Asian men. However, several recent studies have brought into question the role of APOC3 and NAFLD. In a study of 2239 individuals who underwent MR spectroscopy to diagnose NAFLD as a part of the Dallas heart study, no association could be found between APOC3 and hepatic triglyceride content or insulin resistance.[112] A second study using a cohort of southern Europeans with biopsy-proven NAFLD also could not correlate APOC3 with liver disease severity.[113] A possible explanation for the discrepancy in the findings of these studies on APOC3 may relate to the fact that healthy patients with simple steatosis were used in the Petersen study, whereas patients in the other studies were more likely to have more severe liver disease.[114] Nevertheless, at this point the role of APOC3 in the development of NAFLD is in question and remains to be fully determined.

TREATMENT

Given that the primary cause of NAFLD relates to overnutrition, with worse disease associated with the metabolic syndrome, it should be no surprise that the mainstay of treatment should involve diet and exercise to promote weight loss, reduce hepatic TG content, and improve insulin sensitivity. Unfortunately, it is often difficult for patients to adhere to diet and exercise recommendations, necessitating the need to investigate medical and surgical therapies. Adult data have shown that a gradual 6% weight loss can improve insulin resistance and hepatic TG content.[115] Adult studies have also shown that weight loss from caloric restriction and exercise can also improve aminotransferases and histology in patients with NAFLD.[116,117] Pediatric studies in this area are limited but seem to support the adult findings. A 1-year lifestyle-intervention study in 84 pediatric patients with biopsy-proven NAFLD found that in the 68% of patients that were compliant, significant improvements were noted in markers of insulin resistance, aminotransferases, and hepatic lipid content as measured by ultrasound.[118] But improvements might be possible within an even shorter time frame. In a recently published study from Denmark, 117 obese children went to a 10-week camp in which weight loss was induced with dietary intervention and 1 hour of moderate exercise daily. At baseline, 43% of the patients had evidence of fatty liver on ultrasound and 50% had elevated aminotransferases. Of the 71 patients that finished the study, insulin sensitivity, liver steatosis, and aminotransferases all improved significantly, with a mean weight loss of 7.1 kg.[119] A study in adults demonstrates that vigorous activity (defined as energy expenditure greater than 6 times resting expenditure) is more beneficial in preventing NASH than longer intervals of moderate exercise.[120] Although diet and exercise that result in weight loss seem to be beneficial in the treatment of NAFLD in children, lack of intervention standardization has limited scientific knowledge in this area. What types of diet and exercise are most beneficial needs to be determined. A randomized adult study sponsored by the National Institutes of Health (NCT00771108) is underway comparing the effectiveness of low and moderate exercise regimens on NAFLD. Although weight loss is considered beneficial in NAFLD, very rapid weight loss resulting from starvation has been associated with worsening liver disease and should be avoided.[117] In clinical practice, the authors recommend that children with NAFLD follow a low-fat, low–glycemic index diet, consume a minimum of 5 servings of vegetables and fruits per day, minimize television/computer time to 2 hours per day, and participate in daily aerobic exercise for at least 1 hour per day.[121] An added benefit of successful lifestyle intervention is that it will not only treat NAFLD but also reduce the risk for other obesity-related illnesses.

Adherence to lifestyle changes is difficult and made more complicated by lack of scientific evidence on the effectiveness of specific interventions, which is why the development of medications to treat NAFLD has become such a priority. Medications used to treat NAFLD can be divided into 2 major categories: those that treat the metabolic syndrome and those that have a hepatoprotective response. The thiazolidinediones are a class of medications from the former category that have shown promise in adult studies. The thiazolidinediones activate PPARγ, which increases insulin sensitivity and reduces hepatic fat content but often results in weight gain and increased propensity for bone fractures. The safety of thiazolidinediones in children is not established. Antioxidants, such as vitamin E, have been suggested as a possible therapy given the role of reactive oxygen species in NAFLD pathophysiology. A recent randomized controlled trial compared pioglitazone or vitamin E with placebo in a 96-week trial using 247 adult patients with biopsy-proven NASH vitamin E versus placebo for the treatment of nondiabetic patients with nonalcoholic steatohepatitis (PIVENS).[122] Liver biopsy was performed at the end of the trial to assess for histologic changes from the baseline. Although pioglitazone treatment significantly improved individual histologic features of NASH and insulin sensitivity, only vitamin E significantly improved NASH histology based on the designated primary outcome. The findings of a long-anticipated, randomized, placebo-controlled pediatric trial were recently published comparing the effectiveness of the insulin sensitizer, metformin (1000 mg/d), with vitamin E (800 IU daily) validated these results. This trial, abbreviated TONIC (Treatment of NAFLD in Children), recruited children aged 8 to 17 years with biopsy-proven NASH and placed them on either metformin, vitamin E, or placebo for 96 weeks.[123] Although neither vitamin E nor metformin attained the primary outcome of sustained lowering of plasma ALT, treatment with vitamin E resulted in significant resolution of NASH and improvement in the NAFLD activity index. There were no serious adverse events. Taken together with the PIVENS data, there is now strong evidence supporting the use of vitamin E in addition to lifestyle interventions for the treatment of NASH in patients with biopsy-proven disease. However, there are no data on the long-term treatment of NAFLD with vitamin E.

The use of N-3 polyunsaturated fatty acids (LCPUFA) for the treatment of NAFLD has received attention because of their beneficial effects on insulin sensitivity, inflammation, and dyslipidemia. A recent randomized controlled study sought to investigate the effect of docosahexaenoic (DHA) in 60 children with biopsy-proven NAFLD.[124] The study population was divided into 3 groups: DHA 500 mg/d, DHA 250 mg/d, or placebo. After 6 months, hepatic echogenicity and insulin sensitivity were significantly improved in the DHA groups, although there was no change in serum ALT or BMI. The study was limited in that ultrasound was used to quantify liver fat, which is semiquantitative, and there is no evidence that reduction in liver fat fraction modulates progression in NASH. These results, however, warrant further investigation given encouraging adult data.[125,126]

In patients who suffer from extreme obesity and its comorbidities and have failed lifestyle intervention, bariatric surgery has become an increasingly popular option. In those adults with NAFLD who have undergone bariatric surgery, a substantial number have had resolution or significant improvement in their disease.[127–130] Data on the effectiveness of bariatric procedures on adolescent patients are lacking, but with increasing use of these procedures in older children, there is likely be information shortly on whether bariatric surgery provides benefit to adolescents with NASH.

SUMMARY

NAFLD is the most common cause of liver disease in children and its rising prevalence is inextricably linked to the obesity epidemic. The consequences of having the disease include liver dysfunction, cirrhosis, and cardiovascular disease. NAFLD can be seen in all racial groups but seems particularly prevalent in children of American Hispanic ancestry and Asians. The disease is closely linked to the metabolic syndrome that sets the stage for NAFLD by promoting inflammation and hepatic lipid accumulation. Pathologically, children have a distinct form of NASH, with inflammation and steatosis predominant near the portal tract. The different pathology of pediatric NASH implies a different pathophysiology compared with its adult counterpart, which remains to be characterized. Significant advancements have been made in identifying genetic risk factors for the disease, particularly the discovery and characterization of PNPLA3 variants that have been shown to correlate with increased hepatic steatosis and liver injury. Although liver biopsy remains the gold standard for diagnosis and monitoring disease activity, imaging studies and biomarkers have the potential to minimize or replace the use of liver biopsy. The mainstay of treatment of NAFLD remains rational weight loss, but vitamin E has been shown to ameliorate hepatic injury in well-designed adult and pediatric studies. Considerable research remains to identify genetic risk factors, identify environmental risks, and test superior therapeutic interventions.

ACKNOWLEDGMENTS

The authors would like to acknowledge Professor Jay Lefkowitch of the Columbia University Pathology Department for providing histologic images of NAFLD.

REFERENCES

1. Schwimmer JB, Deutsch R, Kahen T, et al. Prevalence of fatty liver in children and adolescents. Pediatrics 2006;118:1388.
2. Centers for Disease Control and Prevention (CDC). Vital signs: state-specific obesity prevalence among adults –- United States, 2009. MMWR Morb Mortal Wkly Rep 2010;59:951.
3. Janssen I, Katzmarzyk PT, Boyce WF, et al. Comparison of overweight and obesity prevalence in school-aged youth from 34 countries and their relationships with physical activity and dietary patterns. Obes Rev 2005;6:123.
4. Ji CY. The prevalence of childhood overweight/obesity and the epidemic changes in 1985-2000 for Chinese school-age children and adolescents. Obes Rev 2008;9(Suppl 1):78.
5. Matthiessen J, Velsing Groth M, Fagt S, et al. Prevalence and trends in overweight and obesity among children and adolescents in Denmark. Scand J Public Health 2008;36:153.
6. Ogden CL, Carroll MD, Curtin LR, et al. Prevalence of high body mass index in US children and adolescents, 2007-2008. JAMA 2010;303:242.
7. Park HS, Han JH, Choi KM, et al. Relation between elevated serum alanine aminotransferase and metabolic syndrome in Korean adolescents. Am J Clin Nutr 2005;82:1046.
8. Roberts EA. Non-alcoholic fatty liver disease (NAFLD) in children. Front Biosci 2005;10:2306.
9. Angulo P. Nonalcoholic fatty liver disease. N Engl J Med 2002;346:1221.
10. Schwimmer JB, Dunn W, Norman GJ, et al. SAFETY study: alanine aminotransferase cutoff values are set too high for reliable detection of pediatric chronic liver disease. Gastroenterology 2010;138:1357.
11. Manco M, Marcellini M, Devito R, et al. Metabolic syndrome and liver histology in paediatric non-alcoholic steatohepatitis. Int J Obes (Lond) 2008;32:381.

12. Rodriguez G, Gallego S, Breidenassel C, et al. Is liver transaminases assessment an appropriate tool for the screening of non-alcoholic fatty liver disease in at risk obese children and adolescents? Nutr Hosp 2010;25:712.

13. Fraser A, Longnecker MP, Lawlor DA. Prevalence of elevated alanine aminotransferase among US adolescents and associated factors: NHANES 1999-2004. Gastroenterology 2007;133:1814.

14. Chiang DJ, Pritchard MT, Nagy LE. Obesity, diabetes mellitus, and liver fibrosis. Am J Physiol Gastrointest Liver Physiol 2011;300:G697.

15. Manco M, Bedogni G, Marcellini M, et al. Waist circumference correlates with liver fibrosis in children with non-alcoholic steatohepatitis. Gut 2008;57:1283.

16. Wiegand S, Keller KM, Robl M, et al. Obese boys at increased risk for nonalcoholic liver disease: evaluation of 16 390 overweight or obese children and adolescents. Int J Obes (Lond) 2010;34(10):1468–74.

17. Chitturi S, Wong VW, Farrell G. Nonalcoholic fatty liver in Asia: firmly entrenched and rapidly gaining ground. J Gastroenterol Hepatol 2011;26(Suppl 1):163.

18. Barshop NJ, Francis CS, Schwimmer JB, et al. Nonalcoholic fatty liver disease as a comorbidity of childhood obesity. Ped Health 2009;3:271.

19. Louthan MV, Theriot JA, Zimmerman E, et al. Decreased prevalence of nonalcoholic fatty liver disease in black obese children. J Pediatr Gastroenterol Nutr 2005;41:426.

20. Petersen KF, Dufour S, Feng J, et al. Increased prevalence of insulin resistance and nonalcoholic fatty liver disease in Asian-Indian men. Proc Natl Acad Sci U S A 2006;103:18273.

21. Schwimmer JB, McGreal N, Deutsch R, et al. Influence of gender, race, and ethnicity on suspected fatty liver in obese adolescents. Pediatrics 2005;115:e561.

22. Schwimmer JB, Behling C, Newbury R, et al. Histopathology of pediatric nonalcoholic fatty liver disease. Hepatology 2005;42:641.

23. Feldstein AE, Charatcharoenwitthaya P, Treeprasertsuk S, et al. The natural history of non-alcoholic fatty liver disease in children: a follow-up study for up to 20 years. Gut 2009;58:1538.

24. Argo CK, Northup PG, Al-Osaimi AM, et al. Systematic review of risk factors for fibrosis progression in non-alcoholic steatohepatitis. J Hepatol 2009;51:371.

25. Ascha MS, Hanouneh IA, Lopez R, et al. The incidence and risk factors of hepatocellular carcinoma in patients with nonalcoholic steatohepatitis. Hepatology 2010;51:1972.

26. Starley BQ, Calcagno CJ, Harrison SA. Nonalcoholic fatty liver disease and hepatocellular carcinoma: a weighty connection. Hepatology 2010;51:1820.

27. Sanyal A, Poklepovic A, Moyneur E, et al. Population-based risk factors and resource utilization for HCC: US perspective. Curr Med Res Opin 2010;26:2183.

28. Kistler KD, Molleston J, Unalp A, et al. Symptoms and quality of life in obese children and adolescents with non-alcoholic fatty liver disease. Aliment Pharmacol Ther 2010;31:396.

29. Argo CK, Caldwell SH. Epidemiology and natural history of non-alcoholic steatohepatitis. Clin Liver Dis 2009;13:511.

30. Schwimmer JB, Pardee PE, Lavine JE, et al. Cardiovascular risk factors and the metabolic syndrome in pediatric nonalcoholic fatty liver disease. Circulation 2008;118:277.

31. Caserta CA, Pendino GM, Amante A, et al. Cardiovascular risk factors, nonalcoholic fatty liver disease, and carotid artery intima-media thickness in an adolescent population in southern Italy. Am J Epidemiol 2010;171:1195.

32. Demircioglu F, Kocyigit A, Arslan N, et al. Intima-media thickness of carotid artery and susceptibility to atherosclerosis in obese children with nonalcoholic fatty liver disease. J Pediatr Gastroenterol Nutr 2008;47:68.

33. Pacifico L, Cantisani V, Ricci P, et al. Nonalcoholic fatty liver disease and carotid atherosclerosis in children. Pediatr Res 2008;63:423.

34. Pacifico L, Anania C, Martino F, et al. Functional and morphological vascular changes in pediatric nonalcoholic fatty liver disease. Hepatology 2010;52:1643.

35. Brunt EM. Pathology of nonalcoholic fatty liver disease. Nat Rev Gastroenterol Hepatol 2010;7:195.

36. Wong VW, Wong GL, Choi PC, et al. Disease progression of non-alcoholic fatty liver disease: a prospective study with paired liver biopsies at 3 years. Gut 2011; 59:969.

37. Carter-Kent C, Yerian LM, Brunt EM, et al. Nonalcoholic steatohepatitis in children: a multicenter clinicopathological study. Hepatology 2009;50:1113.

38. Chen J, Talwalkar JA, Yin M, et al. Early detection of nonalcoholic steatohepatitis in patients with nonalcoholic fatty liver disease by using MR elastography. Radiology 2011;259:749.

39. Schwenzer NF, Springer F, Schraml C, et al. Non-invasive assessment and quantification of liver steatosis by ultrasound, computed tomography and magnetic resonance. J Hepatol 2009;51:433.

40. Schwimmer JB, Celedon MA, Lavine JE, et al. Heritability of nonalcoholic fatty liver disease. Gastroenterology 2009;136:1585.

41. Wong VW, Vergniol J, Wong GL, et al. Diagnosis of fibrosis and cirrhosis using liver stiffness measurement in nonalcoholic fatty liver disease. Hepatology 2010; 51:454.

42. Yoneda M, Mawatari H, Fujita K, et al. Noninvasive assessment of liver fibrosis by measurement of stiffness in patients with nonalcoholic fatty liver disease (NAFLD). Dig Liver Dis 2008;40:371.

43. Nobili V, Vizzutti F, Arena U, et al. Accuracy and reproducibility of transient elastography for the diagnosis of fibrosis in pediatric nonalcoholic steatohepatitis. Hepatology 2008;48:442.

44. Miller MH, Ferguson MA, Dillon JF. Systematic review of performance of noninvasive biomarkers in the evaluation of non-alcoholic fatty liver disease. Liver Int 2011;31:461.

45. Wieckowska A, McCullough AJ, Feldstein AE. Noninvasive diagnosis and monitoring of nonalcoholic steatohepatitis: present and future. Hepatology 2007;46:582.

46. Guha IN, Parkes J, Roderick P, et al. Noninvasive markers of fibrosis in nonalcoholic fatty liver disease: validating the European Liver Fibrosis Panel and exploring simple markers. Hepatology 2008;47:455.

47. Nobili V, Parkes J, Bottazzo G, et al. Performance of ELF serum markers in predicting fibrosis stage in pediatric non-alcoholic fatty liver disease. Gastroenterology 2009;136:160.

48. Alkhouri N, Carter-Kent C, Lopez R, et al. A combination of the pediatric NAFLD fibrosis index and enhanced liver fibrosis test identifies children with fibrosis. Clin Gastroenterol Hepatol 2011;9(2):150–5.

49. Maffeis C, Banzato C, Rigotti F, et al. Biochemical parameters and anthropometry predict NAFLD in obese children. J Pediatr Gastroenterol Nutr 2011. [Epub ahead of print].

50. Shah AG, Lydecker A, Murray K, et al. Comparison of noninvasive markers of fibrosis in patients with nonalcoholic fatty liver disease. Clin Gastroenterol Hepatol 2009;7:1104.

51. Feldstein AE, Wieckowska A, Lopez AR, et al. Cytokeratin-18 fragment levels as noninvasive biomarkers for nonalcoholic steatohepatitis: a multicenter validation study. Hepatology 2009;50:1072.
52. Day CP, James OF. Steatohepatitis: a tale of two "hits"? Gastroenterology 1998; 114:842.
53. Tilg H, Moschen AR. Evolution of inflammation in nonalcoholic fatty liver disease: the multiple parallel hits hypothesis. Hepatology 2010;52:1836.
54. Larter CZ, Chitturi S, Heydet D, et al. A fresh look at NASH pathogenesis. Part 1: the metabolic movers. J Gastroenterol Hepatol 2010;25:672.
55. Cohen JC, Horton JD, Hobbs HH. Human fatty liver disease: old questions and new insights. Science 2011;332:1519.
56. Hu FB, Malik VS. Sugar-sweetened beverages and risk of obesity and type 2 diabetes: epidemiologic evidence. Physiol Behav 2010;100:47.
57. Stanhope KL, Schwarz JM, Keim NL, et al. Consuming fructose-sweetened, not glucose-sweetened, beverages increases visceral adiposity and lipids and decreases insulin sensitivity in overweight/obese humans. J Clin Invest 2009; 119:1322.
58. Nielsen SJ, Popkin BM. Changes in beverage intake between 1977 and 2001. Am J Prev Med 2004;27:205.
59. Abdelmalek MF, Suzuki A, Guy C, et al. Increased fructose consumption is associated with fibrosis severity in patients with nonalcoholic fatty liver disease. Hepatology 2010;51:1961.
60. Abid A, Taha O, Nseir W, et al. Soft drink consumption is associated with fatty liver disease independent of metabolic syndrome. J Hepatol 2009;51:918.
61. Assy N, Nasser G, Kamayse I, et al. Soft drink consumption linked with fatty liver in the absence of traditional risk factors. Can J Gastroenterol 2008;22:811.
62. Vos MB, Ryan C, Patricia B, et al. Correlation of vitamin E, uric acid and diet composition with histologic features of pediatric nonalcoholic fatty liver disease. J Pediatr Gastroenterol Nutr 2011. [Epub ahead of print].
63. Kohli R, Kirby M, Xanthakos SA, et al. High-fructose, medium chain trans fat diet induces liver fibrosis and elevates plasma coenzyme Q9 in a novel murine model of obesity and nonalcoholic steatohepatitis. Hepatology 2010;52:934.
64. Funaki M. Saturated fatty acids and insulin resistance. J Med Invest 2009;56:88.
65. Micha R, Mozaffarian D. Trans fatty acids: effects on metabolic syndrome, heart disease and diabetes. Nat Rev Endocrinol 2009;5:335.
66. Sullivan S. Implications of diet on nonalcoholic fatty liver disease. Curr Opin Gastroenterol 2010;26:160.
67. Obara N, Fukushima K, Ueno Y, et al. Possible involvement and the mechanisms of excess trans-fatty acid consumption in severe NAFLD in mice. J Hepatol 2010;53:326.
68. Tetri LH, Basaranoglu M, Brunt EM, et al. Severe NAFLD with hepatic necroinflammatory changes in mice fed trans fats and a high-fructose corn syrup equivalent. Am J Physiol Gastrointest Liver Physiol 2008;295:G987.
69. Wang D, Wei Y, Pagliassotti MJ. Saturated fatty acids promote endoplasmic reticulum stress and liver injury in rats with hepatic steatosis. Endocrinology 2006;147:943.
70. Vega GL, Chandalia M, Szczepaniak LS, et al. Metabolic correlates of nonalcoholic fatty liver in women and men. Hepatology 2007;46:716.
71. Donnelly KL, Smith CI, Schwarzenberg SJ, et al. Sources of fatty acids stored in liver and secreted via lipoproteins in patients with nonalcoholic fatty liver disease. J Clin Invest 2005;115:1343.

72. Schenk S, Saberi M, Olefsky JM. Insulin sensitivity: modulation by nutrients and inflammation. J Clin Invest 2008;118:2992.
73. Hosogai N, Fukuhara A, Oshima K, et al. Adipose tissue hypoxia in obesity and its impact on adipocytokine dysregulation. Diabetes 2007;56:901.
74. Ye J, Gao Z, Yin J, et al. Hypoxia is a potential risk factor for chronic inflammation and adiponectin reduction in adipose tissue of ob/ob and dietary obese mice. Am J Physiol Endocrinol Metab 2007;293:E1118.
75. Turkay C, Ozol D, Kasapoglu B, et al. Influence of obstructive sleep apnea on fatty liver disease: role of chronic intermittent hypoxia. Respir Care 2011. [Epub ahead of print].
76. Polyzos SA, Kountouras J, Zavos C, et al. The potential adverse role of leptin resistance in nonalcoholic fatty liver disease: a hypothesis based on critical review of the literature. J Clin Gastroenterol 2010;45:50.
77. Choi SS, Syn WK, Karaca GF, et al. Leptin promotes the myofibroblastic phenotype in hepatic stellate cells by activating the hedgehog pathway. J Biol Chem 2010;285:36551.
78. De Minicis S, Seki E, Oesterreicher C, et al. Reduced nicotinamide adenine dinucleotide phosphate oxidase mediates fibrotic and inflammatory effects of leptin on hepatic stellate cells. Hepatology 2008;48:2016.
79. Wang SN, Lee KT, Ker CG. Leptin in hepatocellular carcinoma. World J Gastroenterol 2010;16:5801.
80. Tilg H. The role of cytokines in non-alcoholic fatty liver disease. Dig Dis 2010; 28:179.
81. Arita Y, Kihara S, Ouchi N, et al. Paradoxical decrease of an adipose-specific protein, adiponectin, in obesity. Biochem Biophys Res Commun 1999;257:79.
82. Buechler C, Wanninger J, Neumeier M. Adiponectin, a key adipokine in obesity related liver diseases. World J Gastroenterol 2011;17:2801.
83. Polyzos SA, Kountouras J, Zavos C, et al. The role of adiponectin in the pathogenesis and treatment of non-alcoholic fatty liver disease. Diabetes Obes Metab 2010;12:365.
84. Xu A, Wang Y, Keshaw H, et al. The fat-derived hormone adiponectin alleviates alcoholic and nonalcoholic fatty liver diseases in mice. J Clin Invest 2003;112:91.
85. Miller RA, Chu Q, Le Lay J, et al. Adiponectin suppresses gluconeogenic gene expression in mouse hepatocytes independent of LKB1-AMPK signaling. J Clin Invest 2011;121:2518.
86. Mandal P, Pratt BT, Barnes M, et al. Molecular mechanism for adiponectin-dependent M2 macrophage polarization: link between the metabolic and innate immune activity of full-length adiponectin. J Biol Chem 2011;286:13460.
87. Pisto P, Ukkola O, Santaniemi M, et al. Plasma adiponectin-an independent indicator of liver fat accumulation. Metabolism 2011. [Epub ahead of print].
88. Higuchi N, Kato M, Shundo Y, et al. Liver X receptor in cooperation with SREBP-1c is a major lipid synthesis regulator in nonalcoholic fatty liver disease. Hepatol Res 2008;38:1122.
89. Tsochatzis EA, Papatheodoridis GV, Archimandritis AJ. Adipokines in nonalcoholic steatohepatitis: from pathogenesis to implications in diagnosis and therapy. Mediators Inflamm 2009;2009:831670.
90. Wanless IR, Shiota K. The pathogenesis of nonalcoholic steatohepatitis and other fatty liver diseases: a four-step model including the role of lipid release and hepatic venular obstruction in the progression to cirrhosis. Semin Liver Dis 2004;24:99.

91. Choi SS, Diehl AM. Hepatic triglyceride synthesis and nonalcoholic fatty liver disease. Curr Opin Lipidol 2008;19:295.
92. Yamaguchi K, Yang L, McCall S, et al. Inhibiting triglyceride synthesis improves hepatic steatosis but exacerbates liver damage and fibrosis in obese mice with nonalcoholic steatohepatitis. Hepatology 2007;45:1366.
93. Monetti M, Levin MC, Watt MJ, et al. Dissociation of hepatic steatosis and insulin resistance in mice overexpressing DGAT in the liver. Cell Metab 2007;6:69.
94. Neuschwander-Tetri BA. Hepatic lipotoxicity and the pathogenesis of nonalcoholic steatohepatitis: the central role of nontriglyceride fatty acid metabolites. Hepatology 2010;52:774.
95. Witek RP, Stone WC, Karaca FG, et al. Pan-caspase inhibitor VX-166 reduces fibrosis in an animal model of nonalcoholic steatohepatitis. Hepatology 2009; 50:1421.
96. Bataller R, Brenner DA. Liver fibrosis. J Clin Invest 2005;115:209.
97. Tilg H, Moschen A. Update on nonalcoholic fatty liver disease: genes involved in nonalcoholic fatty liver disease and associated inflammation. Curr Opin Clin Nutr Metab Care 2010;13:391.
98. Romeo S, Kozlitina J, Xing C, et al. Genetic variation in PNPLA3 confers susceptibility to nonalcoholic fatty liver disease. Nat Genet 2008;40:1461.
99. Romeo S, Sentinelli F, Cambuli VM, et al. The 148M allele of the PNPLA3 gene is associated with indices of liver damage early in life. J Hepatol 2010;53:335.
100. Santoro N, Kursawe R, D'Adamo E, et al. A common variant in the patatin-like phospholipase 3 gene (PNPLA3) is associated with fatty liver disease in obese children and adolescents. Hepatology 2010;52:1281.
101. Rotman Y, Koh C, Zmuda JM, et al. The association of genetic variability in patatin-like phospholipase domain-containing protein 3 (PNPLA3) with histological severity of nonalcoholic fatty liver disease. Hepatology 2010;52:894.
102. Sookoian S, Pirola CJ. Meta-analysis of the influence of I148M variant of patatin-like phospholipase domain containing 3 gene (PNPLA3) on the susceptibility and histological severity of nonalcoholic fatty liver disease. Hepatology 2011; 53:1883.
103. Stickel F, Buch S, Lau K, et al. Genetic variation in the PNPLA3 gene is associated with alcoholic liver injury in Caucasians. Hepatology 2011;53:86.
104. Trepo E, Gustot T, Degre D, et al. Common polymorphism in the PNPLA3/adiponutrin gene confers higher risk of cirrhosis and liver damage in alcoholic liver disease. J Hepatol 2011;55(4):906.
105. Wilson PA, Gardner SD, Lambie NM, et al. Characterization of the human patatin-like phospholipase family. J Lipid Res 2006;47:1940.
106. Rae-Whitcombe SM, Kennedy D, Voyles M, et al. Regulation of the promoter region of the human adiponutrin/PNPLA3 gene by glucose and insulin. Biochem Biophys Res Commun 2010;402:767.
107. Huang Y, He S, Li JZ, et al. A feed-forward loop amplifies nutritional regulation of PNPLA3. Proc Natl Acad Sci U S A 2010;107:7892.
108. Qiao A, Liang J, Ke Y, et al. Mouse patatin-like phospholipase domain-containing 3 influences systemic lipid and glucose homeostasis. Hepatology 2011;54(2):509–21.
109. Goran MI, Walker R, Le KA, et al. Effects of PNPLA3 on liver fat and metabolic profile in Hispanic children and adolescents. Diabetes 2010;59:3127.
110. Speliotes EK, Yerges-Armstrong LM, Wu J, et al. Genome-wide association analysis identifies variants associated with nonalcoholic fatty liver disease that have distinct effects on metabolic traits. PLoS Genet 2011;7:e1001324.

111. Petersen KF, Dufour S, Hariri A, et al. Apolipoprotein C3 gene variants in nonalcoholic fatty liver disease. N Engl J Med 2010;362:1082.

112. Kozlitina J, Boerwinkle E, Cohen JC, et al. Dissociation between APOC3 variants, hepatic triglyceride content and insulin resistance. Hepatology 2011;53:467.

113. Valenti L, Nobili V, Al-Serri A. The APOC3 T-455C and C-482T promoter region polymorphisms are not associated with the severity of liver damage independently of PNPLA3 I148M genotype in patients with non-alcoholic fatty liver. J Hepatol 2011. [Epub ahead of print].

114. Romero-Gomez M. APOC3 polymorphisms and non-alcoholic fatty liver disease: resolving some doubts and raising others. J Hepatol 2011. [Epub ahead of print].

115. Sato F, Tamura Y, Watada H, et al. Effects of diet-induced moderate weight reduction on intrahepatic and intramyocellular triglycerides and glucose metabolism in obese subjects. J Clin Endocrinol Metab 2007;92:3326.

116. Musso G, Gambino R, Cassader M, et al. A meta-analysis of randomized trials for the treatment of nonalcoholic fatty liver disease. Hepatology 2010;52:79.

117. Torres DM, Harrison SA. Diagnosis and therapy of nonalcoholic steatohepatitis. Gastroenterology 2008;134:1682.

118. Nobili V, Marcellini M, Devito R, et al. NAFLD in children: a prospective clinical-pathological study and effect of lifestyle advice. Hepatology 2006;44:458.

119. Gronbaek H, Lange A, Birkebaek NH, et al. Effect of a 10-week weight-loss camp on fatty liver disease and insulin sensitivity in obese Danish children. J Pediatr Gastroenterol Nutr 2011. [Epub ahead of print].

120. Kistler KD, Brunt EM, Clark JM, et al. Physical activity recommendations, exercise intensity, and histological severity of nonalcoholic fatty liver disease. Am J Gastroenterol 2011;106:460.

121. Barlow SE. Expert committee recommendations regarding the prevention, assessment, and treatment of child and adolescent overweight and obesity: summary report. Pediatrics 2007;120(Suppl 4):S164.

122. Sanyal AJ, Chalasani N, Kowdley KV, et al. Pioglitazone, vitamin E, or placebo for nonalcoholic steatohepatitis. N Engl J Med 2010;362:1675.

123. Lavine JE, Schwimmer JB, Van Natta ML, et al. Effect of vitamin E or metformin for treatment of nonalcoholic fatty liver disease in children and adolescents: the TONIC randomized controlled trial. JAMA 2011;305:1659.

124. Nobili V, Bedogni G, Alisi A, et al. Docosahexaenoic acid supplementation decreases liver fat content in children with non-alcoholic fatty liver disease: double-blind randomised controlled clinical trial. Arch Dis Child 2011;96:350.

125. Capanni M, Calella F, Biagini MR, et al. Prolonged n-3 polyunsaturated fatty acid supplementation ameliorates hepatic steatosis in patients with non-alcoholic fatty liver disease: a pilot study. Aliment Pharmacol Ther 2006;23:1143.

126. Spadaro L, Magliocco O, Spampinato D, et al. Effects of n-3 polyunsaturated fatty acids in subjects with nonalcoholic fatty liver disease. Dig Liver Dis 2008;40:194.

127. Barker KB, Palekar NA, Bowers SP, et al. Non-alcoholic steatohepatitis: effect of Roux-en-Y gastric bypass surgery. Am J Gastroenterol 2006;101:368.

128. Mattar SG, Velcu LM, Rabinovitz M, et al. Surgically-induced weight loss significantly improves nonalcoholic fatty liver disease and the metabolic syndrome. Ann Surg 2005;242:610.

129. Pardee PE, Lavine JE, Schwimmer JB. Diagnosis and treatment of pediatric nonalcoholic steatohepatitis and the implications for bariatric surgery. Semin Pediatr Surg 2009;18:144.

130. Weiner RA. Surgical treatment of non-alcoholic steatohepatitis and non-alcoholic fatty liver disease. Dig Dis 2010;28:274.

Psychological Complications of Pediatric Obesity

Jillon S. Vander Wal, PhD*, Elisha R. Mitchell, MS

KEYWORDS

• Mental health • Child • Obesity • Pediatrics

In the United States, 16% of children ages 6 to 19 are between the 85th and 95th percentiles of body mass index (BMI) for age and 18.7% are at or above the 95th percentile.[1] Rates of extreme pediatric obesity, defined as a BMI percentile at or above the 99th percentile, are increasing disproportionately faster than rates of obesity.[2,3] The projected annual health care costs associated with increases in pediatric BMI are $14.1 billion annually.[4]

Psychological complications faced by overweight and obese youth are gaining increased recognition. Given heightened health care use among obese youth,[5] pediatricians are in a unique position to assess, identify, and intervene for mental health concerns. The purposes of this article are to review the psychological complications faced by obese youth, to examine models of the interaction between pediatric obesity and psychological complications via systems-level approaches for prevention and intervention, and to provide recommendations for pediatric practice.

PSYCHOLOGICAL COMPLICATIONS

Five comprehensive reviews of the literature on the psychological complications of pediatric obesity have been written, including those by Friedman and Brownell,[6] Hebebrand and Herpertz-Dahlmann,[7] Puder and Munsch,[8] Puhl and Latner,[9] and Wardle and Cooke.[10] Precise rates of psychological complications are uncertain owing to differences in methodology,[8] use of community versus treatment-seeking samples,[10] failure to control for relevant demographic characteristics,[10] and failure to take into consideration additional variables, such as parent psychopathology.[8] Psychological complications with small to moderate associations with child and adolescent obesity include body dissatisfaction, symptoms of depression, loss-of-control eating, unhealthy and extreme weight control behaviors, impaired social relationships, obesity stigma, and decreased health-related quality of life, whereas

Department of Psychology, Saint Louis University, 221 North Grand Boulevard, St Louis, MO 63103, USA
* Corresponding author.
E-mail address: vanderjs@slu.edu

Pediatr Clin N Am 58 (2011) 1393–1401
doi:10.1016/j.pcl.2011.09.008   **pediatric.theclinics.com**

complications with negligible to small associations include low self-esteem, clinically significant depression (of diagnostic severity, associated with significant distress and/or impairment, or inclusive of serious symptomatology), suicide, and full-syndrome eating disorders.[6–11] Additional complications manifested in later life include decreased educational and financial attainment.[4,9]

Associations between pediatric obesity and anxiety disorders are less well documented, although a recent study found modest associations after controlling for age, race, and Tanner Stage,[12] and a Swedish study found that psychosocial stress in the family was associated with increased odds of obesity at age 5.[13] Similarly, the association between child obesity and externalizing disorders, such as attention deficit hyperactivity disorder or oppositional defiant disorder, is less well documented, although recent literature suggests that aggressive and destructive behaviors at 24 months of age were predictive of disproportionate gains in BMI by age 12 among a nationally representative sample,[14] and a Finnish study suggested that conduct problems among boys at age 8 were predictive of disproportionate weight gain by young adulthood, after controlling for hyperactivity and sociodemographic factors.[15]

Overall, the association between child obesity and psychological complications is not as strong as one might suspect; rather, the strength of this association depends on important mediating characteristics, as depicted in **Fig. 1**. Potential demographic mediators include age, gender, race, and ethnicity. For instance, the self-esteem of obese children tends to decrease as they grow older.[7,11] Obese girls tend to have a greater prevalence of body dissatisfaction and low self-esteem than obese boys.[9,10] Self-esteem issues tend to be more prevalent among white than African American or Hispanic girls.[10] Further, some evidence suggests that childhood depression predicts the development of obesity, but that childhood obesity seldom predicts the development of depression.[9,7] This evidence suggests that, for some children, the treatment of childhood depression may help prevent the development of obesity. Unfortunately, the risks associated with pediatric obesity tend to increase over time.[4] Additional characteristics worthy of consideration include maternal mental health and socioeconomic status.[8]

In addition to demographic characteristics, the strength of the association between pediatric obesity and psychological complications may depend on teasing, obesity stigma, and treatment-seeking status. Obese children face greater levels of obesity stigma than nonobese children.[9,10,16,17] Obesity stigma may be evidenced in the form of negative stereotypes (eg, less attractive, less intelligent, less physically

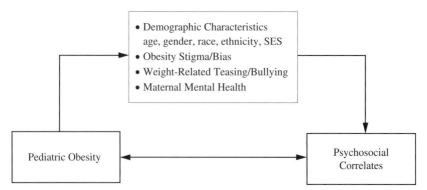

Fig. 1. The associations among pediatric obesity, psychological complications, and mediating characteristics. SES, socioeconomic status.

capable), victimization (ie, physical, verbal, or relational), and social marginalization.[16] Obesity stigma may come from peers, educators, or parents.[4,9] Overweight parents, as well as overweight youth, are just as likely to endorse negative stereotypes as are thin parents and youth,[9] suggesting that with time, obesity stigma may be internalized.

Obesity stigma is associated with adverse effects on self-esteem, depression, and body image; social marginalization; disproportionate weight gain; decreased physical activity; and lower academic achievement, and tends to be more prevalent among girls.[16] Unfortunately, the negative effects of obesity stigma may be self-perpetuating. That is, the negative impact of obesity on academic performance, emotional disturbance, or social difficulties may reinforce stereotypes and negative expectations.[9] Despite increases in the prevalence of youth overweight, obesity stigma appears to be increasing.[17]

An important manifestation of obesity stigma is weight-related teasing and peer victimization. Weight-related teasing is associated with degree of overweight, follows the development of obesity, and tends to increase with age before leveling off during adulthood.[9,11] Weight-related teasing is associated with depression and body dissatisfaction above and beyond gender, ethnicity, or weight status,[18] and is associated with additional psychological complications, including lower self-esteem, suicidality, anxiety, loneliness, binge-eating tendencies, reduced liking of physical activity, and a preference for isolative activities.[4,9,11] The prevalence of psychological complications according to teasing status in a sample of 4746 adolescents reported by Eisenberg and colleagues[18] is provided in **Table 1**. As can be seen, weight-related teasing nearly doubled the rates of psychological complications endorsed.

Obese youth presenting for weight loss treatment have a greater number of psychological complications than population-based samples of obese youth, particularly if they endorse body dissatisfaction.[7,9] Obese youth presenting for weight loss treatment have higher BMIs,[7,10] as well as higher family conflict, ineffective parental styles, and maternal distress,[11] than population-based samples of obese youth, which may be driving the greater prevalence of psychiatric problems. Among severely obese children with BMIs greater than or equal to 40 kg/m^2 presenting for bariatric surgery, 38.7% reported depressive symptomatology in the clinical range and marked impairments in both generic and health-related quality of life.[19]

Weight bias may affect eating behavior by increasing stress, in response to which unhealthy eating may be a common although misguided coping strategy.[7] Further, greater social isolation may result in reduced opportunities for physical activity, greater inactivity, and greater overconsumption of food.[11] Unhealthy weight control

Table 1
Prevalence of mental health concerns among adolescents by weight-based teasing status

Mental Health Concern	Girls		Boys	
	No Teasing, %	Peer/Family Teasing, %	No Teasing, %	Peer/Family Teasing, %
Low body satisfaction	24.1	47.7	10.2	36.3
Low self-esteem	16.0	37.2	8.9	19.3
High depressive symptoms	30.5	55.1	16.6	42.0
Suicidal ideation	24.7	51.1	14.4	34.3
Suicidal attempt (yes)	8.5	24.4	4.2	12.0

Data from Eisenberg ME, Neumark-Sztainer D, Story M. Associations of weight-based teasing and emotional well-being among adolescents. Arch Pediatr Adolesc Med 2003;157:733–8.

behaviors may be driven by obesity stigma, lower perceived acceptance, and relational victimization as a way of fitting in, and may reflect a lack of knowledge of healthy weight control behaviors.[20]

Unfortunately, psychosocial difficulties are associated with decreased weight loss success. Baseline depression,[11,21] loss-of-control eating,[22] greater parental distress,[23] and parent BMI[24] are associated with higher rates of weight loss treatment dropout. Improvements in weight status are associated with improvements in social problems, adjustment, and reductions in maternal distress.[11] Conversely, the presence of fewer psychological complications predicts better long-term weight loss maintenance.[25] Greater social marginalization is associated with increased television viewing, decreased sports participation, and decreased school club participation,[26] which may adversely affect weight status.

MODELS OF PEDIATRIC OBESITY AND PSYCHOLOGICAL COMPLICATIONS

The association between pediatric obesity and psychological complications is clearly multidirectional. As evidenced in the preceding presentation, ecological models that take into consideration individual, psychosocial, physical, and macrolevel environments are best suited for understanding the associations between child obesity and psychosocial difficulties.[11] Wilfley and colleagues[27] applied Bronfenbrenner's model of child development[28] to the treatment and maintenance of pediatric weight loss and regain. The resulting socioecological model addresses the relationships between the child and the child's family, peers, and community, including the child's school and neighborhood.

Consistent with the bioecological paradigm, interventions aimed at the child's family, lifestyle, and broader environment appear to hold the most promise with regard to treating pediatric obesity[29]; however, no single factor has been identified as having a significant impact on the pediatric obesity problem. Lifestyle interventions, defined as any combination of diet, physical activity, and/or behavioral treatments, have produced significant treatment effects compared with no-treatment wait-list control groups, as well as information/education-only control groups.[29]

In an excellent application of this model, Wilfley and colleagues[25] tested two family-based maintenance approaches to childhood weight loss in children ages 7 to 12 with at least one overweight parent: (1) behavioral skills maintenance (BSM), and (2) social facilitation maintenance (SFM). Children in both maintenance groups with fewer initial social problems demonstrated better long-term maintenance compared with controls, with slightly larger effects observed in the SFM group. Consistent with the bioecological theory, these interventions addressed the more immediate family social context, but also the broader peer environment. These findings highlight the importance of addressing these issues before the initiation of weight loss treatment or, at the very least, concurrently. The addition of social facilitation and skills building may prove to be a core improvement to lifestyle intervention programs.

Interpersonal therapy (IPT) has recently been identified as a targeted intervention strategy for the appetitive traits and social environmental factors associated with pediatric obesity.[27] This treatment aids in drawing connections between interpersonal triggers and behavior; eating outcomes are modified through social skills training and role negotiation.[27] IPT was piloted as a randomized treatment to adolescent girls at risk for weight gain with standard health education implemented as a control.[30] IPT resulted in fewer instances of loss-of-control eating episodes, and girls in the IPT group were less likely to increase BMI and BMI percentile over 1 year.

Another promising approach involves the application of multisystemic therapy (MST), a home-based treatment originally designed for the treatment of antisocial behavior, to the treatment of pediatric obesity.[31] Similar to IPT, MST is based in social-ecological theory and works by addressing the multiple systems in which the child is raised, including the family, peers, school, and community. MST was recently piloted as an intervention for obesity among African American adolescents.[31] Results showed significant reductions in percent overweight in the treatment as compared with a control group.

On a broader scale, social policies that encourage after-school programs offering an environment conducive to physical activity and social interaction may counteract both behavioral and social-environmental aspects of childhood obesity.[32] Thus, in addition to social aspects of treatment, an expansion of preventive interventions to include earlier age of intervention[33] and the larger system of family, peers, and community of the child may increase effectiveness of treatment. The social facilitation component of these interventions addresses the crucial mediating factors of weight-related teasing and obesity stigma.

The serious psychological complications of pediatric obesity are an important focus of treatment. Treatments, such as IPT, may prove to be more effective at preventing or treating pediatric obesity than more simple behavioral change strategies focused on either side of the energy balance equation. Consistent with a bioecological model, successful interventions for psychological complications and healthful weight in children must be achieved by engaging in activity that promotes these outcomes on a regular basis over an extended period of time, slowly becoming increasingly complex, with initiation and response in both directions within the environment.[28] Early intervention in the feeding environment, treatments that target the psychological correlates of pediatric obesity, including depression, self-efficacy, appetitive habits (eating in response to stress), and social skills training related to increasing interpersonal effectiveness, are likely to hold promise.

RECOMMENDATIONS FOR PEDIATRICIANS

The challenge of identifying children with obesity-related psychological complications is particularly salient for pediatricians. The medical setting is often the first point of contact for families and can facilitate much-needed early intervention.[27,33] The assessment of BMI must not only include assessment of dietary patterns and physical activity, but environmental and social supports and barriers, opinions on cause and effect of the problems, and self-efficacy and readiness to change.[11,34] It is the responsibility of the pediatrician to recognize the interactions between pediatric obesity and psychological complications and to engage patients and their caregivers accordingly.

The topics of weight and mental health issues must be approached with care and consideration. Evidence suggests that even health care professionals hold biased attitudes toward adult patients[9]—biases that may be extended to younger patients. Biased attitudes may be manifested in a tendency to blame parents for their children's weight status, negative comments on the parents' or child's weight, or failures to listen to parents. Parents may feel guilt, anger, and frustration because they do not know how to help their children, blamed for their children's weight status, or that their concerns and perspectives have been dismissed.[9,35] Parents are instrumental in the provision of their children's physical and social environments and a positive working relationship is essential to their children's physical and mental health.[11,35,36]

Motivational interviewing[37] is a directive therapy by which the professional helps move patients toward greater willingness and likelihood of making changes and implementing recommendations while diminishing resistance. Motivational interviewing has four guiding principles that collectively form the acronym, "rule." The first principle, resist the righting reflex, refers to the ability to refrain from directing or correcting others' ideas and behaviors. The natural reaction of patients is to defend themselves and their choices, which impedes change. The second principle, understanding patient motivations, refers to learning about patients' motivations for change rather than one's own. Personal motivations are stronger than impersonal motivations. The third principle, listening to your patient, involves the ability to understand and reflect back not only patient statements, but their underlying meaning. This understanding improves the ability to elicit changes that families can and will make. The final principle, empower your patient, involves eliciting families' own ideas for change and reinforcing them.

Physicians must objectively evaluate psychological complications among overweight youth and not assume maladjustment.[10,11] Although cue cards and tool kits to aid physicians in communicating with patients and their parents about obesity have been developed,[4] few such resources are available for psychological screenings. In general practice settings with low-risk patients, however, inquiry into the psychological functioning of children and their families is a good starting point. Areas of inquiry and possible conversation starters are provided in **Table 2**.

For moderate-risk patients, the addition of objective screening methods, such as standardized brief screening tools, is appropriate.[10] A variety of self-report measures are available by which to assess individual psychological complications. A better approach may be to administer a brief obesity-specific quality-of-life measure that incorporates the psychological complications described. Sizing Them Up[38] is a 22-item parent-report questionnaire for use with parents of children between the ages of 5 and 18. Sizing Them Up has 6 scales, including emotional functioning, physical functioning, teasing/marginalization, positive social attributes, mealtime challenges, and school functioning. A related scale, Sizing Me Up[39] is a 22-item self-report questionnaire appropriate for use with children between the ages of 5 and 13. Sizing Me Up has 5 subscales, including emotional functioning, physical functioning, social

Table 2
Conversation starters for assessing mental health concerns

Areas to Note	Conversation Starters
Demographics	• Age, gender, socioeconomic status, race, ethnicity
Peer relationships	• How would you describe your child's relationships with his/her peers? with his/her classmates?
Bullying/teasing	• Has your child encountered any difficulties with teasing? with bullying? • Does your child avoid socializing with peers?[a]
Body image	• Does your child have difficulty deciding what to wear? • Does your child express concerns regarding appearance?
Eating	• Does your child eat when not hungry? • Does your child engage in sneak-eating? • Does your child eat when upset?
Self-esteem	• Does your child say he/she isn't good enough? stupid? no good? • Does your child give up easily?
Depression	• Is your child often sad? • Does your child appear to be withdrawn? • Is your child frequently irritable?
Anxiety	• Does your child have difficulties with headaches? stomachaches? • Does your child worry a lot?

[a] May also be associated with depression or anxiety.

avoidance, positive social attributes, and teasing/marginalization. The Lifestyle Behavior Checklist (LBC)[40] is a measure of 26 weight-related problem behaviors among children, appropriate for parents of children between the ages of 4 and 11. The LBC also measures the extent of the problems and parents' confidence in dealing with them. The Impact of Weight on Quality of Life–Kids[41] is a 27-item self-report questionnaire for children between the ages of 11 and 19, with 4 subscales, including physical, emotional, social, and school functioning, as well as a summary score. Finally, a generic measure of health-related quality of life for children between the ages of 2 and 18 and their parents often used in the pediatric obesity area is the 23-item Pediatric Quality of Life Inventory (PedsQL 4.0).[42] The PedsQL measures physical, emotional, social, and school functioning.

More comprehensive screenings for high-risk populations are available and should be used by appropriately trained professionals, preferably in multidisciplinary treatment settings. These tools are most applicable for high-risk children, such as children with BMIs of 40 or greater or for youth presenting for professional weight loss services.[7] One such instrument is the Behavior Assessment System for Children (BASC-2),[43] a broad-based measure of the psychological well-being of children between the ages of 2 and 21. The BASC-2 includes forms appropriate for caregivers, children, adolescents, and teachers; takes about 10 to 30 minutes to complete depending on the reporter and patient age; and is available in English and Spanish. The Child Behavior Checklist[44] is a broad-based measure of behavioral and emotional problems for children between the ages of 1.5 and 18.0; suitable for caregivers, children, adolescents, and teachers; takes about 15 to 20 minutes to complete; and is available in multiple languages.

Mental health referrals may be made through insurance networks. Pediatricians may consider referral to psychologists who can assess for a broad range of physical and mental health conditions and aid in their treatment, as well as associated psychosocial difficulties.[27] Further, psychologists can intervene from a systems-level approach to promote the individual, family, and social-level change needed to promote and maintain weight loss. A psychologist intervening at a systemic level works not only with the child, but with the child's family to promote healthy eating practices, engage in opportunities for physical activity, and establish positive peer interactions at home, with external caretakers, in the child's school, and in the surrounding community. A coordinated interdisciplinary approach with frequent communication is optimal. Psychologists may be found via professional Web sites, including those of the American Psychological Association (http://www.apa.org), Association for Behavioral and Cognitive Therapies (http://www.abct.org), the Obesity Society (http://www.obesity.org), and the National Eating Disorders Association (http://www.edap.org), which contain clinician directories. Doctoral-level training centers, often affiliated with universities, may be low-cost alternatives for families with few resources. Addressing psychological complications associated with pediatric obesity is an important component of treatment success.

REFERENCES

1. Ogden CL, Carroll MD, Curtin LR, et al. Prevalence of high body mass index in US children and adolescents. JAMA 2011;303(3):242–9.
2. Freedman DS, Kettel Khan L, Serdula MK, et al. Racial and ethnic differences in secular trends for childhood BMI, weight, and height. Obesity 2006;14:301–8.
3. Koebnick C, Smith N, Coleman KJ, et al. Prevalence of extreme obesity in a multiethnic cohort of children and adolescents. J Pediatr 2010;157(1):1–6.

4. Maloney AE. Pediatric obesity: a review for the child psychiatrist. Child Adolesc Psychiatr Clin N Am 2010;19:353–70.
5. Hampl SE, Carroll CA, Simon SD, et al. Resource utilization and expenditures for overweight and obese children. Arch Pediatr Adolesc Med 2007;161: 11–4.
6. Friedman MA, Brownell KD. Psychological correlates of obesity: moving to the next research generation. Psychol Bull 1995;117(1):3–20.
7. Hebebrand J, Herpertz-Dahlmann B. Psychological and psychiatric aspects of pediatric obesity. Child Adolesc Psychiatr Clin N Am 2008;18:49–65.
8. Puder JJ, Munsch S. Psychological correlates of child obesity. Int J Obes 2010; 34:s37–43.
9. Puhl RM, Latner JD. Stigma, obesity, and the health of the nation's children. Psychol Bull 2007;133(4):557–80.
10. Wardle J, Cooke L. The impact of obesity on psychological well-being. Best Pract Res Clin Endocrinol Metab 2005;19(3):421–40.
11. Daniels SR, Jacobson MS, McCrindle BW, et al. American Heart Association Childhood Obesity Research Summit Report. Circulation 2009;119:e489–517.
12. Hillman JB, Dorn LD, Huang B. Association of anxiety and depressive symptoms and adiposity among adolescent females, using dual energy x-ray absorptiometry. Clin Pediatr 2010;49(7):671–7.
13. Koch F, Sepa A, Ludvigsson J. Psychological stress and obesity. J Pediatr 2008; 153:839–44.
14. Anderson SE, He X, Schoppe-Sullivan S, et al. Externalizing behavior in early childhood and body mass index from age 2 to 12 years: longitudinal analyses of a prospective cohort study. BMC Pediatr 2010;10:49–56.
15. Duarte CS, Sourander A, Nikolakaros G, et al. Child mental health problems and obesity in early adulthood. J Pediatr 2010;156:93–7.
16. Tang-Peronard JL, Heitmann BL. Stigmatization of obese children and adolescents, the importance of gender. Obes Rev 2008;9:522–34.
17. Latner JD, Stunkard AJ. Getting worse: the stigmatization of obese children. Obes Res 2003;11(3):452–6.
18. Eisenberg ME, Neumark-Sztainer D, Story M. Associations of weight-based teasing and emotional well-being among adolescents. Arch Pediatr Adolesc Med 2003;157:733–8.
19. Zeller MH, Modi AC, Noll JG, et al. Psychosocial functioning improves following bariatric surgery. Obesity 2009;17(5):985–90.
20. Stice E, Presnell K, Shaw H, et al. Psychological and behavioral risk factors for obesity onset in adolescent girls: a prospective study. J Consult Clin Psychol 2005;73(2):195–202.
21. Zeller MH, Kirk S, Claytor R, et al. Predictors of attrition from a pediatric weight management program. J Pediatr 2004;144:466–70.
22. Levine MD, Ringham RM, Kalarchian MA, et al. Overeating among seriously overweight children seeking treatment: results of the Children's Eating Disorder Examination. Int J Eat Disord 2006;39:135–40.
23. Epstein LH, Wisniewski L, Weng R. Child and parent psychological problems influence child weight control. Int J Eat Disord 1994;2:509–15.
24. Jelalian E, Hart CN, Mehlenbeck RS, et al. Predictors of attrition and weight loss in an adolescent weight control program. Obesity 2008;16:1318–23.
25. Wilfley DE, Stein RI, Saelens BE, et al. Efficacy of maintenance treatment approaches for childhood overweight: a randomized controlled trial. JAMA 2007;298:1661–73.

26. Strauss RS, Pollack HA. Social marginalization of overweight children. Arch Pediatr Adolesc Med 2003;157:746–52.
27. Wilfley DE, Vannucci A, White EK. Early intervention of eating- and weight-related problems. J Clin Psychol Med Settings 2010;17:285–300.
28. Bronfenbrenner U. Environments in developmental perspective: theoretical and operational models. In: Friedman SL, Wachs TD, editors. Measuring environment across the lifespan: emerging methods and concepts. Washington, DC: American Psychological Association Press; 1999. p. 3–28.
29. Wilfley DE, Tibbs TL, Van Buren DJ, et al. Lifestyle intervention for the treatment of childhood overweight: a meta-analytic review of randomized controlled trials. Health Psychol 2007;26:521–32.
30. Tanofsky-Kraff M, Marcus MD, Yanovski S, et al. Loss of control eating disorder in children age 12 and younger: proposed research criteria. Eat Behav 2010;9: 360–5.
31. Naar-King S, Ellis D, Kolmodin K, et al. A randomized pilot study of multisystemic therapy targeting obesity in African-American adolescents. J Adolesc Health 2009;45:417–9.
32. Goodman E, Whitaker RC. A prospective study of the role of depression in the development and persistence of adolescent obesity. Pediatrics 2002;109: 497–504.
33. Birch LL, Ventura AK. Preventing childhood obesity: what works? Int J Obes 2009;33:S74–81.
34. Lavizzo-Mourey R. Childhood obesity: what it means for physicians. JAMA 2007; 298(8):920–2.
35. Edmunds LD. Parents' perceptions of health professionals' responses when seeking help for their overweight children. Fam Pract 2005;22:287–92.
36. Rodin RL, Alexander MH, Guillory J, et al. Physician counseling to prevent over-weight in children and adolescents: American College of Preventive Medicine Position Statement. J Public Health Manag Pract 2007;13(6):655–61.
37. Rollnick S, Miller WR, Butler CC. Motivational interviewing in health care: helping patients change behavior. New York: Guilford; 2008.
38. Modi AC, Zeller MH. Validation of a parent-proxy, obesity-specific quality-of-life measure: Sizing Them Up. Obesity 2008;16:2624–33.
39. Zeller M, Modi AC. Development and initial validation of an obesity-specific quality-of-life measure for children: Sizing Me Up. Obesity 2009;17:1171–7.
40. West F, Sanders MR. The lifestyle behavior checklist: a measure of weight-related problem behavior in obese children. Int J Pediatr Obes 2009;4:266–73.
41. Kolotkin RL, Zeller MH, Modi AC, et al. Assessing weight-related quality of life in adolescents. Obesity 2006;14:448–57.
42. Varni JW, Burwinkel TM, Seid M, et al. The PedsQL 4.0 as a pediatric population health measure: feasibility, reliability, and validity. Ambul Pediatr 2003;3:329–41.
43. Reynolds CR, Kamphaus RW. BASC-2: behavioral assessment system for children manual. 2nd edition. Circle Pines (MN): AGS; 2004.
44. Achenbach TM, Rescorla LA. Manual for the ASEBA School-Age Forms and Profiles. Burlington (VT): University of Vermont, Research Center for Children, Youth, and Families; 2001.

Counseling and Behavior Change in Pediatric Obesity

Denise E. Wilfley, PhD*, Andrea E. Kass, MA, Rachel P. Kolko, MA

KEYWORDS

- Pediatric obesity • Socioenvironmental
- Office-based approaches • Health care professionals
- Lifestyle interventions

This article includes a brief summary of important points and objectives for recall:

- Family-based behavioral lifestyle interventions using a socioenvironmental approach produce sustainable weight loss.
- Ideally, providers are actively engaged in tracking children's body mass index (BMI) trajectory and addressing obesity with families.
- By using the socioenvironmental approach, providers can ensure that children receive consistent health messaging and encourage families to implement healthy eating and activity behaviors across contexts.

The obesity epidemic has reached epic proportions in the United States.[1,2] Approximately 70% of adults[3] and 32% of children in the United States are overweight or obese.[1] For children and adolescents, the Center for Disease Control and Prevention (CDC) defines overweight as a BMI (calculated as weight in kilograms divided by height in meters squared) between the 85th and 95th percentiles and obesity as a BMI at or above the 95th percentile for sex and age.[4] The BMI scores and specified percentile distributions are easy and feasible to obtain and serve as indirect measures of body fat.[5] Overweight and obesity are associated with chronic health conditions, heightened psychological distress, increased medical costs, and reduced quality of life.[6–10] As children become heavier, their risk for health problems, such as metabolic syndrome and cardiovascular disease, directly increases, as well.[6,11] Early intervention is essential because elevated childhood height and BMI are robust predictors of young adult BMI,[12] and findings show that children with a BMI above the 85th percentile are more likely to continue to gain weight and to become overweight or

The authors report no financial relationships with commercial interests.
Department of Psychiatry, Washington University School of Medicine, 660 South Euclid Avenue, Campus Box 8134, St Louis, MO 63110, USA
* Corresponding author.
E-mail address: wilfleyd@psychiatry.wustl.edu

Pediatr Clin N Am 58 (2011) 1403–1424
doi:10.1016/j.pcl.2011.09.014
0031-3955/11/$ – see front matter © 2011 Elsevier Inc. All rights reserved.

obese in adolescence than normal-weight children.[13] Although many assume that children will simply grow out of their overweight or obese status, the reality is that childhood overweight and obesity are critical risk factors for overweight and obesity in adulthood,[14] and risk of developing obesity later in life increases with child age and BMI.[13,14] The tendency for overweight or obesity to track across the lifespan starts as young as 9 months and necessitates early intervention because pediatric overweight and obesity do not spontaneously resolve with age.[15,16] **Box 1** provides key reasons why childhood is an ideal point of intervention[16]; in fact, even small weight loss reductions are sufficient for overweight and obese children to satisfy criteria for normal weight. (Goldschmidt AB, Wilfley DE, Paluch RA, et al. Indicated prevention of adult obesity: reference data for weight normalization in overweight children. Submitted for publication.)

The US Preventive Task Force recommends that overweight and obese children receive specialty treatment of moderate to high intensity that includes counseling and other interventions to target diet and physical activity; in addition, parents are expected to play a pivotal role in treatment.[17] A collaborative effort between primary care providers (PCPs) and behavioral interventionists is necessitated to provide consistent health messaging and support for successful weight loss and prevention of excess weight gain. Also, social support is the ultimate driver of sustainable behavior change; it is imperative to promote social facilitation within interventions for pediatric obesity.

The purpose of this article is to (1) discuss current practices and limitations for weight loss intervention in health care settings, (2) describe family-based behavioral interventions and outcome predictors, (3) review successful behavior change strategies for weight loss maintenance and the components of family-based behavioral interventions applied within a socioenvironmental approach, and (4) discuss recommendations for how to best utilize the office environment as a critical point for obesity prevention and treatment across socioenvironmental domains.

OVERVIEW OF OFFICE-BASED COUNSELING APPROACHES: CURRENT PRACTICES

Extending pediatric obesity interventions into common practice relies on identification of settings in which effective programs can be integrated. The health care office environment is ripe for intervention deployment because PCPs routinely meet with children and families, can screen for obesity and heightened weight status, and are

---

Box 1
Advantages of early intervention

Reasons Why Childhood is an Ideal Point of Intervention

- It is more difficult to reverse obesity in adulthood; adult interventions typically lead to only modest weight loss.

- Addressing overweight early can reduce or reverse negative medical and psychosocial sequelae.

- Children's dietary and exercise habits are not fully ingrained and are more amenable to change.

- Children are still growing taller, which might make it easier to achieve a reduction in overweight percentage even while maintaining weight.

- Traditional universal prevention programs (eg, in-school physical activity) do not yield significant weight reductions, necessitating a more intensive approach.

often the first line of care. In 2003, the American Academy of Pediatrics (AAP) published expert guidelines for the screening and monitoring of pediatric obesity.[18] This report encourages PCPs to track BMI percentile and promote healthy eating and activity behaviors. In 2007, the guidelines were updated with more intensive recommendations for obesity treatment and prevention.[5]

A significant proportion of PCPs report being unaware of these guidelines[19] or do not report regular implementation.[20] Some providers are able to incorporate the recommendations into practice,[20] especially after training,[21] although it is unclear whether PCPs sustain these behaviors in the long term.[22] Among PCPs who used current criteria for identifying overweight or obese children, many reported concerns that they lacked adequate skills to address the problem,[23] their counseling was ineffective, or adequate treatment strategies do not exist.[20,24–26] One study found that nearly all PCPs used visual assessment to determine children's obesity status, but only half actually computed BMI percentile.[20,25] Results from a separate survey revealed that most (71%) PCPs engaged in discussions with families about increasing healthy behaviors of overweight or obese children, but few (19%) provided families with the necessary tools to implement the changes, although only a limited number of providers followed up with families about their behavior changes.[23] In studies that report on children's weight change outcome as a result of brief provider counseling, findings generally point to nonsignificant reductions in BMI.[27–30]

However, despite a lack of weight change, some PCP interventions have led to increased healthy behaviors (eg, improved nutrition and physical activity patterns).[31,32] There is promise that PCPs are able to successfully incorporate behavior change principles into practice; given that effective intervention methods have been established but not implemented into routine care, there is a need for a more targeted intensive approach that unifies families, providers, and behavioral interventionists.[21]

UNDERSTANDING MOTIVATION IN PARENTS

Identifying families in need of intervention, connecting them with appropriate services, and checking on their progress represent central roles of PCPs. To maximize the integration of care across settings, it is ideal for PCPs to engage parents in conversations to assess their motivation and to evaluate their current needs and resources.

Given their crucial role in child weight loss success, it is important to address parents' confidence in their ability to do well in a weight loss intervention.[33,34] Gaining an understanding of parent motivation may be particularly relevant for PCPs because some PCPs rate lack of parental involvement as a common barrier to pediatric obesity treatment.[23] A recent study assessed 3 components of motivation: readiness (to change a specific behavior), importance (of making the change), and confidence (in their ability to make the change).[33] Parental confidence was the strongest predictor of treatment completion and child weight loss. Braet and colleagues[34] showed that parents' motivation at baseline predicted treatment completion. In addition, an intervention designed to increase and maintain motivation for continued weight loss behaviors was efficacious.[35] Thus, it may be useful to assess and increase parents' motivating factors to optimize their likelihood of completing treatment and losing weight; motivational interviewing skills (eg, reflective listening and a nonjudgmental stance) can be used to help individuals assess the benefits and drawbacks to a decision and make a positive choice toward behavior change.

Specifically, providers can talk with parents to learn what is reinforcing to them about losing weight and their ability to implement the intervention strategies.[36] Questions such as, "What concerns do you have about your family's ability to implement healthy behaviors in the home?" can help parents to articulate their motivation and readiness for participation in a weight loss intervention.[5] Providers are encouraged to help parents to map out a network of support by identifying individuals in their social circle, as well as peers and caretakers in their children's social circle, who will support or possibly hinder their weight loss efforts. Capitalizing on supportive resources is helpful to families in the long term. It is important to discuss potential barriers to treatment success with parents (eg, busy schedules, lack of motivation, previous weight loss failures). This dialogue identifies strategies to increase and maintain families' motivation throughout the intervention.

PREDICTORS OF SUSTAINABLE BEHAVIOR CHANGE FOR PEDIATRIC OBESITY

Once providers identify families in need of intervention, it is imperative to choose effective intervention strategies as well as to consider specific factors that predict outcome.

Family-Based Behavioral Lifestyle Interventions

Lifestyle interventions are active treatments that modify overweight and obese children's daily practices (eg, improved dietary intake and physical activity); by capitalizing on daily living, behavior changes are better sustained over time.[37] A lifestyle intervention uses an organic strategy in which behavioral goals are tracked and made progressively more comprehensive and families learn to problem solve barriers. Providers can encourage patients to meet with a specialist and participate in a behavioral weight loss program that emphasizes weekly monitoring, skill building, goal setting, and evaluating progress over time. Such a comprehensive approach is in contrast to an education-only intervention condition in which information is presented to families to help them make changes. Numerous randomized controlled trials (RCTs) and meta-analyses have shown that active lifestyle interventions are superior to no-treatment control or education-only conditions (**Table 1**).[38] A recent meta-analysis found that lifestyle interventions yield an average decrease in overweight percentage of 8.9% compared with education-only controls that yield an average increase of 2.7% at follow-up.[38]

Family-based behavioral weight loss treatments (FBTs) are lifestyle interventions that are typically regarded as the first line of treatment of childhood overweight and obesity due to their empirically demonstrated efficacy[39–45] and relative safety compared with pharmacotherapy or bariatric surgery.[40] Recent work indicates that children receiving a multicomponent FBT demonstrated significant decreases in overweight percentage and improvements in related comorbidities, whereas those receiving usual care did not exhibit changes in overweight percentage.[46] Furthermore, positive outcomes of FBT are not limited to changes in child weight; this approach produces significant reductions in blood pressure and cholesterol levels[47] as well as psychosocial health benefits.[43,48,49]

The Importance of Parental Involvement

The rationale for parental involvement in treatment is 2-fold. Parental obesity has been identified as a significant risk factor for childhood obesity,[50] with one study reporting that children with obese parents are at a 2- to 3-fold increased risk for being obese themselves in adulthood.[14] This concordance of parent-child weight status, likely due to shared genetic and environmental factors, suggests a strong parental influence on the weight status of their offspring and could have a powerful positive impact on FBTs. FBTs recognize that children's weight-related behaviors are developed and

Table 1
Recent reviews and meta-analyses of pediatric weight loss studies

Author	Type of Review and Number of Studies	Target Population	Conclusions
American Dietetic Association,[48] 2006	Review of 29 RCTs and 15 other types of studies	Overweight children (aged 2–12 y) and adolescents (aged 13–18 y)	Positive effects for multicomponent family-based programs, especially for children aged 5–12 y
Latzer et al,[103] 2008	Review of 80 articles	Overweight children and adolescents (aged 2–19 y)	Behavioral modification strategies have a modest short-term efficacy, family and parents improve treatment outcome
McGovern et al,[58] 2008	Meta-analysis of 61 randomized trials	Overweight children and adolescents (aged 2–18 y)	Small to moderate treatment effects of combined lifestyle interventions on BMI
Snethen et al,[104] 2006	Meta-analysis of 7 interventions	Overweight children (aged 6–16 y, with an overall mean age not older than 12 y)	Multicomponent lifestyle interventions that include parental involvement can be effective in assisting children to lose weight
Tsiros et al,[93] 2008	Review of 34 RCTs	Overweight or obese adolescents (aged 12–19 y)	Lifestyle interventions with behavior/cognitive-behavioral components are promising, particularly for long-term maintenance
Wilfley et al,[38,61] 2007	Meta-analysis of 14 RCTs	Overweight youth (aged ≤19 y)	Lifestyle interventions produce significant changes in weight status in the short term with encouraging results for the persistence of effects

Abbreviation: RCT, randomized controlled trial.

maintained within the context of the family[51]; therefore, lifestyle interventions aim to capitalize on the influence parents can have over the weight-related behaviors of their young children and the structure of the family environment.[52,53]

Parents or caregivers are necessary partners in pediatric weight loss[53,54] because of their role as key agents of change and the impact of parent behavior change on child weight outcomes. Parents are conceptualized in a helper or facilitator role and taught to encourage children to exercise and make healthy choices as well as to modify the shared home environment.[52] Parental involvement is supported by behavioral economics theory, which suggests that individuals choose behaviors that are less effortful and highly reinforcing. Therefore, inducing child behavior change is contingent upon parents providing healthful reinforcing alternatives while limiting access to less healthy options. Social cognitive theory[55] also provides a strong argument for parental inclusion in treatment, as it posits that modeling is a potent contributor to intervention success because children learn through observing their parents' behaviors. In addition, the benefits of parents and children modeling healthier behaviors in the shared home environment may generalize to at-risk siblings.[41] Overall, harnessing parental influence has the potential to improve the weight status of the entire family by creating an environment that supports healthy lifestyles. The most effective interventions for pediatric obesity incorporate multiple components and hinge upon parental involvement.

In addition to utilizing the evidence-based approaches shown to elicit successful weight loss in youth, it is important for providers to be mindful of key factors that predict sustainable behavior change and address them accordingly (**Table 2**).

Early Treatment Response for Children

Sustainable behavior change is associated with early treatment response; specifically, recent work highlights that children who lose weight by week 8 of a weight loss intervention have the greatest likelihood of sustained success.[56] It is important for providers to encourage weight loss early in the intervention to maximize the potential for long-term success.

Treatment Response for Parents

Children whose parents respond to treatment are more likely to perform well in a weight loss intervention.[57] Parents and caregivers play a pivotal role in treatment success[58] in that they serve as role models and are most often in charge of household decisions; they have the greatest capacity to implement treatment strategies and provide stimulus control.[59] Thus, providers ideally encourage parents and caregivers to actively engage in their own healthy behavior changes along with their children to ensure that children are receiving optimal support for healthful eating and activity.

Social Functioning

Heightened social problems (eg, loneliness, jealousy, susceptibility to teasing) predict greater weight regain after FBT.[60] In addition, children with higher levels of social problems evidence poorer weight loss maintenance.[61] Young people who experience social problems or rejection may be more likely to use food as a coping mechanism[62] and less likely to engage in physical activity.[63] Obese children are less likely to join teams and physical activities and are more likely to experience concerns about physical competence[63] and be perceived as less athletic than nonobese peers.[64] Identifying children with social problems allows providers to effectively tailor treatment goals as well as help families to develop social support for sustainable behavior change.[61]

Table 2
Specific predictors of sustainable behavior change

Predictor	Intervention Target
Children's early treatment response	• Encourage early weight loss (ie, by wk 8 of the intervention)
Parents' treatment response	• Promote parental behavior changes and weight loss • Discuss strategies for restructuring the home environment to maximize healthful options
Social functioning	• Evaluate social skills and identify target areas (eg, making friends, coping with teasing) • Encourage parents to set up healthy active get-togethers with peers and facilitate their children's social skill development
Built environment	• Identify specific aspects of the built environment that may promote (eg, parks, open spaces) or hinder (eg, fast-food restaurants) weight loss success • Determine how to capitalize on available resources or develop plans to increase access to healthful resources
Poor satiety responsiveness	• Encourage parents to replace unhealthy food/activity with healthy options • Discuss how to increase awareness of hunger/satiety cues • Promote meal regularity and healthy meal patterns
High food reinforcement	• Discuss the importance of eating only when hungry • Identify alternative sources of reinforcement • Encourage parents to limit access to unhealthy food items
Binge or loss of control Eating	• Encourage parents to regulate eating patterns • Facilitate improvement of emotion regulation skills and body esteem • Identify ways to enhance supportive interpersonal relationships as alternatives to food
Impulsivity	• Discuss how to improve self-control and planning skills • Use stimulus control; maximize access to healthy food items and minimize access to unhealthy food items and sedentary behaviors

Built Environment

Specific aspects of the built environment are associated with increased rates of obesity, including limited accessibility to parks and open spaces and increased accessibility to fast-food restaurants.[65,66] Recent research suggests that the built environment affects children's weight loss success in FBTs; access to parks and open spaces predicted greater weight loss success at 2-year follow-up, whereas reduced access to parks and greater access to supermarkets and convenience stores predicted poorer outcome. (Epstein LH, Raja S, Oluyomi T, et al. Activity and eating built environments influence child weight loss over two years. Submitted for publication.) Thus, it is important for providers to consider the built environment when identifying intervention goals and determining how to best capitalize on available resources.

Appetitive Traits

When examining predictors that enhance sustainability, it is equally important to consider factors that increase vulnerability to weight gain and therefore may be barriers to weight loss. Appetitive traits, such as poor satiety responsiveness,[67–69] high food reinforcement,[70] binge or loss of control eating,[71,72] and impulsivity,[73] are heritable factors associated with increased energy intake, excess weight gain, and obesity risk among youth and adults.[23,74–83] The presence of these traits may hinder treatment response, and, as a result, addressing these weight-related liabilities through early detection and targeted intervention is critical. The primary mechanism for addressing these traits is training parents to help their children by shifting the environment and teaching them critical skills related to eating. Overall, PCPs should encourage parents of children who have difficulties in these domains to help their children to (1) regulate their portion sizes, (2) delay gratification for food (eg, limit access to unhealthy food items to decrease temptation), (3) differentiate between hunger and emotional states, and (4) seek alternate activities other than eating if they are not hungry. Using stimulus control enhances children's potential for success as well.

Encouraging early treatment response and parent response, inquiring about social functioning and associated problems, capitalizing on resources in the built environment, and identifying and targeting appetitive traits maximize treatment success and the long-term sustainability of these results. The presence of any of these factors indicates vulnerability for continued weight gain and need for higher intensity treatment; providers are encouraged to increase the frequency of visits for families who present with these identified factors.

BEHAVIORAL MODIFICATION TECHNIQUES THAT WORK ACROSS THE SOCIOENVIRONMENTAL CONTEXTS
Intervening Within a Socioenvironmental Framework

Interventions that utilize a socioenvironmental approach are efficacious for weight loss because they extend the focus of behavior change beyond the individual to encompass the home, peer, and community contexts.[84–86] Interventions are most potent when embedded within the contexts of parents and children's lives (ie, where they live, learn, play) and when they devote sufficient time to the mastery and practice of strategies for implementing healthful behaviors.[87] Given the ease with which old behavior patterns are cued, interventions need to be intensive enough and need to facilitate repeated practice across contexts so that newly learned patterns become ingrained and entrenched.

Unhealthy eating and activity patterns have increased, and rapid changes in our diet over the past 200 years have led to significant increases in consumption of highly processed food items and refined grains, sugars, and fats.[88] Messages encouraging unhealthy choices are ubiquitous in our culture, such that children are barraged with obesogenic cues. Children repeatedly see billboards for fast food, walk near desserts for lunch in the cafeteria, and receive packaged sweets and juice after sports games. Promotion of physical activity has decreased; excluding gym class from the curriculum is a common response to budget cuts, and the convenience of handheld video game devices gives way to increased sedentary activity. Given the myriad environmental prompts, weight loss is an uphill battle; individuals may be able to lose weight, but they often have difficulty sustaining these effects.[40] Thus, the cross-contextual approach of the socioenvironmental model optimizes treatment success because it addresses eating and activity cues and behaviors across contexts and brings the family and social network together to support individuals as they make healthy behavior changes. For example, parents aiming to increase the availability and range of healthy meal options would first be prompted to have a conversation with their children and family members about offering healthy meal options at home. Parents would then be encouraged to talk with friends about serving healthy meal options during get-togethers with their children or themselves. In addition, parents would be advised to advocate with coworkers so that healthy meal options are offered in office settings and with school teachers so that healthy meal options are served in the classroom. Parents would be encouraged to solicit support from organizers of community events (eg, girl/boy scout troop leader, person responsible for food after a community-based run) to offer healthy food options. This example of comprehensive support across levels demonstrates how families may maximize opportunities for increasing healthy default options. As families become more adept at implementing these strategies, they become increasingly empowered to extend their healthy behaviors into new situations.

In a standard behavioral weight loss intervention, the treatment emphasis and responsibility for behavior change are placed solely on the individual. The socioenvironmental model increases the duration and extends the scope of standard behavioral weight loss treatment by focusing on practicing skills and infusing support across contexts. This framework encourages behavior change via continued practice of newly learned behaviors throughout a variety of settings. In standard behavioral weight loss intervention, individuals are encouraged to increase their daily physical activity (eg, go for a run); the socioenvironmental approach builds on this by promoting that individuals engage in physical activities such as joining sports teams at school, doing physical activity fitness classes with friends, and training for community-based runs (eg, 5-km events) with their family. Beyond relying on individual willpower and self-regulatory skills, using the socioenvironmental framework promotes an increased awareness of environmental cues and advocacy for making sustainable healthful changes. For instance, parents will be able to recognize that their usual drive home contains many fast-food restaurants that prompt their children to ask for snacks and will be able to select an alternate route to avoid the prompts altogether. Recent evidence supports this approach as a strategy to achieve sustainable weight loss in children and adults.[61,84,85,89] Given that weight regain is common following standard treatment,[40,90,91] efforts to reverse the obesity epidemic hinge on incorporating these targets into weight loss interventions.

Delivery of the socioenvironmental model for youth and families

Wilfley and colleagues have developed, evaluated, and refined Social Facilitation Maintenance (SFM), a socioenvironmental family-based framework for promoting long term weight maintenance in youth and families.[61,89] SFM builds on previous work to focus on addressing social skills and capitalizing on social support for healthy behaviors. Wilfley and colleagues[61] found that SFM was associated with sustained weight loss compared with a behavioral weight loss intervention and control condition. More recently, biosimulation modeling revealed that the SFM approach of increased duration (eg, 1 year) likely yields better weight loss maintenance over the long term.[89]

The application of the socioenvironmental intervention in clinical settings provides necessary encouragement of healthful behaviors so that children receive more integrated messages and support for weight loss.[92] Given their role in treating children and discussing health-related targets with families, providers can work in concert with public health and community initiatives to educate, support, and follow-up with families about behavior change implementation. The breadth of the obesity epidemic warrants that individuals across the health care profession actively engage in interventions to combat this problem.

Applying the Socioenvironmental Approach

Several behavioral modification techniques are effective in promoting healthy weight control within each context across the socioenvironmental domains (ie, family/home, peer, and community). **Box 2** provides recommendations from the AAP

Box 2
Recommendations from the AAP to address pediatric obesity in the primary care setting

For providers to implement in primary care settings

- Routinely document BMI and assess children for obesity.
- Deliver messages about healthy eating and activity behaviors to all children and families, regardless of children's weight status.
- Establish practice procedures for addressing overweight and obesity (eg, determine, medical assessments to review, and flag charts of overweight and obese children to indicate need for intervention).
- Involve and train interdisciplinary teams.
- Audit charts to identify current practices and goals for improvement, and assess improvement over time.

For providers to discuss with families

- Limit sugar-sweetened beverages.
- Increase vegetables and fruits (at least 9 servings per day).
- Limit television and other screen time (no television for children younger than 2 years, less than 2 hours per day for children older than 2 years), and remove televisions from children's sleeping areas.
- Eat breakfast every day.
- Limit meals eaten out at restaurants.
- Increase family meals (parents and children eat together).
- Limit portion sizes.

---

regarding PCP behaviors to implement within the primary care setting as well as specific energy balance behaviors for PCPs to recommend to families.[5] As health care offices infuse these changes in routine clinical practice, it is recommended that an evaluation system becomes established to measure how effectively providers are incorporating these changes.

Fig. 1 depicts specific health behaviors across the socioenvironmental domains that PCPs can help families to implement. Although these strategies focus on pediatric approaches, they are applicable across the age spectrum. As families begin to infuse these changes across their everyday contexts, providers should remind parents and children that progress may be gradual. Supportive, yet persistent, monitoring and praise help families continue to stay on track with their behavior change goals.

Family/home context

The socioenvironmental approach encourages families to implement behaviors and solicit social support in each relevant context. **Box 3** provides a detailed list of specific behaviors providers can discuss with parents to facilitate sustainable weight loss. Within the family/home context, it is critical for families to monitor their eating and activity behaviors. Full monitoring, or the use of food and exercise diaries to document energy consumption (ie, caloric intake) and energy expenditure (ie, 10-minute bouts of activity), is helpful for identifying current behaviors and determining areas for improvement. Awareness is crucial for behavior change; for instance, full monitoring reveals sources of excess energy intake or misconceptions about the healthfulness of the food items consumed, thereby allowing clinicians and families the opportunity to alter these behaviors.

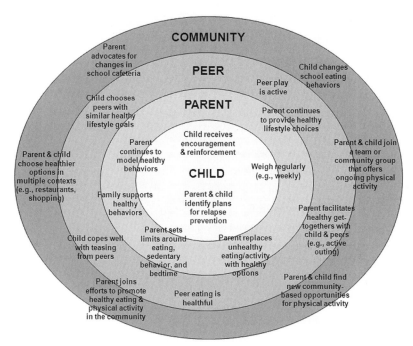

Fig. 1. Socioenvironmental model and recommendations for providers to make across domains.

Weight loss is achieved during a state of negative energy balance or when energy expenditure is greater than energy consumption. As described in **Box 1**, healthy eating behaviors, such as increased fruit and vegetable consumption and decreased portion sizes as well as improved activity patterns are key components of effective weight control interventions[93] Given that providers have limited time in session to distill information to families, easy-to-explain tools are helpful, particularly for children. For example, the Traffic Light Plan (TLP)[43] is a user-friendly guide that codes food items and activities into RED, YELLOW, or GREEN categories. The TLP encourages children and families to limit RED food items, which are low-nutrient energy-dense food items high in fat and/or sugar, and RED activities, which are sedentary behaviors that do not burn calories (eg, "screen" time leisure activities, such as watching television, playing videogames, talking/texting on the phone, or using the computer). Furthermore, the TLP promotes the replacement of RED food items and activities with GREEN food items, which are healthful nutrient-dense food items low in fat and calories, and GREEN activities, which are moderate to intense physical activities).

Another critical monitoring skill to promote within the family/home context is regular weighing (eg, at the same time each week) to keep track of families' weight trajectory. Weight measurements provide important objective data regarding their recent behaviors. Families can also get into the habit of having conversations about connecting behaviors to weight change, which is an important evaluative skill.

To help children achieve a negative energy balance, parenting behaviors are crucial. It is recommended that providers work with parents to routinely implement the following strategies:

1. Modeling: parents demonstrate how to make healthy choices and thus serve as models to their children, family members, friends, and community members.

Box 3
Parental involvement in family-based behavioral interventions

Supporting healthy eating behaviors

Increase low–energy density food items.

- Plan for healthy meals.
- Shop for nutritious food items (fruits, vegetables, "good" fats, high fiber).
- Prepare healthy meals.
- Serve fruits and vegetables at meals and for snacks.

Decrease high–energy density food items.

- Limit high–energy density food items at home.
- Limit access to fast-food restaurants.
- Limit eating away from the kitchen and dining room.
- Replace sugar-sweetened beverages with water, or serve low-fat milk products at home.

Improve meal patterns.

- Establish the routine of 3 meals and 1 to 2 planned healthy snacks per day.
- Serve healthy portion sizes.
- Involve the child in preparing meals.
- Cook traditionally unhealthy food items in a healthier way (eg, baking instead of frying)

Supporting physical and lifestyle activity

Increase physical activity.

- Make a weekly activity schedule.
- Provide equipment and clothing for exercise.
- Set up active play dates with the child's peer group.
- Join a local community recreation center.
- Use local parks and playgrounds.

Increase lifestyle activity.

- Plan fun activities for the family.
- Model for and encourage children to take the stairs instead of escalators or elevators.
- Walk instead of drive with family, when possible.

Decrease time spent in sedentary behaviors.

- Limit the child's television and computer time to 2 h/d.

Supporting healthful behavior change

Use behavior modification strategies.

- Set goals for weight and behavioral change targets.
- Create a family-based rewards system.
- Engage in self-monitoring and logging.
- Use stimulus control strategies in the shared home environment.

Target changes in the parent.

- Focus on weight loss in parents.
- Model healthful behaviors for the child.

Provide support for the child.

- Hold family meetings.
- Review self-monitoring logs.
- Praise healthy behaviors.
- Encourage healthy behaviors, and minimize attention to unhealthy behaviors.
- Explain the family-based behavioral intervention to family and friends.
- Solicit support from family and friends to maximize prompts for healthy eating and activity across contexts.

2. Stimulus control: it is necessary for parents to remove prompts for unhealthy food items and activity equipment (eg, removing chips and cookies from the home or from within easy reach for children, keeping videogame equipment on a high shelf in the closet) and increase the availability of prompts for healthy food items and activity (eg, placing fruits in a basket on the kitchen counter, keeping sneakers by the door) at home.

3. Limit setting: parents can set house rules to target reduction of specific behaviors, such as amount of unhealthy food items consumed or time spent watching television. This structure helps families to establish healthy patterns around eating (eg, planning for and eating breakfast, lunch, dinner, and 1–2 snacks every day), activity (eg, incorporating a daily walk after dinner), and sleep (eg, setting electronic curfews, the time by which all electronics must be turned off, and bedtimes).

Clinical skills also include helping parents to problem solve barriers to behavior implementation and identify plans for high-risk situations (eg, an upcoming birthday party that will only serve unhealthy food items). In addition, it is important to recommend to parents that they establish a no-tolerance policy for teasing and an open environment for healthful discussions about body image because these represent common issues for the overweight or obese youth.[8,64,94–97]

Inherent within behavior modification strategies is the identification of goals. Providers can help families accomplish their goals consistently by encouraging them to establish a system of reinforcement. Use of a behavioral rewards system is effective for reinforcing weight loss and attainment of healthy behaviors.[98] However, it is important to ensure that reinforcement patterns encourage healthy behaviors, as this is not always the case. For instance, when parents reward children with dessert or only spend time with them while watching television, they are reinforcing unhealthy choices. Instead, explaining to parents that they should reward children with alternate nonfood reinforcers (eg, activities they like to do or social events, such as going swimming, instead of candy or television shows) promotes the implementation of healthful behaviors. Praise is also a powerful reinforcer for positive behaviors. Thus, PCPs are encouraged to remind families to use reinforcement techniques to replace unhealthy behaviors with healthier options, which will ultimately help them to establish sustainable changes.

Peer context

The peer context provides unique opportunities for intervention, given that friends are important sources of social support, both as models of healthy eating and sources of alternate reinforcement. Studies demonstrate that overweight and obese children are more likely to make healthy eating choices when they are with peers who make healthy choices.[99-101] In addition, spending time with friends is a viable alternative to other types of reinforcers, including eating unhealthy food articles.[102] To reduce the amount of food children eat and provide an alternate reinforcer, providers should encourage parents to schedule active healthy get-togethers with their children's peers, capitalizing on friendships with peers who already do healthy behaviors. Clinicians can also help families to develop advocacy plans for peers, such as only serving healthy options at events and asking friends to make healthy food items as well. As is critical within the family/home context, providers should recommend to parents that they promote a healthy environment with friends in terms of teasing (eg, establish a no-tolerance policy for teasing).

Community context

Within the community context, families should be encouraged to use available resources and advocate for improved healthful options. For instance, clinicians can help families to become aware of neighborhood facilities and services, such as through the local community center, that promote healthy behaviors. Joining a physical activity–oriented team or club offers multiple benefits, including increased time spent being physically active, identification of a network of peers who engage in physical activity that is of interest to the child, and development of an alternate reinforcer to eating or sedentary behavior. Families should be encouraged to avoid unhealthy restaurants (eg, fast food) or other venues in which it is difficult to make healthy choices. As families become more skilled in implementing these changes, they should also be encouraged to advocate for healthful changes in the local community regarding eating (eg, serving skim milk at school or low-fat deli sandwiches as work) and activity (eg, vigorous intensity games during gym class or access to stairs in addition to elevators). By developing support for healthy options throughout the community, families optimize their local resources and are better able to maintain healthy weight control habits.

USING THE OFFICE ENVIRONMENT AND RESOURCES TO PROMOTE OBESITY PREVENTION

In effective lifestyle interventions, parents and children work with a behavioral specialist and attend regular treatment sessions, with options for phone sessions and e-mail check-ins interspersed throughout the intervention. Families participate in group (45 minutes) and individual (30 minutes) sessions during each appointment; this format provides families with peer support through the group setting and a tailored intervention via the individual sessions. To optimize support at home, additional family members are encouraged to attend as well.

Although these effective interventions have been established, recommended practices have not been implemented into routine practice. Thus, it is critical to extend beyond traditional settings and have providers work in concert with behavioral interventionists to provide integrated care and reinforce messaging across contexts. For instance, providers are in a prime position to identify at-risk families and make referrals for specialized weight loss intervention. Providers can then follow up with families once every 3 months to regularly track children's health outcomes. Providers can support the behavioral interventionists in establishing a unified treatment program for families by facilitating parents' use of community resources and encouraging children's development of positive social ties. Such collaborative effort is necessary to most effectively promote healthy behaviors, address families' weight trajectories, and eliminate obesity.

Optimally, office policies and practices ensure that staff members are equipped to confront weight-related problems. It is important for staff to be educated in behavior change principles so that they gain an understanding of how to help families to implement healthy strategies in their homes and communities. Office-based trainings can include the importance of early intervention, with instruction on how to appropriately and effectively intervene with parents and children and provide referrals.[22] In addition, it is advantageous for staff to be educated in diversity awareness, as cultural differences may affect families' values regarding weight status, body ideals, and parenting behaviors, and socioeconomic barriers (eg, family finances and spending practices, access to community resources) may affect the intervention strategies that families are willing or able to implement. Ideally, providers learn families' stances on these issues to tailor their recommendations appropriately. Ongoing training and supervision in stigma awareness and reduction may be of benefit as well.

Concerted efforts to (1) reduce providers' skepticism regarding the efficacy of weight loss interventions and (2) increase reimbursement for the provision of obesity-related services will increase the likelihood that providers will engage families in weight loss interventions.[22] Offering Continuing Medical Education training opportunities, making accessible medical journals (eg, *Pediatrics*), and increasing access to medically relevant Web sites (eg, AAP, CDC) are useful avenues for increasing providers' knowledge of AAP recommendations.[20]

When addressing weight-related problems with families, it is imperative for staff to remain empathetic and use reflective listening. Ideally, staff are trained to engage in open discussion with families about making healthy eating and activity changes, particularly as discomfort surrounding these conversations is a reported barrier for providers to address this issue.[22] These conversations typically focus on understanding a family's health behaviors as well as their social network, with the goal of identifying sources of support for making healthy changes. Skills clinicians teach families to include how to engage in healthy eating, meal planning, self-monitoring, and the tools for implementing these changes across the socioenvironmental contexts.

As mentioned earlier, the regularity of doctor's appointments places PCPs in an ideal position to track and monitor children's progress over time. Structuring appointments to allow time to calculate children's BMI, review their weight trajectory, and discuss families' progress in implementing healthy strategies optimizes intervention. Routine assessment of metabolic profiles and tracking risk for obesity-related health consequences is also imperative; this recommendation is in line with the AAP guidelines for addressing pediatric obesity.[5,18] It is crucial for staff to engage families about their weight goals and help families to problem solve potential barriers. Discussing ways to maintain social support or seek avenues for developing healthy social ties is encouraged as well. Overall, it is important that sessions focus on increasing families' skills for at-home implementation of behavior change strategies.

It is recommended for obesity prevention that providers calculate BMI and address weight status with all families. Providers are encouraged to talk with parents of children who are of normal weight to confirm whether they are currently engaging in healthy eating and activity behaviors; PCPs can promote the implementation or maintenance of these practices as needed and address any areas of concern to prevent the development of obesity. Noting family histories of overweight or obesity, obesity-related health problems, or gestational diabetes mellitus helps providers to screen for children at elevated risk for obesity. By using a universal approach, providers encourage healthy eating and activity practices and reduce risk for excessive weight gain among all families.

Promoting healthy lifestyles does not need to be limited to conversations between health professionals and patients; the office environment itself provides substantial opportunities to promote healthy lifestyle behaviors by making healthy resources and relevant prompts accessible and visible. First, offices can promote healthy life-style activities, such as emphasizing the use of stairs, increasing office walkability, and making breastfeeding rooms accessible. Second, healthy eating can be encour-aged by removing vending machines, providing water fountains, and enforcing healthy standards for office meals (eg, healthy staff lunches). Third, prompts for healthy local events and resources, such as farmers' markets and community events for running, walking, or biking, can be made available in waiting rooms and hallways. It would be ideal for take-home materials with strategies for implementing behavior change to be made accessible. Last, staff can set a positive example by modeling healthy behaviors (eg, by not making unhealthy food visible, drinking water, walking during lunch breaks). In doing so, families receive consistent healthful messaging that extends beyond the appointment session in that the office environment models the infusion of healthy prompts across contexts.

SUMMARY AND FUTURE DIRECTIONS

The pressing pediatric obesity epidemic warrants immediate attention and a collective effort across health care professionals. This article provides an overview of current PCP counseling practices, evidence-based recommendations for addressing pedi-atric obesity and eliciting behavior change, and encouragement to providers to imple-ment these strategies in the primary care setting to help children lose weight and prevent excess weight gain.

By intervening early, providers are in a prime position to help families instill healthy habits. The earlier the intervention, the more potent providers can be; for instance, it is less likely that children become obese if parents never get into the habit of giving soda to their children.

Importantly, awareness of the discussed strategies represents only the first step. Implementing these changes with every family, at every visit, is critical for curbing the widespread problem of pediatric obesity. Researchers and clinicians must estab-lish ongoing open communication about the adoption of behavioral interventions and methods for training health professionals in these strategies. Future work is required to determine the optimal way to connect community resources to health care settings, including the use of social media and online forums for intervention. Building collabo-rative partnerships provides consistent health messaging and establishes greater referral services, thereby enhancing opportunities for families to embed healthy behaviors across all areas of their lives. Researching models and utilizing stakeholder (eg, PCP) input on how best to disseminate this work lays necessary groundwork for widespread implementation. Through the employment of behavior change strategies into everyday clinical practice, providers will be in a prime position to affect sustain-able weight loss outcomes and promote healthier young people.

REFERENCES

1. Ogden CL, Carroll MD, Curtin LR, et al. Prevalence of high body mass index in US children and adolescents, 2007-2008. JAMA 2010;303(3):242–9.
2. Ogden CL, Carroll MD, Curtin LR, et al. Prevalence of overweight and obesity in the United States, 1999-2004. JAMA 2006;295(13):1549–55.
3. Flegal KM, Carroll MD, Ogden CL, et al. Prevalence and trends in obesity among US adults, 1999-2008. JAMA 2010;303(3):235–41.
4. Kuczmarski RJ, Ogden CL, Grummer-Strawn LM, et al. CDC growth charts: United States. Adv Data 2000;(314):1–27.

5. Barlow SE. Expert committee recommendations regarding the prevention, assessment, and treatment of child and adolescent overweight and obesity: summary report. Pediatrics 2007;120(Suppl 4):S164–92.

6. August GP, Caprio S, Fennoy I, et al. Prevention and treatment of pediatric obesity: an endocrine society clinical practice guideline based on expert opinion. J Clin Endocrinol Metab 2008;93(12):4576–99.

7. Hampl SE, Carroll CA, Simon SD, et al. Resource utilization and expenditures for overweight and obese children. Arch Pediatr Adolesc Med 2007;161(1):11–4.

8. Dietz WH. Medical consequences of obesity in children and adolescents. In: Fairburn CG, Brownell KD, editors. Eating disorders and obesity: a comprehensive handbook. 2nd edition. New York: Guilford Press; 2002. p. 473–6.

9. BeLue R, Francis LA, Colaco B. Mental health problems and overweight in a nationally representative sample of adolescents: effects of race and ethnicity. Pediatrics 2009;123(2):697–702.

10. Luppino FS, de Wit LM, Bouvy PF, et al. Overweight, obesity, and depression: a systematic review and meta-analysis of longitudinal studies. Arch Gen Psychiatry 2010;67(3):220–9.

11. Weiss R, Dziura J, Burgert TS, et al. Obesity and the metabolic syndrome in children and adolescents. N Engl J Med 2004;350(23):2362–74.

12. Stovitz SD, Pereira MA, Vazquez G, et al. The interaction of childhood height and childhood BMI in the prediction of young adult BMI. Obesity (Silver Spring) 2008;16(10):2336–41.

13. Nader PR, O'Brien M, Houts R, et al. Identifying risk for obesity in early childhood. Pediatrics 2006;118(3):e594–601.

14. Whitaker RC, Wright JA, Pepe MS, et al. Predicting obesity in young adulthood from childhood and parental obesity. N Engl J Med 1997;337(13):869–73.

15. Moss BG, Yeaton WH. Young children's weight trajectories and associated risk factors: results from the Early Childhood Longitudinal Study-Birth Cohort. Am J Health Promot 2011;25(3):190–8.

16. Wilfley DE, Vannucci A, White EK. Family-based behavioral interventions. In: Freemark M, editor. Pediatric obesity: etiology, pathogenesis, and treatment. New York: Humana Press; 2010. p. 281–302.

17. Barton M. Screening for obesity in children and adolescents: US Preventive Services Task Force recommendation statement. Pediatrics 2010;125(2):361–7.

18. Krebs NF, Jacobson MS. Prevention of pediatric overweight and obesity. Pediatrics 2003;112(2):424–30.

19. Rhodes ET, Ebbeling CB, Meyers AF, et al. Pediatric obesity management: variation by specialty and awareness of guidelines. Clin Pediatr (Phila) 2007;46(6):491–504.

20. Klein JD, Sesselberg TS, Johnson MS, et al. Adoption of body mass index guidelines for screening and counseling in pediatric practice. Pediatrics 2010;125(2):265–72.

21. Young PC, DeBry S, Jackson WD, et al. Improving the prevention, early recognition, and treatment of pediatric obesity by primary care physicians. Clin Pediatr (Phila) 2010;49(10):964–9.

22. Dorsey KB, Mauldon M, Magraw R, et al. Applying practice recommendations for the prevention and treatment of obesity in children and adolescents. Clin Pediatr (Phila) 2010;49(2):137–45.

23. Holt N, Schetzina KE, Dalton WT 3rd, et al. Primary care practice addressing child overweight and obesity: a survey of primary care physicians at four clinics in southern Appalachia. South Med J 2011;104(1):14–9.

24. Rausch JC, Perito ER, Hametz P. Obesity prevention, screening, and treatment: practices of pediatric providers since the 2007 expert committee recommendations. Clin Pediatr (Phila) 2011;50(5):434–41.

25. Flower KB, Perrin EM, Viadro CI, et al. Using body mass index to identify overweight children: barriers and facilitators in primary care. Ambul Pediatr 2007; 7(1):38–44.

26. Spivack JG, Swietlik M, Alessandrini E, et al. Primary care providers' knowledge, practices, and perceived barriers to the treatment and prevention of childhood obesity. Obesity (Silver Spring) 2010;18(7):1341–7.

27. Wake M, Baur LA, Gerner B, et al. Outcomes and costs of primary care surveillance and intervention for overweight or obese children: the LEAP 2 randomised controlled trial. BMJ 2009;339:b3308.

28. Schwartz RP, Hamre R, Dietz WH, et al. Office-based motivational interviewing to prevent childhood obesity: a feasibility study. Arch Pediatr Adolesc Med 2007;161(5):495–501.

29. Taveras EM, Gortmaker SL, Hohman KH, et al. Randomized controlled trial to improve primary care to prevent and manage childhood obesity: the high five for kids study. Arch Pediatr Adolesc Med 2011;165(8):714–22.

30. McCallum Z, Wake M, Gerner B, et al. Outcome data from the LEAP (Live, Eat and Play) trial: a randomized controlled trial of a primary care intervention for childhood overweight/mild obesity. Int J Obes (Lond) 2007;31(4): 630–6.

31. Perrin EM, Finkle JP, Benjamin JT. Obesity prevention and the primary care pediatrician's office. Curr Opin Pediatr 2007;19(3):354–61.

32. Perrin EM, Jacobson Vann JC, Benjamin JT, et al. Use of a pediatrician toolkit to address parental perception of children's weight status, nutrition, and activity behaviors. Acad Pediatr 2010;10(4):274–81.

33. Gunnarsdottir T, Njardvik U, Olafsdottir AS, et al. The role of parental motivation in family-based treatment for childhood obesity. Obesity (Silver Spring) 2011; 19(8):1654–62.

34. Braet C, Jeannin R, Mels S, et al. Ending prematurely a weight loss programme: the impact of child and family characteristics. Clin Psychol Psychother 2010; 17(5):406–17.

35. West DS, Gorin AA, Subak LL, et al. A motivation-focused weight loss maintenance program is an effective alternative to a skill-based approach. Int J Obes (Lond) 2011;35(2):259–69.

36. Chang MW, Nitzke S, Guilford E, et al. Motivators and barriers to healthful eating and physical activity among low-income overweight and obese mothers. J Am Diet Assoc 2008;108(6):1023–8.

37. Faith MS, Saelens BE, Wilfley DE, et al. Behavioral treatment of childhood and adolescent obesity: current status, challenges, and future directions. In: Thompson JK, Smolak L, editors. Body image, eating disorders, and obesity in youth: assessment, prevention, and treatment. Washington, DC: American Psychological Association; 2001. p. 313–39.

38. Wilfley DE, Tibbs TL, Van Buren DJ, et al. Lifestyle interventions in the treatment of childhood overweight: a meta-analytic review of randomized controlled trials. Health Psychol 2007;26(5):521–32.

39. Epstein LH. Family-based behavioral intervention for obese children. Int J Obes Relat Metab Disord 1996;20:14–21.

40. Epstein LH, Myers MD, Raynor HA, et al. Treatment of pediatric obesity. Pediatrics 1998;101(3):S554–70.

41. Epstein LH, Paluch R, Roemmich JN, et al. Family-based obesity treatment: then and now. Twenty-five years of pediatric obesity treatment. Health Psychol 2007; 26(4):381–91.
42. Epstein LH, Valoski AM, Koeske R, et al. Family-based behavioral weight control in obese young children. J Am Diet Assoc 1986;86:481–4.
43. Epstein LH, Valoski AM, Wing RR, et al. Ten-year follow-up of behavioral, family-based treatment for obese children. JAMA 1990;264(19):2519–23.
44. Epstein LH, Valoski AM, Wing RR, et al. Ten-year outcomes of behavioral family based treatment for childhood obesity. Health Psychol 1994;13:373–83.
45. Epstein LH, Wing RR, Woodall K, et al. Effects of family-based behavioral treatment on obese 5-8 year old children. Behav Ther 1985;16:205–12.
46. Kalarchian MA, Levine MD, Arslanian SA, et al. Family-based treatment of severe pediatric obesity: randomized, controlled trial. Pediatrics 2009;124(4): 1060–8.
47. Pratt CA, Stevens J, Daniels S. Childhood obesity prevention and treatment: recommendations for future research. Am J Prev Med 2008;35(3):249–52.
48. ADA. Position of the American Dietetic Association: individual-, family-, school-, and community-based interventions for pediatric overweight. J Am Diet Assoc 2006;106(6):925–45.
49. Tanofsky-Kraff MH, Hayden-Wade HA, Cavazos P, et al. Pediatric overweight treatment and prevention. In: Anderson R, editor. Overweight: etiology, assessment, treatment, and prevention. Champaign (IL): Kuman Kinetics; 2003. p. 155–76.
50. Hunt MS, Katzmarzyk PT, Perusse L, et al. Familial resemblance of 7-year changes in body mass and adiposity. Obes Res 2002;10:507–17.
51. Golan M, Weizman A. Familial approach to the treatment of childhood obesity: conceptual model. J Nutr Educ 2001;33(2):102–7.
52. Young KM, Northern JJ, Lister KM, et al. A meta-analysis of family-behavioral weight-loss treatments for children. Clin Psychol Rev 2007;27:240–9.
53. Davison KK, Birch LL. Childhood overweight: a contextual model and recommendations for future research. Obes Rev 2001;(2):159–71.
54. Kitzmann KM, Beech BM. Family-based interventions for pediatric obesity: methodological and conceptual challenges from family psychology. J Fam Psychol 2006;20(2):175–89.
55. Bandura A. Social foundations of thought and action: a social cognitive theory. Englewood Cliffs (NJ): Prentice-Hall; 1986.
56. Goldschmidt AB, Stein RI, Saelens BE, et al. Importance of early weight change in a pediatric weight management trial. Pediatrics 2011;128(1):e33–9.
57. Wrotniak BH, Epstein LH, Paluch RA, et al. Parent weight change as a predictor of child weight change in family-based behavioral obesity treatment. Arch Pediatr Adolesc Med 2004;158(4):342–7.
58. McGovern L, Johnson JN, Paulo R, et al. Clinical review: treatment of pediatric obesity: a systematic review and meta-analysis of randomized trials. J Clin Endocrinol Metab 2008;93(12):4600–5.
59. Golan M, Fainaru M, Weizman A. Role of behaviour modification in the treatment of childhood obesity with the parents as the exclusive agents of change. Int J Obes Relat Metab Disord 1998;22(12):1217–24.
60. Epstein LH, Wisniewski L, Weng R. Child and parent psychological problems influence child weight control. Obes Res 1994;2(6):509–15.
61. Wilfley DE, Stein RI, Saelens BE, et al. Efficacy of maintenance treatment approaches for childhood overweight: a randomized controlled trial. JAMA 2007;298(14):1661–73.

62. DeWall CN, Bushman BJ. Social acceptance and rejection: the sweet and the bitter. Curr Dir Psychol Sci 2011;20(4):256–60.

63. Jefferson A. Breaking down barriers-examining health promoting behaviour in the family. Kellogg's Family Health Study 2005. Nutr Bull 2006;31:60–4.

64. Zeller MH, Reiter-Purtill J, Ramey C. Negative peer perceptions of obese children in the classroom environment. Obesity (Silver Spring) 2008;16(4):755–62.

65. Wolch J, Jerrett M, Reynolds K, et al. Childhood obesity and proximity to urban parks and recreational resources: a longitudinal cohort study. Health Place 2011;17(1):207–14.

66. Oreskovic NM, Winickoff JP, Kuhlthau KA, et al. Obesity and the built environment among Massachusetts children. Clin Pediatr (Phila) 2009;48(9):904–12.

67. Wardle J, Carnell S. Appetite is a heritable phenotype associated with adiposity. Ann Behav Med 2009;38(Suppl 1):25–30.

68. Carnell S, Wardle J. Appetitive traits and child obesity: measurement, origins and implications for intervention. Proc Nutr Soc 2008;67(4):343–55.

69. Carnell S, Wardle J. Appetitive traits in children. New evidence for associations with weight and a common, obesity-associated genetic variant. Appetite 2009; 53(2):260–3.

70. Temple JL, Legierski CM, Giacomelli AM, et al. Overweight children find food more reinforcing and consume more energy than do nonoverweight children. Am J Clin Nutr 2008;87(5):1121–7.

71. Tanofsky-Kraff M, Yanovski SZ, Wilfley DE, et al. Eating-disordered behaviors, body fat, and psychopathology in overweight and normal-weight children. J Consult Clin Psychol 2004;72(1):53–61.

72. Goldschmidt AB, Aspen VP, Sinton MM, et al. Disordered eating attitudes and behaviors in overweight youth. Obesity (Silver Spring) 2008;16(2):257–64.

73. Nederkoorn C, Braet C, Van Eijs Y, et al. Why obese children cannot resist food: the role of impulsivity. Eat Behav 2006;7(4):315–22.

74. Tanofsky-Kraff M, Han JC, Anandalingam K, et al. The FTO gene rs9939609 obesity-risk allele and loss of control over eating. Am J Clin Nutr 2009;90(6):1483–8.

75. Wardle J, Llewellyn C, Sanderson S, et al. The FTO gene and measured food intake in children. Int J Obes (Lond) 2009;33(1):42–5.

76. Birch LL, Fisher JO. Development of eating behaviors among children and adolescents. Pediatrics 1998;101(3 Pt 2):539–49.

77. Jansen A, Theunissen N, Slechten K, et al. Overweight children overeat after exposure to food cues. Eat Behav 2003;4(2):197–209.

78. Mirch MC, McDuffie JR, Yanovski SZ, et al. Effects of binge eating on satiation, satiety, and energy intake of overweight children. Am J Clin Nutr 2006;84(4): 732–8.

79. Tanofsky-Kraff M, McDuffie JR, Yanovski SZ, et al. Laboratory assessment of the food intake of children and adolescents with loss of control eating. Am J Clin Nutr 2009;89(3):738–45.

80. Butte NF, Cai G, Cole SA, et al. Metabolic and behavioral predictors of weight gain in Hispanic children: the Viva la Familia Study. Am J Clin Nutr 2007; 85(6):1478–85.

81. Hill C, Saxton J, Webber L, et al. The relative reinforcing value of food predicts weight gain in a longitudinal study of 7–10-y-old children. Am J Clin Nutr 2009; 90(2):276–81.

82. Seeyave DM, Coleman S, Appugliese D, et al. Ability to delay gratification at age 4 years and risk of overweight at age 11 years. Arch Pediatr Adolesc Med 2009; 163(4):303–8.

83. Tanofsky-Kraff M, Yanovski SZ, Schvey NA, et al. A prospective study of loss of control eating for body weight gain in children at high risk for adult obesity. Int J Eat Disord 2009;42(1):26–30.

84. Glass TA, McAtee MJ. Behavioral science at the crossroads in public health: extending horizons, envisioning the future. Soc Sci Med 2006;62(7):1650–71.

85. Huang TT, Drewnosksi A, Kumanyika S, et al. A systems-oriented multilevel framework for addressing obesity in the 21st century. Prev Chronic Dis 2009; 6(3):A82.

86. Kumanyika SK, Obarzanek E, Stettler N, et al. Population-based prevention of obesity: the need for comprehensive promotion of healthful eating, physical activity, and energy balance: a scientific statement from American Heart Association Council on Epidemiology and Prevention, Interdisciplinary Committee for Prevention (formerly the Expert Panel on Population and Prevention Science). Circulation 2008;118(4):428–64.

87. Bouton ME. Context, ambiguity, and unlearning: sources of relapse after behavioral extinction. Biol Psychiatry 2002;52(10):976–86.

88. Cordain L, Eaton SB, Sebastian A, et al. Origins and evolution of the Western diet: health implications for the 21st century. Am J Clin Nutr 2005; 81(2):341–54.

89. Wilfley DE, Van Buren DJ, Theim KR, et al. The use of biosimulation in the design of a novel multilevel weight loss maintenance program for overweight children. Obesity (Silver Spring) 2010;18(Suppl 1):S91–8.

90. Jeffery RW, Drewnowski A, Epstein LH, et al. Long-term maintenance of weight loss: current status. Health Psychol 2000;19(Suppl 1):5–16.

91. Wadden TA, Butryn ML, Byrne KJ. Efficacy of lifestyle modification for long-term weight control. Obes Res 2004;12(Suppl):151S–62S.

92. Dietz W, Lee J, Wechsler H, et al. Health plans' role in preventing overweight in children and adolescents. Health Aff (Millwood) 2007;26(2):430–40.

93. Tsiros MD, Sinn N, Coates AM, et al. Treatment of adolescent overweight and obesity. Eur J Pediatr 2008;167(1):9–16.

94. Goldfield A, Chrisler JC. Body stereotyping and stigmatization of obese persons by first graders. Percept Mot Skills 1995;81(3 Pt 1):909–10.

95. Gortmaker SL, Must A, Perrin JM, et al. Social and economic consequences of overweight in adolescence and young adulthood. N Engl J Med 1993;329(14): 1008–12.

96. Hayden-Wade HA, Stein RI, Ghaderi A, et al. Prevalence, characteristics, and correlates of teasing experiences among overweight children vs. non-overweight peers. Obes Res 2005;13(8):1381–92.

97. Striegel-Moore RH, Schreiber GB, Lo A, et al. Eating disorder symptoms in a cohort of 11 to 16-year-old black and white girls: the NHLBI growth and health study. Int J Eat Disord 2000;27(1):49–66.

98. Dietz WH, Robinson TN. Clinical practice. Overweight children and adolescents. N Engl J Med 2005;352(20):2100–9.

99. Salvy SJ, Coelho JS, Kieffer E, et al. Effects of social contexts on overweight and normal-weight children's food intake. Physiol Behav 2007;92(5):840–6.

100. Salvy SJ, Kieffer E, Epstein LH. Effects of social context on overweight and normal-weight children's food selection. Eat Behav 2008;9(2):190–6.

101. Salvy SJ, Romero N, Paluch R, et al. Peer influence on pre-adolescent girls' snack intake: effects of weight status. Appetite 2007;49(1):177–82.

102. Romero ND, Epstein LH, Salvy SJ. Peer modeling influences girls' snack intake. J Am Diet Assoc 2009;109(1):133–6.

103. Latzer Y, Edmunds L, Fenig S, et al. Managing childhood overweight: behavior, family, pharmacology, and bariatric surgery interventions. Obesity 2008;17: 411–23.
104. Snethen JA, Broome ME, Cashin SE. Effective weight loss for overweight children: a meta-analysis of intervention studies. J Pediatr Nurs 2006;21:45–56.

Practical Approaches to the Treatment of Severe Pediatric Obesity

C.M. Lenders, MD, MS, ScD[a,b,*], K. Gorman, MS, RD, LDN[c],
A. Lim-Miller, MSW, LICSW[c], S. Puklin, BS[d], J. Pratt, MD[b,e]

KEYWORDS
- Pediatrics • Severe obesity • Assessment • Pharmacotherapy
- Weight loss surgery • Behavior treatment

Pediatric obesity is a major public health threat. Obese children and adolescents are at increased risk for a wide range of medical and surgical conditions **Fig. 1**. These conditions may affect both their quality of life and life expectancy. The rapidly progressive nature of type 2 diabetes mellitus (T2DM) within the first 5 years of obesity diagnosis is particularly concerning. Because health risk increases with degree of obesity, it is crucial that one identify and counsel adolescents who may be eligible for more aggressive obesity treatment.[1]

DEFINITION OF SEVERE OBESITY

Defining a child as obese is only useful if that definition helps to predict morbidity or mortality. Most complications of obesity are associated with body fat and not muscle mass. Using Body Mass Index (BMI, weight/height^2), therefore, is a solid attempt at estimating adiposity. BMI is an adequate screening method at a population level.

[a] Nutrition and Fitness for Life Program (Pediatric Obesity), Department of Pediatrics, Boston University School of Medicine, Boston Medical Center, Vose Hall 3, 88 East Newton Street, Boston, MA 02118, USA
[b] Harvard Medical School, Boston, MA 02118, USA
[c] Nutrition and Fitness for Life Program (Pediatric Obesity), Department of Pediatrics, Boston Medical Center, Vose Hall 4, 88 East Newton Street, Boston, MA 02118, USA
[d] Boston University School of Medicine, Boston Medical Center, Vose Hall 5, 88 East Newton Street, Boston, MA 02118, USA
[e] Weight Loss Surgery Program, Department of Surgery, Massachusetts General Hospital, 15 Parkman Street, WAC 460, Boston, MA 02114-3117, USA
* Corresponding author. Nutrition and Fitness for Life Program (Pediatric Obesity), Department of Pediatrics, Boston University School of Medicine, Boston Medical Center, Vose Hall 3, 88 East Newton Street, Boston, MA 02118.
E-mail address: Carine.Lenders@bmc.org

Pediatr Clin N Am 58 (2011) 1425–1438
doi:10.1016/j.pcl.2011.09.013
0031-3955/11/$ – see front matter Published by Elsevier Inc.

pediatric.theclinics.com

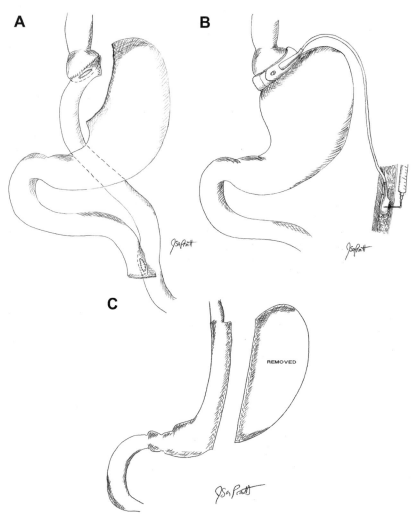

Fig. 1. Current weight loss surgery procedures. (*A*) The route -en-Y gastric bypass. (*B*) The adjustable gastric band. (*C*) The sleeve gastrectomy.

However, its strength as an indicator of pediatric adiposity decreases with younger children (birth to 12 years). There is also variation in BMI by ethnicity/race. Currently there is no valid measure to define children as having severe obesity.[2]

Barlow and the Expert Committee (2007) proposed to use a BMI cut off point at the 99th percentile among adolescents, which corresponds to a BMI of about 30–31 kg/m^2 for those 10 to 12 years old and a BMI of about 34 kg/m^2 for adolescents age 14 to 16 years, given its association with higher cardiovascular risk.[3–5] As will be described, a more conservative approach has been proposed for weight loss surgery.[1,6]

EVALUATION OF ASSOCIATED COMORBIDITIES

Even though the cause of obesity is typically idiopathic (>95%), the next most important step for the medical assessment of obesity is the exclusion of potential underlying syndromic and endocrine conditions. The presence of complications associated with obesity is based on history, physical examination, and laboratory tests (**Table 1**). Screening for short stature (most overweight children are average height or tall for their age), developmental delay, dysmorphic features, and abnormal genitalia help rule out many genetic and endocrine causes of pediatric obesity. As in ambulatory care pediatric weight clinics, the consultations with multidisciplinary specialty weight management programs may also include other pediatric specialties such as sleep disorder, gastroenterology, endocrinology, pulmonary/allergy, ophthalmology, otolaryngology (ORL), neurology, orthopedics, genetics, and psychiatry. Although referrals to comprehensive specialty weight management programs are recommended for severe obesity, there is a lack of published guidelines besides those for weight loss surgery[6,7] and for the treatment of the hospitalized obese pediatric patient.[2]

SPECIAL CONSIDERATIONS FOR BEHAVIOR RECOMMENDATIONS

As evidence is scarce, and more aggressive treatment is not readily available for all children and adolescents, behavior change is typically the main focus of specialty clinics treating pediatric obesity. Lower functioning families, such as those described as having poor parenting skills or experiencing multiple stressors and conflicts due to their socioeconomic difficulties, need interventions that focus first on basic parenting and conflict resolution skills before addressing lifestyle behaviors.[8] Identifying potential barriers to treatment of obesity and helping families move from their current stage toward readiness of action is imperative before behavior modification. This article will highlight key areas of assessment and treatment used in multidisciplinary specialty weight management programs.

Assessment

The first step toward creating change includes a comprehensive psychosocial assessment that targets areas of behavior and functioning. These areas include readiness and motivation to change, family functioning, parenting style, feeding practices, sedentary and activity practices, sleep hygiene, cultural beliefs, and psychiatric as well as developmental and environmental conditions that may interfere with feasibility and effectiveness of an intervention.[9–11]

Motivation and readiness to change

Barlow (2007) states, "a weight management program for a parent or an adolescent who is not ready to change may be not only futile but also harmful, because an unsuccessful program may diminish the child's self-esteem and impair future efforts to improve weight."[3] Some of the questions included in assessment of the motivation of patients and parents include: why they want a change, how they perceive success or failure in previous attempts, how they think this would affect their life in the future, and how committed they are to change (based on the readiness to change scale). The Stages of Change Model developed by Prochaska and DiClementi is adapted to facilitate dialog about readiness for change with patients and families, while aspects of motivational interviewing will facilitate change in families' readiness to change.[10]

Family functioning/parenting style

Family functioning is evaluated by examining how members of a family manage daily routines, how parenting roles are fulfilled, and how members of a family communicate and connect emotionally with each other. Children of authoritarian parents (strict disciplinarians) are at higher risk of obesity when compared with children of authoritative parents (parents who set boundaries but are respectful of their child's opinions).[12]

Table 1
Complications associated with obesity in children and youth

Body System	Relevant History and Examination	Diagnostic Tests
Cardiovascular		
Dyslipidemia	Family history: xanthomas	Fasting or nonfasting lipid profile
Hypertension	Family history: 14% children with persistent high blood pressure have left ventricular hypertrophy	SBP and/or BP >90th percentile
Endocrine		
Type 2 DM	High thirst, urination, appetite, fatigue, acanthosis, blurred vision, skin/GU infections, family history	Elevated hemoglobin A1C or OGTT
Polycystic ovary syndrome	Amenorrhea, acne, hirsutism, acanthosis	Testosterone (total, free), TSH, prolactin, 17-OH progesterone, option: ovaries US, luteinizing hormone/follicle stimulating hormone
Gastroenterology		
Constipation	Scybalous, pebble-like, hard stools most of the time or firm stools 2 or more times/wk, abdominal/rib pain	Rectal examination, abdominal radiograph, no evidence of structural, endocrine, or metabolic disease
Fecal soiling	At least 12 wks: large bowel movement <2×/wk & retentive posturing	Rectal examination, abdominal radiograph
GERD	Overfeeding, vomiting, chest pain/burning, asthma	PH probe if treatment trial fails
High ALT	Abdominal pain, nausea, vomiting, asymptomatic	ALT/AST ≥2–3× normal, repeat, referral to GI
Orthopedic		
Blount disease	One/both knees, deformity, intra-articular instability	Radiograph, orthopedic referral
Slipped capital femoral epiphysis	Often painless limp, knee pain, flexed hip in external rotation	Radiograph, rapid orthopedic referral
Other	Flat feet, leg length discrepancy, spinal deformity	Orthopedic referral
Neuropsychiatric		
Pseudotumor cerebrei	Blurred vision, headaches	Fundi examination, lumbar puncture
Sleep disturbances	Difficult to focus, to learn, or to perform daily activities, excessive daytime sleepiness, irritability, easy frustration, and difficulty with impulses and emotions (may be attributed to hyperactivity)	Sleep hygiene

Sleep apnea	Snoring, witnessed apnea, cyanosis, concern with child's breathing, restless sleep, daytime somnolence, enuresis, Can lead to right ventricular hypertrophy and right ventricular failure	High RBC, metabolic alkalosis; polysomnography, ear nose and throat evaluation
Binge eating	Large amount of food in discrete time period (eg, 2 h), lack of control, distressed by binging, sneaking/hoarding food, excessive concern with body shape and weight, persists for at least 3 months, no compensatory behaviors	Eating Attitudes Test—Child Version (chEAT) Eating Disorder Inventory-C (preteens and teens), QEWP-A (adolescent version), Eating Disorder Examination (ChEDE) – interview. Use ChEDE-Q-self-report
Compulsive overeating	Characterized by episodic binge eating, may also include uses of purging or restrictive eating, fear of not being able to stop eating, depressed mood, food can become 1° mood regulator	See above
Night eating syndrome	Little/no appetite for breakfast, most caloric intake at night, leaves bed to snack at night, anxious, sleep disturbance, persists at least 2 months	N/A for children or adolescents, screen for symptoms present
Depression	Depressed mood, low self-esteem, anhedonia, irritability, hopelessness, hx of suicide ideation, sleep disturbance, fatigue, diminished concentration	CDI
Anxiety	Excessive worry, sleep disturbance, tantrums/crying, obsessive thoughts, fatigue, low self-esteem, avoidance, history of trauma, rule out social phobia and separation anxiety	CBCL
Weight teasing	Target of name-calling, ridicule, put-downs, verbal insults, can occur at home and at school	Teasing and Bullying Survey (TABS-C)—Bodin (2004) (still in research stage)

Abbreviations: ALT, alanine aminotransferase; AST, aspartate aminotransferase; DM, diabetes mellitus; FSH, follicle-stimulating hormone; GERD, gastroesophageal reflux disease; GI, gastrointestinal; GU, genitourinary; N/A, not applicable; OGTT, oral glucose tolerance test; RBC, red blood cell; TSH, thyrotropin; US, ultrasound.

Adapted from Lenders C, Oliver L, Lakhani S, et al. Pediatric obesity medicine. In: Augustyn M, Zuckerman B, Caronna E, editors. Zuckerman and Parker's handbook of developmental and behavioral pediatrics. 3rd edition. Lippincott Williams & Wilkins; 2011; and Lenders C, Meyers A, Oh H. A clinical guide to pediatric ambulatory weight management. In: Apovian C, Lenders C, editors. A clinical guide for management of overweight and obese children and adults. Boca Raton (FL): CRC press; 2007. p. 197–238.

High family and parental stress affect parental consistency and ability to model healthy lifestyle behaviors.[8]

Feeding practices
When evaluating families with obese children, special attention is given to the family's relationship with food. Ellyn Satter's division of responsibility in feeding is considered the gold standard by dietitians and behavioral health professionals alike. Satter emphasizes that "parents are responsible for the what, when, and where of feeding. Children are responsible for the how much and whether of eating" (**Table 2**).[13] What the family eats is also being evaluated when assessing feeding practices. Dietitians often use a combination of 24-hour recalls, food frequency questions, and food diaries to assess dietary and nutrient intake in specialty weight management clinics.

Sleep schedules
Assessing sleep hygiene has become an integral part of the assessment of routine behaviors associated with obesity. Irregular sleep schedules and shorter sleep duration are linked to greater obesity risk.[11] In fact, a meta-analysis of short sleep duration and obesity noted that the association between sleep disturbance and obesity may be due to changes in hormones and inflammation.[14]

Cultural considerations
Equally important to behavioral considerations are cultural beliefs about weight and food. There is limited research on relationships between obesity and cultural beliefs; however it is known that "some cultures value a more full-bodied appearance," and see this type of appearance as a sign of good health rather than a health problem.[1] Cultural traditions around food and food preparation can affect weight gain. An important example is the way food is prepared; in some cultures traditional preparation of

Table 2
Assessing and addressing child feeding behaviors

Assessments	Recommended Behaviors
Is the child offered meals and snacks at the same times each day? Or, are patterns of feeding unpredictable?	Meals and snacks should be scheduled to occur at the same time each day and should be 2–4 hours apart
Is the child allowed to graze on either food or caloric beverages between meals?	Children should be allowed only water between scheduled meals and snacks
Does the family eat together on a regular basis? What is considered acceptable mealtime behavior?	Families should sit at the table and eat together as often as possible. Families should engage in pleasant mealtime conversations
Who decides what food will be offered, parent or child?	The parent is responsible for deciding what food will be offered. Parents should not short-order cook to meet the likes of each family member
Is the child ever forced to eat certain foods? Is the child ever restricted to only a certain amount of some foods?	Children should never be forced to eat nor should they be restricted. Healthy children are able to regulate their own hunger
Is food ever used for non-nutritive purposes, such as rewards, bribes, or punishment?	Food should not be used for bribing or punishing children

Data from Refs.[3,13,15]

vegetables is with high amounts of fat and salt. In these cultures, vegetables are not traditionally served steamed or lightly sautéed. Also important are the food behaviors of other family members with whom the child spends a significant amount of time outside of the household (eg, grandparents). Children observe the way in which these members eat and will often mimic their behaviors. Understanding each family's beliefs and traditions around food can help shape an individualized intervention that is sensitive to a family's cultural food norms.

Psychiatric or developmental condition

Experts recommend screening for depression, anxiety, eating disorders, post-traumatic stress disorder, trauma, developmental disabilities, and other major psychiatric disorders before weight management intervention, as they may affect eating patterns and physical activity.[15] Recent studies among severely obese children ages 8 to 12 years with binge-eating behavior show decreased success in family-based programs.[16] Children on the autism spectrum may have atypical physical activity and eating patterns that are uniquely associated with the development of obesity[17] and may affect weight management. In addition, several psychiatric medications may affect body metabolism and food intake, and thus weight gain. Therefore, collaboration with mental health providers and referral to appropriate mental health services should be included in the care of obese children.[10,18,19]

Environmental conditions—socioeconomic and food security

Assessing access to nutritious food and safe living environment are key components to understanding the functioning of the patient and family. There is increasing evidence that food insecurity is a risk factor for adolescent obesity.[20] The disease burden associated with obesity is greatest among underserved populations and minorities,[21] especially among individuals living in neighborhoods identified as unsafe.[22]

Management/Treatment

Although studies in the clinical setting are becoming more common,[23,24] they rarely focus on severely obese children. Based on an intent-to-treat analysis, 1 recent randomized case control study of 192 morbidly obese children (BMI >97th percentile) ages 8 to 12 years showed a 7.6% decrease in child percent overweight (percent over the median BMI for age and sex) at 6 months versus a 0.7% decrease with usual care, as well as a significant improvement in metabolic markers.[25] In that study, patients who attended at least 75% of the sessions were also found to maintain weight loss 18 months after the intervention. Unfortunately, there is a lack of studies that address the structural characteristics of pediatric weight management programs, even among severely obese children.

The US Preventive Services Task Force indicated that moderate-to-high intensity (approximately 25 hours of contact over 6 months) was needed to detect significant outcomes among obese children and adolescents.[24] This recommendation is based using outcome data from studies with various designs rather than randomized case control trials, and is thus not evidenced-based. Although more successful programs typically tend to offer weekly or biweekly visits over a period of 4 to 12 months, comparisons between studies are difficult, as contact hours may include contact with mental health, dietitian, physiotherapists, and physicians separately or combined at each visit. Furthermore, there is a lack of evidence on the intensity of treatment needed during the maintenance phase. To the best of the authors' knowledge, there is a lack of comparison between individual versus group treatment, especially according to minority and socioeconomic status. Although weight loss success among pediatric individuals with higher degree of obesity is still controversial,[26,27] promising results are emerging from clinics serving minority and lower socioeconomic populations.[28,29]

Once family function and parenting styles have been addressed, and underserved families have been connected to appropriate social resources (such as Supplemental Nutrition Program for Women, Infants and Children [WIC], Supplemental Nutrition Assistance Program [SNAP, formerly Food Stamps], local food pantries and soup kitchens, Head Start, fuel assistance, and Temporary Assistance for Needy Families (TANF), clinicians can shift focus to food and physical activity behaviors. The recommended behaviors for obese children that are used in ambulatory and specialty clinics are based on the same principles (see **Table 2**). The team targets lifestyle behaviors to reduce weight gain (**Box 1**).

Data on the best dietary and physical activity approach for the treatment of pediatric obesity are emerging. The effect of diet composition on weight measures and metabolic markers is significant in short-term but not long-term studies of obese adolescents.[30,31] Similar findings over time have been observed with meal replacement therapy.[32] Compared with a control diet alone, Berkowitz and colleagues[32] showed that a control diet with meal replacement therapy significantly improved short-term weight loss (6.3 $\pm$ 0.6% versus 3.8 $\pm$ 0.8% reduction in BMI), but its continued use did not improve the maintenance of weight measure loss at 5 to 12 months. Therefore, select dietary approaches may be considered in patients who require acute weight loss. The Expert Committee[3] recommends moderate-to-vigorous activity for at least 60 minutes a day, and more recently the American Academy of Pediatrics also provided recommendations for strength training among adolescents and preadolescents.[33] There is increasing evidence, especially from the adult literature, that strength training increases metabolic rate and improves body composition.[34]

Given that the dietary approach may not be critical to weight and metabolic outcomes in a weight management program, that there is increasing evidence that routine behaviors such as sedentary activities, physical activities, and sleeping activities affect weight change, and that families have difficulties changing many behaviors at once,[10] the specialty team will encourage families and their adolescents to focus on 1 or 2 changes at time, in either an individual or a group setting, until all are achieved.

Box 1
Targeted lifestyle behaviors

Reduce sugar-sweetened beverages with goal of completely eliminating.

Consume $\geq$9 servings of fruits and vegetables every day.

Decrease TV time to $\leq$2 h/d.

Eat breakfast every day.

Prepare more meals at home instead of purchasing restaurant food.

Be physically active for $\geq$1 h/d.

Achieve regular uninterrupted nightly sleep of >8 hours per night.

Data from Barlow SE. Expert Committee. Expert committee recommendations regarding the prevention, assessment, and treatment of child and adolescent overweight and obesity: summary report. Pediatrics 2007;120(Suppl 4):S164-92; and Spruyt K, Molfese D, Gozal D. Sleep duration, sleep regularity, body weight, and metabolic homoeostasis in school-aged children. Pediatrics 2011;127;e345.[3,11]

Group treatment in a tertiary care facility may be more challenging for underserved populations needing access to more flexible schedules, such as those offered in individualized treatment. As pointed out in this article, there are multiple barriers to the management and treatment of severe pediatric obesity. The most important role of a multidisciplinary specialty weight management team is to thoroughly assess families and recognize that each obstacle must be identified and addressed before and during lifestyle interventions.

MEDICAL THERAPIES

Current options for the pharmacologic treatment of obesity are limited but may have some clinical utility in adults and adolescents. In general, the medications demonstrate only modest efficacy (BMI loss ranging between 1–3 kg/m^2) and have a range of adverse effects.[23] Two drugs were approved by the US Food and Drug Administration (FDA): sibutramine for adolescents age 16 years and older and orlistat for adolescents age 12 years and older.[35,36] However, in October 2010, Meridia (sibutramine) was removed from the US market following findings from a European clinical trial data that indicated an increased risk of heart attack and stroke among adults.[37] Although metformin is frequently prescribed by physicians to treat outpatient pediatric obesity, its use is only approved by the FDA for children age 10 years and older with T2DM. In fact, long-term findings from a recent randomized clinical trial of metformin to treat adolescent obesity were rather disappointing, and showed that metformin could even exacerbate weight gain at discontinuation.[38] Currently, there is not enough evidence for long-term safety and efficacy of medications for weight management among children and adolescents. The use of pharmacologic doses of select nutrients and other drugs to improve weight measures and metabolic markers is under study and beyond the scope of this article.

The authors will briefly describe the mechanism of action and side effects of 2 drugs that are commonly prescribed among US obese adolescents: orlistat and metformin.[23,36] Orlistat has been recommended as an adjunct therapy to behavior modification and may be especially beneficial for patients who consume foods cooked in restaurants, have difficulties adhering to a diet lower in fat, and suffer of hypertension, diabetes, or hypercholesterolemia. Orlistat is an inhibitor of gastrointestinal (GI) lipases including pancreatic lipase. At a dose of 120 mg three times a day, orlistat prevents 30% of fat absorption. As a result, orlistat reduces total dietary fat and calorie intake and therefore has a beneficial effect on weight (about 2–3 kg/m^2 loss in BMI) and metabolic markers. A supplement of fat-soluble vitamins is recommended 2 to 3 hours before or after the medication. Alli (orlistat 60 mg) is now available over the counter. Main adverse effects include oily spotting, liquid stools, fecal urgency, flatulence, and abdominal cramping. This explains why orlistat is not popular among adolescents. Finally, this drug is contraindicated among individuals with malabsorptive syndrome and cholestasis.

Metformin has been recommended in the treatment of adolescents with T2DM.[38] Metformin has been especially recommended as an adjunct therapy among obese adolescents with T2DM, and may be useful in adolescents with polycystic ovary syndrome and prediabetes, but more studies are needed. At a dose of 500 mg (850 mg XR (extended release)) up to a maximum of 2500 mg/d, metformin activates the adenosine monophosphate (AMP)-activated protein kinase (AMPK), which results in the inhibition of liver gluconeogenesis and lipid biosynthesis and the stimulation of glucose uptake by the muscle. Metformin is an antihyperglycemiant that improves insulin sensitivity without affecting insulin secretion, and to some extent weight measures (about 1 kg/m² BMI loss), but its overall effect on serum metabolic markers is less clear.[38] A supplement of multivitamin and calcium is recommended to improve B12 absorption during metformin treatment. Metformin is available as Glucophage, Glucophage XR (extended release), or generic. Common adverse effects include diarrhea, flatulence, abdominal discomfort, and headaches. Metformin is contraindicated among patients with kidney or liver disease, as cases of lactic acidosis have been described. In summary, GI adverse effects are the most common for both orlistat and metformin, and both drugs affect vitamin absorption.

Surgical Options

There is increasing evidence that obesity surgery is safe and effective in children and may decrease the long-term risks associated with excess weight and related comorbidities.[7,9] The benefit of surgery must be weighed against the risk of the patient remaining obese and the progression of their comorbidities. This can be particularly difficult in noncompliant adolescents with type 2 diabetes, advanced nonalcoholic steatohepatitis (NASH), severe obstructive sleep apnea (OSA), or pseudotumor cerebri, where timing of surgery is extremely important to prevent permanent end organ injury.

New criteria have been recommended for patient selections.[7,8] The Betsy Lehman recommendations for patient selection were based on evidence that all adolescents with a BMI >40 kg/m² had a BMI greater than the 99th percentile,[1] and all adolescents with a BMI greater than the 99th percentile remained obese adults.[4] These data and the natural BMI curve during teenage years allow for the use of a fixed BMI cutoff of point of 35 kg/m² with severe comorbidities and 40 kg/m² with other comorbidities to be a more conservative approach for the younger adolescents (12–14 years old), to match the adult cut-offs as children reach 18 years old, and to identify individuals at higher health risk. Serious comorbidities were defined as T2DM, moderate-to-severe OSA, NASH, or pseudotumor cerebri. Other comorbidities included mild OSA, mild NASH, hypertension, dyslipidemia, and significantly impaired quality of life.

Besides age (12–18 years old) and BMI (>35 kg/m2 plus serious co-morbidity or BMI >40 kg/m² plus other co-morbidities), other selection criteria also include Tanner stage 4 or 5, skeletal maturity (completed at least 95% of growth only if planning a diversional or malabsorptive operation), lifestyles (demonstrates ability to understand what dietary and physical activity changes will be required for optimal postoperative outcomes), and psychological status (evidence of mature decision making with appropriate understanding of risks vs benefits, evidence of appropriate social support without evidence of abuse and neglect, underlying psychiatric condition under treatment, patient and family ability and motivation to comply with recommended pre- and postoperative treatment including office visits and regular medications intake).[6]

A multidisciplinary team should determine which patients are appropriate for surgery and should be involved in educating and supporting patients through the process. The team should include a pediatrician, either specialized in pediatric obesity or other related subspecialties, psychologist, dietitian, bariatric surgeon, and program coordinator. Other important specialties consider including are exercise physiologists, social services, nursing, gynecology, and child life specialists.

Selecting the appropriate operation in children is similar to selecting the appropriate operation in adults. However, there are significantly fewer data about which operation has the best long-term outcomes. Until there are better ways to select the procedure based on the type of obesity, one will need to continue to use other criteria. Each procedure has its own set of risks and benefits, and the ultimate decision must be weighed based on the patient's comorbidities, severity of his or her obesity, ability to follow-up and comply with treatment, and preference.

There are currently 3 surgical approaches commonly used among adolescents (**Fig. 1**). The Roux-en-Y gastric bypass, the adjustable gastric band, and the sleeve gastrectomy. The gastric bypass is the preferred surgical procedure among adolescent bariatric surgeons because it has the most long-term data in adults and adolescents.[8,39] This operation involves the reduction of the stomach reservoir to a 30 cc pouch and bypassing the proximal intestine. There is increasing evidence that early introduction of food into the more distal small intestine affects appetite and basal metabolic rate via neurohormonal signaling, and thus contributes to weight loss.[40,41] Early outcomes after Roux en Y gastric bypass in adolescents are similar to those of adults with rapid resolution of type 2 diabetes, sleep apnea, and reflux even before weight loss. Patients generally loose 65% of their excess body weight, and patients maintain at least 50% excess body weight loss at 15 years.[42] Complication rates in adolescents appear to be equal to or lower than in adults. However, the risk of vitamin deficiencies, anemias, and ulcers is significant in this population known for noncompliance.

As opposed to the Roux-en-Y procedure, the band is a purely restrictive procedure. Bands have been used in adolescents with excellent 3- to 5-year outcomes.[7] They require frequent follow-up for adjustments. Long-term outcomes are unknown among adolescents; however, the reoperation rate in adults is close to 40% at 10 years. Thus, the FDA disapproved its use in adolescents (June 2011).

Laparoscopic sleeve gastrectomy has been performed as a standalone procedure in the United States since 2002. It is considered a safe operation, where 75% of the stomach volume is removed by partial gastrectomy of the greater curve of the stomach. Long-term outcomes of sleeve are not known in either adults or adolescents; however, the lack of vitamin deficiencies, anemia, and ulcer disease even in the setting of noncompliance makes this operation an attractive option in adolescents. Weight loss outcomes in adults show 50% to 65% excess body weight loss at 5 years.[39] This operation is in no way reversible; however, conversion to a Roux-en-Y gastric bypass is possible, and this can be used for weight regain or reflux, which are the 2 most common complications of this operation.

Based largely on expert opinion but also on evidence from the literature, surgery for the treatment of obesity in adolescents should be used in patients who are emotionally mature or significantly impaired by comorbidities and meet the weight criteria. In the absence of solid data to support one operation over the other, choice of procedure should take into account the patient and family preference and the likelihood of compliance with long-term follow-up. A multidisciplinary team and a strong pre- and postoperative program are imperative. Pediatric programs should also have a transition plan to an adult program for longterm follow-up with an adult bariatric surgeon.

ACKNOWLEDGMENTS

The Nutrition and Fitness for Life program members (CL, KG, ALM, SP) at the Boston Medical Center thank the New Balance Foundation and the Allen Foundation for their clinical and educational activities support.

REFERENCES

1. Lenders CM, Wright JA, Apovian CM, et al. Weight loss surgery eligibility according to various BMI criteria among adolescents. Obesity (Silver Spring) 2009; 17(1):150–5.

2. Jesuit C, Dillon C, Compher C. American Society for Parenteral and Enteral Nutrition (A.S.P.E.N.) Board of Directors, Lenders CM.A.S.P.E.N. Clinical guidelines: nutrition support of hospitalized pediatric patients with obesity. JPEN J Parenter Enteral Nutr 2010;34(1):13–20.

3. Barlow SE. Expert Committee. Expert committee recommendations regarding the prevention, assessment, and treatment of child and adolescent overweight and obesity: summary report. Pediatrics 2007;120(Suppl 4):S164–92.

4. Freedman DS, Khan LK, Serdula MK, et al. Racial and ethnic differences in secular trends for childhood BMI, weight, and height. Obesity (Silver Spring) 2006;14:301–8.

5. Pemberton VL, McCrindle BW, Barkin S, et al. Report of the National Heart, Lung and Blood Institute's working Group on Obesity and Other Cardiovascular Risk Factors in Congenital Heart Disease. Circulation 2010;121(9):1153–9.

6. Pratt JS, Lenders CM, Dionne EA, et al. Best practice updates for pediatric/adolescent weight loss surgery. Obesity (Silver Spring) 2009;17(5):901–10.

7. Inge TH. Bariatric surgery for morbidly obese adolescents: is there a rational for early intervention? Growth Horm IGF Res 2006;16(Suppl A):S15–9.

8. Kitzmann KM, Beech BM. Family-based interventions for pediatric obesity: methodological and conceptual challenges from family psychology. J Fam Psychol 2006;20(2):175–89.

9. Lenders C, Oliver L, Lakhani S, et al. Pediatric obesity medicine. In: Augustyn M, Zuckerman B, Caronna E, editors. Zuckerman and Parker's Handbook of Developmental and Behavioral Pediatrics. 3rd edition. Philadelphia (PA): Lippincott Williams & Wilkins; 2011. p. 288–94.

10. Lakhani S, Marino M, Rivinus, et al. Behavioral health considerations for the management of pediatric obesity in primary care. In: Apovian C, Lenders C, editors. A clinical guide for management of overweight and obese children and adults. Boca Raton (FL): CRC press; 2007. p. 239–69.

11. Spruyt K, Molfese D, Gozal D. Sleep duration, sleep regularity, body weight, and metabolic homoeostasis in school aged children. Pediatrics 2011;127:e345.

12. Rhee KE, Lumeng JC, Appugliese DP, et al. Parenting styles and overweight status in first grade. Pediatrics 2006;117(6):2047–54.

13. Satter E. Your child's weight: helping without harming: birth through adolescence. Madison (WI): Kelcy Press; 2005.

14. Cappuccio FP, Taggart FM, Kandala NB, et al. Meta-analysis of short sleep duration and obesity in children and adults. Sleep 2008;31(5):619–26.

15. Lenders C, Meyers A, Oh H. A clinical guide to pediatric ambulatory weight management. In: Apovian C, Lenders C, editors. A clinical guide for management of overweight and obese children and adults. Boca Raton (FL): CRC press; 2007. p. 197–238.

16. Wildes JE, Marcus MD, Kalarchian MA, et al. Self-reported binge eating in severe pediatric obesity: impact on weight change in a randomized controlled trial of family-based treatment. Int J Obes (Lond) 2010;34(7):1143–8.

17. Curtin C, Anderson SE, Must A, et al. The prevalence of obesity in children with autism: a secondary data analysis using nationally representative data from the national survey of children's health. BMC Pediatr 2010;10(11):1–5.

18. Taner Y, Törel-Ergür A, Bahçivan G, et al. Psychopathology and its effect on treatment compliance in pediatric obesity patients. Turk J Pediatr 2009;51(5):466–71.

19. Zametkin AJ, Zoon CK, Klein HW, et al. Psychiatric aspects of child and adolescent obesity: a review of the past 10 years. J Am Acad Child Adolesc Psychiatry 2004;43(2):518–25.

20. Casey PH, Simpson PM, Gossett JM, et al. The association of child and household food insecurity with childhood overweight status. Pediatrics 2006;118(5): e1406–13.
21. Winkleby MA, Robinson TN, Sundquist J, et al. Ethnic variation in cardiovascular disease risk factors among children and young adults: findings from the Third National Health and Nutrition Examination Study. 1988–1994. JAMA 1999;281: 1006–13.
22. Burdette H, Wadden T, Whitaker R. Neighborhood safety, collective efficacy, and obesity in women with young children. Obesity (Silver Spring) 2006;14:518–25.
23. Oude Luttikhuis H, Baur L, Jansen H, et al. Interventions for treating obesity in children. Cochrane Database Syst Rev 2009;1:CD001872.
24. Whitlock EP, O'Connor EA, Williams SB, et al. Effectiveness of weight management interventions in children: a targeted systematic review for the USPSTF. Pediatrics 2010;125(2):e396–418.
25. Kalarchian MA, Levine MD, Arslanian SA, et al. Family-based treatment of severe pediatric obesity: randomized, controlled trial. Pediatrics 2009;124(4):1060–8.
26. Knöpfli BH, Radtke T, Lehmann M, et al. Effects of a multidisciplinary inpatient intervention on body composition, aerobic fitness, and quality of life in severely obese girls and boys. J Adolesc Health 2008;42(2):119–27.
27. Hughes AR, Stewart L, Chapple J, et al. Randomized, controlled trial of a best-practice individualized behavioral program for treatment of childhood overweight: Scottish Childhood Overweight Treatment Trial (SCOTT). Pediatrics 2008;121(3):e539–46.
28. Skelton JA, DeMattia LG, Flores G. A pediatric weight management program for high-risk populations: a preliminary analysis. Obesity (Silver Spring) 2008;16(7): 1698–701.
29. Lenders C, Heinrick JR, DeBiasse M, et al. Secondary prevention of obesity among children 5 and under. Available at: http://experimentalbiology.org/eb2011archive/content/upload/file/2011%20Sunday%20Posters.pdf. Accessed July 30, 2011.
30. Sacks FM, Bray GA, Carey VJ, et al. Comparison of weight-loss diets with different compositions of fat, protein, and carbohydrates. N Engl J Med 2009; 360(9):859–73.
31. Demol S, Yackobovitch-Gavan M, Shalitin S, et al. Low-carbohydrate (low & high-fat) versus high-carbohydrate low-fat diets in the treatment of obesity in adolescents. Acta Paediatr 2009;98(2):346–51.
32. Berkowitz RI, Wadden TA, Gehrman CA, et al. Meal replacements in the treatment of adolescent obesity: a randomized controlled trial. Obesity (Silver Spring) 2011; 19(6):1193–9.
33. American Academy of Pediatrics. Council on Sports Medicine and Fitness. Strength training in children and adolescents. Pediatrics 2008;121(4):835–40.
34. Strasser B, Schobersberger W. Evidence for resistance training as a treatment therapy in obesity. J Obes 2011.
35. Berkowitz R, Fujioka K, Daniels S, et al. Effects of sibutramine treatment in obese adolescents. A randomized trial. Ann Intern Med 2006;145:81–90.
36. Thearle M, Aronne LJ. Pharmacologyc therapy for obesity and overweight in adults and adolescents. In: Apovian C, Lenders C, editors. A clinical guide for management of overweight and obese children and adults. Boca Raton (FL): CRC press; 2007. p. 98–122.
37. Abbott Laboratories agrees to withdraw its obesity drug Meridia. Available at: http://www.fda.gov/NewsEvents/Newsroom/PressAnnouncements/ucm228812.htm. Accessed July 28, 2011.

38. Wilson DM, Abrams SH, Aye T, et al. Glaser Pediatric Research Network Obesity Study Group. Metformin extended release treatment of adolescent obesity: a 48-week randomized, double-blind, placebo-controlled trial with 48-week follow-up. Arch Pediatr Adolesc Med 2010;164(2):116–23.

39. Brandt ML, Harmon CM, Helmrath MA, et al. Morbid obesity in pediatric diabetes mellitus: surgical options and outcomes. Nat Rev Endocrinol 2010;6(11):637–45.

40. De Carvalho CP, Martin DM, Souza AL, et al. GLP-1 and andiponectin: effect of weight loss after dietary restriction and gastric bypass in morbidly obese patients with normal and abnormal glucose metabolism. Obes Surg 2009;19(3):313–20.

41. Sjöström L, Narbro K, Sjöström CD, et al. Effects of bariatric surgery on mortality in Swedish obese subjects. N Engl J Med 2007;357(8):741–52.

42. D'Hondt M, Vannesete S, Pottel H. Laproscopic sleeve gastrectomy as a single-stage procedure for the treatment of morbid obesity and the resulting quality of life, resolution of comorbidities, food tolerance, and 6-year weight loss. Surg Endosc 2011;25(8):2498–504.

Strategies for Pediatric Practitioners to Increase Fruit and Vegetable Consumption in Children

Sonia A. Kim, PhD*, Kirsten A. Grimm, MPH, Ashleigh L. May, PhD,
Diane M. Harris, PhD, MPH, Joel Kimmons, PhD,
Jennifer L. Foltz, MD, MPH

KEYWORDS
- Fruit • Vegetable • Consumption • Provider strategies
- Children • Diet

Choices individuals make around what, where, and how much they eat and drink are influenced by many factors. Various socioecological models have been proposed to explain how these multiple factors of influence can shape individual behavior.[1,2] The framework proposed by Story and colleagues[1] groups these factors into 4 main levels: individual (eg, skills, preferences), social environment (eg, social support), physical environment (eg, retail and food service opportunities in settings such as schools, worksites, early care and education, and the broader community), and macrolevel influences (eg, systems-level factors such as social norms, food marketing, and food production). Health care providers traditionally have focused on individuals and individual factors to improve patient health, such as knowledge about the importance of healthy behaviors and improved self-efficacy to make healthy choices.[3] However, there is growing recognition that a focus on the individual is not sufficient and strategies acting at multiple levels are needed to improve health, including diet quality. This recognition has led the public health community, including health care providers, to augment individually focused strategies with policy, systems, and environmental approaches.[3,4] These methods emphasize the importance of

We have no financial relationships relevant to this article. The findings and conclusions in this report are those of the authors and do not necessarily represent the official position of the Centers for Disease Control and Prevention.

Division of Nutrition, Physical Activity, and Obesity, National Center for Chronic Disease Prevention and Health Promotion, Centers for Disease Control and Prevention, 4770 Buford Highway Northeast, MS K-25, Atlanta, GA 30341-3717, USA

* Corresponding author.

E-mail address: SKim3@cdc.gov

Pediatr Clin N Am 58 (2011) 1439–1453
doi:10.1016/j.pcl.2011.09.011
0031-3955/11/$ – see front matter Published by Elsevier Inc.

pediatric.theclinics.com

a coordinated, systems-wide approach that engages individuals, families, communities, organizations, health professionals, and policymakers. This broad approach recognizes that, although individuals are responsible for their own health, opportunities need to be available in order for individuals to make healthy choices.

Establishing healthy eating habits early in life may have lifelong impacts on individuals. Dietary exposures and practices in early childhood and youth predict dietary behaviors in adolescence and adulthood.[5–7] The pediatric practitioner can positively influence fruit and vegetable (FV) consumption of children by considering all levels of the socioecological model. Through counseling during clinic visits, the practitioner may be able to directly influence the food choices of caregivers and their children. Practitioners can also recommend community resources to improve access to healthier foods, such as FV, and be community advocates for these resources. By creating a healthy environment in the clinical setting, practitioners can provide healthy options for patients, families, and employees, and serve as role models for the community.

This article reviews the importance of FV consumption, recommended intakes for children, and strategies by which pediatric practitioners can influence FV consumption of children where they live, access care, play, and learn. These strategies are summarized in **Box 1**.

FV provide many important nutrients, including potassium, folate, fiber, vitamin A, vitamin C, vitamin K,[2] and many phytochemicals.[8] Higher intake of FV is associated with a decreased risk for many chronic diseases including heart disease,[9] stroke,[10] diabetes,[11] and some cancers.[12] In addition, replacing energy-dense foods with FV may assist in healthy weight management.[13] This benefit is especially important given the childhood obesity epidemic in the United States, where 32% of children 2 to 19 years old are overweight or obese (defined as body mass index [BMI] for age equal to or greater than the 85th percentile) and 17% are obese (BMI for age equal to or greater than the 95th percentile).[14] The *Expert Committee Recommendations on the Prevention, Assessment, and Treatment of Child and Adolescent Overweight and Obesity* states that pediatric weight management and behavioral counseling should include encouraging families to consume recommended levels of FV.[15]

Because of the many benefits of FV consumption, the *Dietary Guidelines for Americans, 2010* (DGA 2010) recommends increased consumption of FV for all Americans 2 years and older, and emphasizes the importance of eating a variety of these foods, specifically mentioning dark green, orange, and red vegetable subgroups.[2] DGA 2010 stresses the importance of whole food sources (fresh, frozen, canned, and dried), rather than juice, because juice may contain less fiber and other important nutrients.[2] When juice is consumed, it should be 100% fruit or vegetable juice. The American Academy of Pediatrics (AAP) recommends no more than 120 to 180 mL (4–6 ounces) of 100% juice daily for children 1 to 6 years of age and no more than 240 to 360 mL (8–12 ounces) daily for children 7 to 18 years of age.[16]

The US Department of Agriculture's (USDA) food guide, MyPlate, highlights the importance of FV as part of a healthy diet with its key message of "Make half your plate fruits and vegetables." MyPlate's FV recommendations are based on an individual's caloric requirements, which depend on age, sex, and physical activity level. Among sedentary youth, recommendations range from 1 cup of fruit and 1 cup of vegetables for boys and girls 2 to 3 years old, to 1.5 cups of fruit and 2.5 cups of vegetables for girls 14 to 18 years old and 2 cups of fruit and 3 cups of vegetables for boys 14 to 18 years old (individuals with higher levels of physical activity need more). Caregivers and practitioners can refer to MyPlate (www.MyPlate.gov) for individualized FV recommendations, information on serving sizes, and an overall healthy eating plan.

Box 1
Opportunities for pediatric practitioners to influence children's fruit and vegetable (FV) consumption

Patient-level interventions: assess, counsel, and provide resources

- Promote caregiver behaviors that encourage FV consumption by children (specific topics and strategies that may be suggested to caregivers are summarized in **Box 2**).
- Give a FV prescription at clinic visits (available at: http://www.aap.org/obesity/letsmove/index.cfm).
- Integrate assessment of, and counseling on, FV consumption into clinical practice. The American Academy of Pediatrics provides a guide for coding that can be useful for billing purposes.
- Engage individuals external to the medical practice who offer support and connections to community resources.
- Be familiar with resources that promote healthy behaviors, such as food assistance programs (eg, Special Supplemental Nutrition Program for Women, Infants and Children [WIC], WIC Farmers Market Nutrition Program [FMNP], and the Supplemental Nutrition Assistance Program [SNAP]), farmers markets, cooking classes, and community gardens.
- Develop referral guides to these community resources.

Community-level interventions: advocate for and support change

- Influence policies and environments where children play and learn through advocacy, community involvement, and collaborations with local and state health departments, schools, early care and education (ECE), recreation facilities, and community organizations.
- Support school district policies and programs that increase the quality and quantity of nutritious foods offered through the school environment and engage kids in nutrition education and experiential learning activities. Examples include school salad bars (eg, *Let's Move! Salad Bars to Schools*), gardens, the HealthierUS School Challenge, and school wellness policies and committees.
- Support programs and policies that incentivize retail outlets to sell nutritious foods and to locate in underserved neighborhoods.
- Learn how to advocate for community change with resources such as The National Initiative for Children's Healthcare Quality Be Our Voice Campaign (http://www.nichq.org/advocacy/obesity_resources/toolkit.html) and the American Academy of Pediatrics' Policy Opportunities Tool (http://www.aap.org/obesity/matrix_1.html).

Health care facility-level interventions: create an environment supportive of FV consumption

- Be a role model for patients and the community through practices and offerings at health care facilities.
- Provide healthy food options for patients, guests, and employees.
- Host a farmers markets or community-supported agriculture program for employees and the community.
- Create guidelines for increasing FV in vending, food service venues, hospital shops, and inpatient meals.
- Consult the *Health and Sustainability Guidelines for Federal Concessions and Vending Operations* for FV guidelines: (available at: http://www.cdc.gov/chronicdisease/resources/guidelines/food-service-guidelines.htm).

Few children and adolescents consume the recommended amounts of FV. Nationally representative findings from the 1999 to 2002 National Health and Nutrition Examination Survey (NHANES) found that children aged 2 to 5 years met recommendations for fruit intake, but not for vegetable intake, with an average consumption of 1.29 cup equivalents and 0.76 cup equivalents of fruit and vegetables, respectively. Among children aged 6 to 11 years, mean fruit intake was 0.99 cup equivalents and mean vegetable intake was 0.98 cup equivalents.[17] In a separate study of NHANES 1999 to 2002 data, 56.0% of adolescents consumed less than 1 serving of FV daily.[18] The 2003 to 2004 NHANES showed that among adolescents (12–18 years old), median intakes were 0.51 cups of fruit and 1.21 cups of vegetables, and only 6.2% of adolescents met calorie-specific recommendations for fruit intake and 5.8% for vegetable intake.[19]

Although FV consumption is low among children and adolescents 2 to 18 years of age in all sociodemographic groups (sex, age, race/ethnicity, and household income), there are some differences among groups.[17] Findings from NHANES 1999 to 2002 showed that fruit intake was higher among younger compared with older children, among Mexican-Americans compared with non-Hispanic whites, and among those living in households with an income greater than 350% of the federal poverty level versus those living in households with an income between 130% and 350% of the federal poverty level. Vegetable intake was higher among boys than girls and higher among older compared with younger children; however, there was no difference in consumption by either race/ethnicity or household income.[17]

PATIENT-LEVEL INTERVENTIONS: THE HEALTH CARE VISIT

The Expert Committee on the Prevention, Assessment, and Treatment of Child and Adolescent Overweight and Obesity recommends that health care providers conduct a focused assessment of behaviors that have the strongest evidence for association with energy balance and that are modifiable, including the number of FV servings consumed each day.[15] At a minimum, this assessment should be done at each well-child visit and include ability and readiness to change.

In addition to assessment, health care providers should advise caregivers to encourage consumption of the recommended amounts of FV by children and the whole family.[15] Specific ways that caregivers can influence children's FV consumption are discussed later and summarized in **Box 2**. Materials for caregivers and patients to take home (eg, healthy snack ideas and handouts on incorporating FV into the child's diet)[20] can reinforce and elaborate on provider advice. The Expert Committee recommends that providers reinforce and build on health promotion messaging campaigns that are already being delivered in the community (eg, the 5-2-1-0 message) because patients may recognize and identify with them.[15] Toolkits, such as the 5-2-1-0 Keep ME Healthy toolkit,[21] are helpful to streamline, standardize, and coordinate assessment and counseling for busy health care providers and physician extenders. A "FV prescription" written on a prescription pad to document and emphasize the importance of consuming recommended FV servings each day can be provided at clinic visits and is available as part of the First Lady Michelle Obama's *Let's Move! In the Clinic Initiative* resources.[22] Lifestyle and weight management issues should be addressed with all patients, regardless of presenting weight, at least once a year.[15]

Practitioners can connect patients with financial and community resources that may be useful in helping children make and sustain health behavior changes. Food assistance programs such as the Special Supplemental Nutrition Program for Women, Infants and Children (WIC) recently added FV vouchers to the regular benefits. In addition, most states and many Indian Tribal Organizations participate in the WIC Farmers Market Nutrition Program (FMNP) which provides coupons for fresh FV. These coupons can be used to purchase FV from eligible farmers, farmers markets, or roadside stands. There are many community programs that provide financial incentives to those who use Supplemental Nutrition Assistance Program (SNAP) (formerly known as food stamps)

Box 2
Strategies pediatric practitioners can advise caregivers to use to encourage fruit and vegetable (FV) consumption in children

Individual level: getting kids involved

- Garden. Planting seeds and watching the plants grow teaches kids many lessons, and they are thrilled when they can eat their homegrown produce. If space is limited, try growing tomatoes, peppers, and herbs.
- Cook with your kids. Allow them to help choose the recipes and plan meals featuring FV.
- Take kids to a local farm or community garden to see where their food comes from. Some farms even let you pick your own FV to purchase and take home.
- Cut FV into interesting shapes and let children dip their vegetables in a favorite sauce or dip. Kids love to interact and have fun with their food.

Social environment: positive feeding interactions among caregivers and children

- Expose children to a variety of FV. Do not be discouraged if your child does not like a new food at first. It may take 10 exposures or more before a child accepts a new food.
- Guide children's eating by setting reasonable limits, but avoid controlling feeding practices (eg, overly pressuring and overly restricting food).
- Eat together regularly as a family.
- Provide a variety of healthy options and allow children to explore. Do not worry if they do not eat every food you offer.
- Role model healthy behaviors. Let your children see you eating FV during meal and snack times.

Physical environment: FV readily available to children during meals and snacks

- Make FV more accessible than less healthy snacks by having them washed, cut, and ready to eat in a bowl on a counter, or at eye level in the refrigerator. Try not only carrot and celery sticks but red and green pepper strips, broccoli florets, and cucumber slices.
- Incorporate chopped, sliced, and shredded vegetables in dishes such as pasta, chili, soups, casseroles, and pizza.
- Try fresh FV in season when they are tastier and lower in cost.
- Try canned, frozen, and dried fruits and vegetables because they are easily stored.
- Incorporate fruits and vegetables throughout the day, and make FV half the plate:
  - At breakfast, top cereal with fruit or add fruit to pancakes.
  - At lunch, try salad as a main dish or add vegetables to sandwiches.
  - Dinner can be offered as courses, with salad as an appetizer and fruit as a dessert.
  - Pack FV for kids to take to school, early care and education (ECE), the playground or pool, or to camp for meals and snacks.
- Provide FV when bringing snacks for classroom activities and sports events instead of soda, chips, and cookies; ask other caregivers to do the same.
- Get involved at your child's school or early care and education (ECE) center. Encourage staff to offer FV at meals and snacks and to provide opportunities for children to work with FV through cooking, gardening, and farm-to-school programs.

---

benefits at farmers markets. Nutrition assistance programs provide enrolled individuals with resources and opportunities to participate in cooking classes,[23,24] which may improve food preparation knowledge and skills and increase the healthier food choices of participants.[25] Additional community resources may include information about local farmers markets,[26] community gardens,[27] and farm-to-school activities.[28] The health care provider can identify these and other community resources that promote healthy behaviors, develop referral guides, and engage individuals external to the practice, such as registered dieticians[29] or community health workers, who offer support and connection to such resources.[30]

Incorporating assessment, counseling, and community resource provision into pediatric practice is important but challenging and may require changes in health care provider offices and in health care systems.[15] The Expert Committee endorses the use of the chronic care model as the basis for a health care practice that integrates patient self-management, health care, and community resources to provide more comprehensive and useful care.[15,31] Because reimbursement and billing methods are important in this health care approach, AAP provides a guide for coding. For example, a patient identified with overweight or obesity (International Classification of Diseases, 9th Revision, Clinical Modification [ICD-9-CM] codes 278.01, 278.02) during a well-child check could return for a visit with a physician extender for a health and behavior assessment (Current Procedural Terminology [CPT] code 96150) or medical nutrition therapy (97802) visit.[32]

Counseling Topics: Factors that Influence Children's FV Intake

The following strategies are organized by the first 3 levels of the socioecological model (individual, social environment, and physical environment). This article focuses primarily on the home setting; however, other settings in which children typically spend time are also discussed, such as school and early care and education (ECE, which includes pre-K, Head Start, child care centers, and family homes).

Individual level

Knowledge of recommendations Dietary counseling should include discussion of FV recommendations for families. Although knowledge alone is not sufficient to alter dietary behaviors among children and adolescents,[33,34] it has been associated with higher FV intake in children. Two observational studies of the determinants of FV intake among 11-year-old children in several European countries found positive associations with FV intake among those with knowledge of national recommendations.[35,36] A review of studies from the United States and Europe examining the determinants of FV consumption and FV interventions among children 6 to 12 years old found evidence of a positive association between knowledge of FV recommendations and FV intake.[37]

Taste preferences Children's and adolescents' taste preferences are associated with FV intake. A 2006 review found that, in all studies identified that analyzed the influence of taste preferences (n = 11), there was a positive association with intake of fruit and/or vegetables.[38] Research suggests that infants have a genetic predisposition to prefer certain tastes, such as those that are sweet, and therefore may initially reject food that tastes bitter, including vegetables.[39] However, such preferences may be altered as children become more familiar with foods through multiple exposures (10 or more),[40] modeling by parents and caregivers, and positive experiences with these foods.[39,41] Pediatric practitioners can advise caregivers to provide opportunities, such as those discussed later, for children's FV preferences to develop.

Hands-on experiences: gardening and cooking Practitioners can advise caregivers to engage children in hands-on experiences, such as growing and preparing FV. These experiences may help children cultivate a lasting, healthy relationship with food, and a lifetime of healthy eating behaviors. Youth participation in gardening can positively influence FV consumption and related factors,[42] such as willingness to taste fruits and/or vegetables[43]; increased knowledge of, positive attitudes toward, and preferences for fruits and/or vegetables[43–45]; and improved availability of FV at home.[46] Although most evidence linking gardening to FV consumption has focused on youth settings outside the home (eg, school, after school, and community settings) and in conjunction with nutrition education, home gardening may also be an effective way to encourage children's FV consumption. A telephone survey in rural Missouri found that parents and their preschool children who frequently ate homegrown produce ate significantly more FV than those who rarely or never ate it.[47] Increased frequency of eating homegrown FV was also associated with more home availability of produce, preschooler's preference for FV, and parental role modeling of eating FV. Involvement in community gardens has also been associated with increased FV intake among adults,[48] thus families could consider community gardening as well. Additional experiential activities that caregivers may share with their children to promote FV include visiting farmers markets and farms (eg, pick-your-own farms) and participation in community-supported agriculture to receive produce boxes on a regular basis.

Involvement in the selection of, preparation of, and cooking of FV increases children's exposure to, and familiarity with, these foods, 2 important factors in the development of food preferences.[39,49] A cross-sectional study of middle school and high school students found that students who frequently assisted with dinner preparations had higher intakes of FV, fiber, folate, and vitamin A, as well as lower intakes of less healthy foods.[50] Developing children's cooking skills may have lasting impacts as they become independent adults. A cross-sectional study of young adults 18 to 23 years old, found that more frequent food preparation was associated with higher FV intake.[51]

Social environment
Caregiver feeding practices Caregiver-child interactions around food, meals, and nourishment can have a major impact on children's food preferences,[52] their ability to regulate food intake,[53] and FV consumption.[54] Caregiver feeding practices, such as pressure to finish all food provided, may be rooted in historical threats of undernutrition and the economic significance of food, both of which may be less relevant in contemporary society. For example, overnutrition is a growing problem among youth, with 32% of youth being overweight or obese.[14] The percentage of disposable income spent on food has decreased from 21% in 1950 to 9% in 2010.[55] Pediatric practitioners should be aware of the historical and cultural meanings of food, and feeding and parenting practices used among the racial/ethnic groups they serve.

Child feeding is a reciprocal interaction between children and caregivers in which each party has a distinct role. Caregivers are responsible for determining what, where, and when children are served to eat, whereas children determine how much and whether or not they do eat.[56] A caregiver's role is to establish clear eating guidelines that support children in making healthy choices, not to overly restrict or pressure children to eat certain foods or all the food served.

In attempts to ensure healthful eating patterns in their children, caregivers may use controlling strategies, such as restriction or pressuring to eat. However, these strategies often have unintended, negative effects when used with preschool-aged children.[41] Restriction refers to limiting children's access to certain foods, usually foods deemed unhealthy, such as sweets and energy-dense snacks. In general, evidence indicates that overly restricting foods consumed by preschool children, especially those that are highly palatable, often leads to increased selection and consumption of the restricted foods when they are available.[57] Research indicates that this feeding practice disrupts children's ability to self-regulate their food intake,[58] which may lead to overconsumption and excess weight gain over time. Appropriate clinical advice to caregivers is to make FV readily available and provide children with opportunities to experience and consume foods in moderation without overly restricting foods deemed to be less healthy. As with restriction, pressuring children to eat is also counterproductive. Studies of preschool children have shown that pressuring children to eat (eg, ignoring comments regarding satiety, begging them to eat) is associated with negative feelings toward,[59] and low consumption of, the pressured foods. In contrast, feeding practices such as encouraging children to try new foods,[60] encouraging children to eat FV (eg, offering praise or congratulations for trying FV), and providing children with a variety of healthy food options have been linked to healthy dietary patterns among children.[41]

Caregivers may use controlling behaviors in response to individual characteristics of their children, such as neophobia (fear or reluctance to try new foods). Feeding practices that may help overcome or lessen food neophobia include breastfeeding[61] and repeated exposure to,[40,62] and parental modeling of, eating[63,64] the refused foods.

Caregiver influence on FV consumption through feeding practices may be especially salient during early childhood but become less important as children's autonomy increases and they begin to exert more developmentally appropriate control over their own eating. Among children aged 6 to 18 years, evidence indicates that neither parental restriction nor parental pressure to eat is associated with children's FV intake.[65] However, caregivers can still positively affect their children's FV consumption in a variety of ways, including modeling healthy eating habits.

Role modeling Caregivers are important role models in shaping children's dietary intake, including FV consumption.[63,64] Pediatric practitioners should advise caregivers that their personal healthy behaviors have the potential to positively shape their children's food preferences and behaviors. Parental FV intake is positively associated with children's FV intake,[35,66] which may be a result of parental modeling. Although this relationship may be mediated by other factors such as FV availability, practitioners should encourage caregivers to increase their own consumption of FV as a way to encourage the consumption of such foods among children. Thus, intervention programs and other resources that promote FV intake among adults may subsequently be helpful in improving children's FV intake.[67]

Family meals The Expert Committee advises practitioners to encourage parents to eat family meals with their children. A 2011 meta-analysis found that children and adolescents who shared family meals 3 or more times per week were more likely to eat healthy foods (including FV) than those who shared fewer family meals (increased odds of 24%).[68] In addition, regular family meals can have positive long-term benefits on FV consumption.[69] During family meals, caregivers have an opportunity to repeatedly expose children to a variety of FV and to model and encourage healthy eating behaviors. Furthermore, family meals have been associated with a host of other benefits for children, including academic achievement, language development, and reduced risk for substance abuse and eating disorders.[70] Research suggests that television viewing during family meals has a negative impact on FV consumption and therefore should be avoided.[71,72] Thus, pediatric practitioners should encourage caregivers not only to increase the frequency of family meals but also to promote the quality of the family meal experience through positive mealtime interactions.

Physical environment
Availability and accessibility Caregivers can create a supportive environment for children to make healthy choices by ensuring that a variety of FV are available in the home, easily accessible (eg, washed, cut, at eye level in the refrigerator), and served to

children during meals and snacks. Availability and accessibility are positively associated with FV intake in children and adolescents[37,38] and may be able to overcome low taste preferences. For example, a study of middle school and high school students found that, even when children's taste preferences for FV were low, greater home availability was associated with higher intake.[73] The amount of FV in the home compared with less healthy foods may also be an important factor in consumption. A recent cross-sectional study found that the ratio of more-healthful to less-healthful foods and FV availability and accessibility in the home were both positively associated with higher intake of FV among children and adolescents.[74] Thus pediatric practitioners can assist caretakers in understanding the importance of their role as gatekeepers who control the foods that are brought into the home.[41,75]

Practitioners should encourage caregivers to serve a variety of FV prepared in appealing ways to their children during meals and snacks. Current recommendations encourage individuals to fill half their plates with FV during meals,[76] which can be done in a variety of ways, such as topping cereal with fruit, serving a salad with dinner, and adding vegetables to pastas. In addition, caregivers should be advised to pack FV for children to take to school, ECE, community venues such as pools, playgrounds, and sporting events, and other places where children spend time outside the home, because this may influence them to eat more FV.[35,77–80] Caregivers can also encourage and support efforts to make FV more available within these settings.

COMMUNITY-LEVEL INTERVENTIONS: SUPPORTING A HEALTHY COMMUNITY

FV consumption is more likely when healthier choices are made easier for individuals. Children and families may have difficulty making healthy choices without an environment that is supportive of FV consumption. FV access, affordability, and availability are important in each place a child spends time, from the home to community venues, ECE, and schools. Health care providers are in a position to influence change in the community. Through advocacy, community involvement, and collaborations with local and state health departments, schools, recreation facilities, and community organizations, pediatric practitioners can influence policies and environments where children play and learn.[81] For example, providers can support school district policies (eg, implementation of salad bars) that increase the quality and quantity of nutritious foods in schools, advocate for programs and policies that incentivize retail outlets to sell FV and to locate in underserved neighborhoods, and engage faith-based leaders on nutrition issues.[29] In addition to *Let's Move! In the Clinic*, the First Lady Michelle Obama's *Let's Move! Initiative*, which is dedicated to addressing the problem of childhood obesity, offers multiple opportunities for health care providers to support increases in children's and communities' access to FV in many settings. For example, *Let's Move! Salad Bars to Schools* has a goal of placing 3000 salad bars in schools in 3 years; *Let's Move! Childcare* encourages child care providers and parents to improve the quality of nutrition and physical activity in ECE settings, and *Let's Move! In Indian Country* aims to improve the health of American Indian and Alaskan Native children by focusing on early childhood, healthy schools, healthy communities, and physical activity.[82] Programs such as the National Initiative for Children's Healthcare Quality (NICHQ) Be Our Voice campaign[29] offer technical assistance to aid health care providers in supporting policy and environmental changes by providing sample letters, training, and techniques for advocating for community change. AAP offers the Policy Opportunities Tool, which identifies specific practice-level, community, school, state and federal strategies that health care providers can support to create healthier environments.[83] Although this tool is designed for health care professionals who have experience in advocacy, AAP also offers additional resources to members, including an AAP Advocacy Guide, the AAP Online Resident Advocacy Modules, and live training opportunities.

HEALTH CARE FACILITY-LEVEL INTERVENTIONS: SUPPORTING A HEALTHY CLINICAL ENVIRONMENT

The third sphere in which health care providers can influence FV consumption is within the clinical setting in which they work. Practitioners can promote healthy lifestyles and food choices and serve as positive examples for patients, employees, and the broader community by modeling healthy behaviors and by influencing their organizations' policies and practices.[84]

Health care facilities' offerings can affect patients' perceptions of healthy food options. For example, in a study of 3 children's hospitals, respondents who attended the hospital with a fast food restaurant were more likely to have consumed fast food on the day of the survey and to rate the food as healthy, than those who attended the 2 hospitals without fast food restaurants.[85] Focus group research has found that patients think that food served in the hospital should be a model for a healthy diet.[86]

Practitioners can promote healthy lifestyles and food choices by providing access to affordable FV for patients, guests, employees, and the wider community through policy and environmental initiatives. For example, health care facilities can adopt policies to ensure that FV are available in vending machines, food service venues, health care facility shops, and hospital inpatient food service. Pricing strategies that allow FV to be offered at lower cost than less healthy items and point-of-purchase nutrition information may enhance these policies and further increase consumption of FV at health care facilities. The federal government has developed worksite guidelines that include recommendations for FV and can be applied at health care facilities.[87] In addition, some health care facilities are increasing access to FV by incorporating fresh, local produce into health care foodservice,[88] and hosting farmers markets and community-supported agriculture programs for patients, families, employees, and the community.[89] AAP provides a broad range of additional practice-level policy strategies for a comprehensive approach to obesity prevention that supports healthy, active living for children and families.[83]

SUMMARY

Pediatric practitioners can promote increased FV consumption by children by considering all levels of the socioecological model. This article presents strategies for how practitioners can encourage parents and caregivers to create an environment supportive of making healthier choices through experiential activities such as gardening and cooking; positive feeding interactions that expose children to a variety of FV, focus on whole forms of FV, and limit 100% juice; role modeling of healthy behaviors; and ensuring that FV are easily available in the home and other settings where children spend time. To effect lasting change, ideas are also presented for how health care providers can move beyond patient-level interactions and work to positively influence FV consumption by advocating for and supporting policy and environmental changes in health care facilities, schools, and other community settings.

REFERENCES

1. Story M, Kaphingst KM, Robinson-O'Brien R, et al. Creating healthy food and eating environments: policy and environmental approaches. Annu Rev Public Health 2008;29(1):253–72.

2. U.S. Department of Agriculture and U.S. Department of Health and Human Services. Dietary guidelines for Americans, 2010. Washington, DC: US Government Printing Office; 2010.

3. Frieden TR. A framework for public health action: the health impact pyramid. Am J Public Health 2010;100(4):590–5.

4. Glanz K, Lankenau B, Foerster S, et al. Environmental and policy approaches to cardiovascular disease prevention through nutrition: opportunities for state and local action. Health Educ Behav 1995;22(4):512–27.

5. Kelder SH, Perry CL, Klepp KI, et al. Longitudinal tracking of adolescent smoking, physical activity, and food choice behaviors. Am J Public Health 1994;84(7):1121–6.

6. Lien N, Lytle LA, Klepp KI. Stability in consumption of fruit, vegetables, and sugary foods in a cohort from age 14 to age 21. Prev Med 2001;33(3):217–26.

7. Wang Y, Bentley ME, Zhai F, et al. Tracking of dietary intake patterns of Chinese from childhood to adolescence over a six-year follow-up period. J Nutr 2002; 132(3):430–8.

8. Nebeling L. Phytochemicals: the color of a healthy diet. Pediatric Basics:The Journal of Pediatric Nutrition and Development 2002;98:2–9.

9. He FJ, Nowson CA, Lucas M, et al. Increased consumption of fruit and vegetables is related to a reduced risk of coronary heart disease: meta-analysis of cohort studies. J Hum Hypertens 2007;21:717–28.

10. He FJ, Nowson CA, MacGregor GA. Fruit and vegetable consumption and stroke: meta-analysis of cohort studies. Lancet 2006;367(9507):320–6.

11. Montonen J, Knekt P, Jarvinen R, et al. Dietary antioxidant intake and risk of type 2 diabetes. Diabetes Care 2004;27(2):362–6.

12. Food, nutrition, physical activity, and the prevention of cancer: a global perspective. World Cancer Research Fund, American Institute for Cancer Research (Washington, DC); 2007.

13. Rolls BJ, Ello-Martin JA, Tohill BC. What can intervention studies tell us about the relationship between fruit and vegetable consumption and weight management? Nutr Rev 2004;62(1):1–17.

14. Ogden CL, Carroll MD, Curtin LR, et al. Prevalence of high body mass index in US children and adolescents, 2007-2008. JAMA 2010;303(3):242–9, 2009. 2012.

15. Barlow SE, Expert Committee. Expert committee recommendations regarding the prevention, assessment, and treatment of child and adolescent overweight and obesity: summary report. Pediatrics 2007;120(Suppl 4):S164–92.

16. American Academy of Pediatrics Committee on Nutrition. The use and misuse of fruit juice in pediatrics. Pediatrics 2001;107(5):1210–3.

17. Lorson BA, Melgar-Quinonez HR, Taylor CA. Correlates of fruit and vegetable intakes in US children. J Am Diet Assoc 2009;109(3):474–8.

18. Foltz JL, Cook SR, Szilagyi PG, et al. US adolescent nutrition, exercise, and screen time baseline levels prior to national recommendations. Clin Pediatr (Phila) 2011;50(5):424–33.

19. Kimmons J, Gillespie C, Seymour J, et al. Fruit and vegetable intake among adolescents and adults in the United States: percentage meeting individualized recommendations. Medscape J Med 2009;11(1):26.

20. Produce for Better Health Foundation. Fruits and veggies; more matters. Available at: www.fruitsandveggiesmorematters.org. Accessed July 11, 2011.

21. Keep ME Healthy 5210. Maine Center for Public Health; 2007. Available at: http://www.mcph.org/major_activities/keepmehealthy.htm. Accessed July 11, 2011.

22. American Academy of Pediatrics. Prevention and treatment of child overweight and obesity, Spotlight: White House Obesity Initiative. Available at: http://www.aap.org/obesity/whitehouse/index.html. Accessed July 7, 2011.

23. California WIC. Cooking Live! Program. Available at: http://www.sandiegowic.org/Default.aspx?alias=www.sandiegowic.org/cookinglive. Accessed July 28, 2011.

24. United States Department of Agriculture. SNAP-Ed Connection, Resource Library. Available at: http://snap.nal.usda.gov/nal_display/index.php?info_center=15&tax_level=4&tax_subject=261&topic_id=1243&level3_id=6213&level4_id=10045. Accessed July 28, 2011.

25. Eat Smart New York, NYS SNAP-Ed annual report. New York State - Office of Temporary and Disability Assistance (New York); 2010.

26. Local Harvest. Available at: http://www.localharvest.org. Accessed August 17, 2011.

27. American Community Gardening Association. Available at: http://www.communitygarden.org. Accessed August 22, 2011.

28. National Farm to School Network. Available at: http://www.farmtoschool.org. Accessed August 22, 2011.

29. Mobilizing healthcare professionals in the fight against childhood obesity, advocacy resource guide. National Initiative for Children's Healthcare Quality; 2010. Available at: http://www.nichq.org/advocacy/obesity_resources/toolkit.html. Accessed July 7, 2011.

30. Etz RS, Cohen DJ, Woolf SH, et al. Bridging primary care practices and communities to promote healthy behaviors. Am J Prev Med 2008;35(5 Suppl 1):S390–7.

31. Bodenheimer T, Wagner EH, Grumbach K. Improving primary care for patients with chronic illness. JAMA 2002;288(14):1775–9.

32. Obesity and related co-morbidities coding fact sheet for primary care pediatricians. Elk Grove Village (IL): American Academy of Pediatrics; 2006.

33. Axelson ML, Federline TL, Brinberg D. A meta-analysis of food- and nutrition-related research. J Nutr Educ 1985;17(2):51–4.

34. Contento IR, Manning AD, Shannon B. Research perspective on school-based nutrition education. Journal of Nutrition Education 1992;24(5):247–59.

35. De Bourdeaudhuij I, te Velde S, Brug J, et al. Personal, social and environmental predictors of daily fruit and vegetable intake in 11-year-old children in nine European countries. Eur J Clin Nutr 2008;62(7):834–41.

36. Wind M, de Bourdeaudhuij I, te Velde SJ, et al. Correlates of fruit and vegetable consumption among 11-year-old Belgian-Flemish and Dutch schoolchildren. J Nutr Educ Behav 2006;38(4):211–21.

37. Blanchette L, Brug J. Determinants of fruit and vegetable consumption among 6–12-year-old children and effective interventions to increase consumption. J Hum Nutr Diet 2005;18(6):431–43.

38. Rasmussen M, Krolner R, Klepp KI, et al. Determinants of fruit and vegetable consumption among children and adolescents: a review of the literature. Part I: Quantitative studies. Int J Behav Nutr Phys Act 2006;3:22.

39. Birch LL. Development of food preferences. Annu Rev Nutr 1999;19:41–62.

40. Sullivan SA, Birch LL. Infant dietary experience and acceptance of solid foods. Pediatrics 1994;93(2):271–7.

41. Savage JS, Fisher JO, Birch LL. Parental influence on eating behavior: conception to adolescence. J Law Med Ethics 2007;35(1):22–34.

42. Robinson-O'Brien R, Story M, Heim S. Impact of garden-based youth nutrition intervention programs: a review. J Am Diet Assoc 2009;109(2):273–80.

43. Morris J, Neustadter A, Zidenberg-Cherr S. First-grade gardeners more likely to taste vegetables. Calif Agr 2001;55(1):43–6.

44. Lineberger S, Zajicek J. School gardens: can a hands-on teaching tool affect students' attitudes and behaviors regarding fruit and vegetables? HortTechnology 2000;10(3):593–6.

45. Morris JL, Zidenberg-Cherr S. Garden-enhanced nutrition curriculum improves fourth-grade school children's knowledge of nutrition and preferences for some vegetables. J Am Diet Assoc 2002;102(1):91–3.

46. Heim S, Bauer KW, Stang J, et al. Can a community-based intervention improve the home food environment? parental perspectives of the influence of the delicious and nutritious garden. J Nutr Educ Behav 2011;43(2):130–4.

47. Nanney MS, Johnson S, Elliott M, et al. Frequency of eating homegrown produce is associated with higher intake among parents and their preschool-aged children in rural Missouri. J Am Diet Assoc 2007;107(4):577–84.

48. McCormack LA, Laska MN, Larson NI, et al. Review of the nutritional implications of farmers markets and community gardens: a call for evaluation and research efforts. J Am Diet Assoc 2010;110(3):399–408.

49. Burchett H. Increasing fruit and vegetable consumption among British primary schoolchildren: a review. Health Educ 2003;103(2):99–109.

50. Larson N, Story M, Eisenberg M, et al. Food preparation and purchasing roles among adolescents: associations with sociodemographic characteristics and diet quality. J Am Diet Assoc 2006;106(2):211–8.

51. Larson NI, Perry CL, Story M, et al. Food preparation by young adults is associated with better diet quality. J Am Diet Assoc 2006;106(12):2001–7.

52. Birch L, Zimmerman S, Hind H. The influence of social-affective context on the formation of children's food preferences. Child Dev 1980;51:856–61.

53. Wolf A, Bray GA, Popkin BM. A short history of beverages and how our body treats them. Obes Rev 2008;9(2):151–64.

54. Tak NI, Te Velde SJ, Brug J. Are positive changes in potential determinants associated with increased fruit and vegetable intakes among primary schoolchildren? Results of two intervention studies in the Netherlands: the Schoolgruiten Project and the Pro Children Study. Int J Behav Nutr Phys Act 2008;5:21.

55. USDA Economic Research Service. Food Consumer Price Index (CPI) and Expenditure Tables. Available at: http://www.ers.usda.gov/Briefing/CPIFoodAndExpenditures/Data/Expenditures_tables. Accessed August 10, 2011.

56. Satter E. Your child's weight: helping without harming (from birth through adolescence). Madison (WI): Kelcy Press; 2005.

57. Fisher JO, Birch LL. Restricting access to palatable foods affects children's behavioral response, food selection, and intake. Am J Clin Nutr 1999;69(6):1264–72.

58. Johnson SL, Birch LL. Parents' and children's adiposity and eating style. Pediatrics 1994;94(5):653–61.

59. Galloway AT, Fiorito LM, Francis LA, et al. 'Finish your soup': counterproductive effects of pressuring children to eat on intake and affect. Appetite 2006;46(3):318–23.

60. Bante H, Elliott M, Harrod A, et al. The use of inappropriate feeding practices by rural parents and their effect on preschoolers' fruit and vegetable preferences and intake. J Nutr Educ Behav 2008;40(1):28–33.

61. Mennella JA, Jagnow CP, Beauchamp GK. Prenatal and postnatal flavor learning by human infants. Pediatrics 2001;107(6):E88.

62. Wardle J, Cooke LJ, Gibson EL, et al. Increasing children's acceptance of vegetables; a randomized trial of parent-led exposure. Appetite 2003;40(2):155–62.

63. Cullen KW, Baranowski T, Rittenberry L, et al. Child-reported family and peer influences on fruit, juice and vegetable consumption: reliability and validity of measures. Health Educ Res 2001;16(2):187–200.

64. Young EM, Fors SW, Hayes DM. Associations between perceived parent behaviors and middle school student fruit and vegetable consumption. J Nutr Educ Behav 2004;36(1):2–8.

65. Pearson N, Biddle S, Gorely T. Family correlates of fruit and vegetable consumption in children and adolescents: a systematic review. Public Health Nutr 2008;12: 267–83.

66. Hanson NI, Neumark-Sztainer D, Eisenberg ME, et al. Associations between parental report of the home food environment and adolescent intakes of fruits, vegetables and dairy foods. Public Health Nutr 2005;8(1):77–85.

67. Haire-Joshu D, Elliott MB, Caito NM, et al. High 5 for Kids: the impact of a home visiting program on fruit and vegetable intake of parents and their preschool children. Prev Med 2008;47(1):77–82.

68. Hammons AJ, Fiese BH. Is frequency of shared family meals related to the nutritional health of children and adolescents? Pediatrics 2011;127(6): e1565–74.

69. Burgess-Champoux TL, Larson N, Neumark-Sztainer D, et al. Are family meal patterns associated with overall diet quality during the transition from early to middle adolescence? J Nutr Educ Behav 2009;41(2):79–86.

70. Fiese B, Schwartz M. Reclaiming the family table: Mealtimes and child health and wellbeing: Society for Research in Child Development. Social Policy Report 2008; 22(4):3–19.

71. Boutelle KN, Birnbaum AS, Lytle LA, et al. Associations between perceived family meal environment and parent intake of fruit, vegetables, and fat. J Nutr Educ Behav 2003;35(1):24–9.

72. Fitzpatrick E, Edmunds LS, Dennison BA. Positive effects of family dinner are undone by television viewing. J Am Diet Assoc 2007;107(4):666–71.

73. Neumark-Sztainer D, Wall M, Perry C, et al. Correlates of fruit and vegetable intake among adolescents. Findings from Project EAT. Prev Med 2003;37(3):198–208.

74. Ding D, Sallis JF, Norman GJ, et al. Community food environment, home food environment, and fruit and vegetable intake of children and adolescents. J Nutr Educ Behav 2011. [Epub ahead of print].

75. Wansink B. Nutritional gatekeepers and the 72% solution. J Am Diet Assoc 2006; 106(9):1324–7.

76. United States Department of Agriculture. Available at: http://www.choosemyplate. gov. Accessed August 22, 2011.

77. Bere E, Klepp KI. Changes in accessibility and preferences predict children's future fruit and vegetable intake. Int J Behav Nutr Phys Act 2005;2:15.

78. Bere E, Veierod MB, Klepp KI. The Norwegian School Fruit Programme: evaluating paid vs. no-cost subscriptions. Prev Med 2005;41(2):463–70.

79. Di Noia J, Contento IR. Fruit and vegetable availability enables adolescent consumption that exceeds national average. Nutr Res 2010;30(6):396–402.

80. Hearn M, Baranowski T, Baranowski J, et al. Environmental influences on dietary behavior among children: availability and accessibility of fruits and vegetables enable consumption. J Health Educ 1998;29:26–32.

81. Dietz W, Lee J, Wechsler H, et al. Health plans' role in preventing overweight in children and adolescents. Health Affairs (Millwood) 2007;26(2):430–40.

82. Let's move! America's move to raise a healthier generation of kids. Available at: http://www.letsmove.gov/programs. Accessed August 22, 2011.

83. American Academy of Pediatrics. The Policy Opportunities Tool. Available at: http://www.aap.org/obesity/matrix_1.html. Accessed August 22, 2011.
84. American Academy of Pediatrics. The Policy Opportunities Tool - fruits and vegetables/practice. Available at: http://www.aap.org/obesity/practice_5.html. Accessed August 22, 2011.
85. Sahud HB, Binns HJ, Meadow WL, et al. Marketing fast food: impact of fast food restaurants in children's hospitals. Pediatrics 2006;118(6):2290–7.
86. Watters CA, Sorensen J, Fiala A, et al. Exploring patient satisfaction with foodservice through focus groups and meal rounds. J Am Diet Assoc 2003;103(10): 1347–9.
87. Centers for Disease Control and Prevention. Health and sustainability guidelines for federal concessions and vending operations. Available at: http://www.cdc. gov/chronicdisease/resources/guidelines/food-service-guidelines.htm. Accessed July 25, 2011.
88. Sachs E, Feenstra G. Emerging local food purchasing initiatives in northern California hospitals. Agricultural Sustainability Institute; 2008. Available at: http:// www.sarep.ucdavis.edu/CDPP/fti/Farm_To_Hospital_WebFinal.pdf. Accessed July 20, 2011.
89. Farmers markets and CSAs on hospital grounds. Going green: a resource kit for pollution prevention in health care. Arlington (VA): Health Care Without Harm; 2007. Available at: http://www.noharm.org/lib/downloads/food/Food_and_Food_ Purchasing.pdf. Accessed July 7, 2011.

The Role of Added Sugars in Pediatric Obesity

Jean A. Welsh, PhD, MPH, RN[a],*, Solveig A. Cunningham, PhD[b]

KEYWORDS

- Sugar • Weight • Obesity • Child • Nutrition • Carbohydrates
- Cardiovascular disease

Added sugars, caloric sweeteners added at the table or during the processing or preparation of foods,[1] are a major contributor of calories to the US diet. Recent estimates indicate that 14.6% of the total energy consumed by Americans ages 2 years and older comes from added sugars.[2] This level is higher than that estimated for 1977–1978 (13.1%),[3] and, although substantially lower than the 18.9% estimated for 1999 to 2000,[2] it exceeds recommended guidelines.[4,5] The largest contributors of added sugars to American's diets are sugar-sweetened beverages (SSBs), and adolescents are the highest consumers.[2,6] As the consumption of added sugars has been associated with obesity[7,8] as well as other unfavorable diet and health consequences,[9–13] it is important for pediatricians to be aware of the evidence that supports these associations and to be knowledgeable regarding strategies that they may use in counseling high-risk patients and their families.

SUGAR SWEETENERS IN THE FOOD SUPPLY

Sugar-containing sweeteners have been used to improve the taste of foods and beverages for thousands of years, but only natural-occurring sweeteners such as honey and only very small amounts of high-priced refined sugar or "white gold" from cane, were available until the 1800s, so consumption was low.[14] In the United States after the Civil War, with improved methods for extracting sugar from beets as well as cane, the price began to decline, and consumption of refined sugars began to increase dramatically.[14] Since then, sugars added to foods and beverages to improve their taste as well their texture, appearance, and shelf life[15] have become ubiquitous in the food supply.

---

[a] Department of Pediatrics, Emory University School of Medicine, 2015 Uppergate Drive, Northeast, Atlanta, GA 30322, USA
[b] Hubert Department of Global Health, Rollins Schools of Public Health, Emory University, Atlanta, GA 30322, USA
* Corresponding author.
E-mail address: jwelsh1@emory.edu

Pediatr Clin N Am 58 (2011) 1455–1466
doi:10.1016/j.pcl.2011.09.009
0031-3955/11/$ – see front matter © 2011 Elsevier Inc. All rights reserved.   **pediatric.theclinics.com**

While chemically and physiologically there appears to be little difference between sugars that occur naturally and those that are added to foods, in 2000, the US Dietary Guidelines began to use the term "added sugars" to increase awareness that some foods provide energy but generally contribute few vitamins or nutrients.[16] "Added sugars", as defined in the 2005 US Dietary Guidelines, include all sugars and syrups used as ingredients in processed and prepared food as well as those added at the table.[1] Sugars that occur naturally in foods, such as fructose in fruits and lactose in milk, are not included in this definition unless they are used as a food additive.

As fructose is the sweetest of all naturally occurring sugars,[17] it and the sugars and syrups that contain it are commonly used in the processing and preparation of foods. Sucrose (fructose bonded to glucose, obtained primarily from beets and cane) and high-fructose corn syrup (HFCS, a solution of free fructose and glucose made from processed corn starch) are the most commonly consumed sweeteners in the United States.[18] As food manufacturers are not required by the US Food and Drug Administration (FDA) to provide information on the amount of added sugar in processed foods,[19] consumers will not find this information on a product's Nutrition Facts Panel on the food label (where information on the caloric, total sugar, and other important nutrient content appear). To determine if a processed food contains added sugars, consumers must read the ingredients list on the food label, where all forms of sugar and other additives will be listed, in order by weight. The names of several different sugar sweeteners that might be found on food labels 1,[20,21] are listed in **Table 1**.

Naturally occurring sugars, which are those that are intrinsic to foods, are found in fruits and vegetables and in milk and other dairy products. These sources of naturally occurring sugars also contain beneficial nutrients such as fiber, protein, and calcium. In contrast, added sugars are consumed primarily in foods and beverages that are high in energy and low in essential nutrients, such as sugar-sweetened beverages (SSBs) and desserts. A comparison of the sugar and other nutrient content of

Table 1	
Names of added sugars that may be found on food labels	
Examples of Added Sugars	
Agave nectar	High-fructose corn syrup (HFCS)
Brown sugar	Honey
Anhydrous dextrose	Invert sugar
Cane juice	Lactose
Corn sweetener	Maltose
Corn syrup	Malt syrup
Corn syrup solids	Maple syrup
Dextrose	Molasses
Dextrin	Raw sugar
Evaporated cane juice	Sorghum
Fructose	Sucrose
Fruit juice concentrates[a]	Sugar (white)
Glucose	Syrup

[a] Reconstituted fruit juice concentrate is categorized by US Department of Agriculture (USDA) as a fruit. The categorization of a fruit juice concentrates used in mixed foods varies by source with some categorizing them as a fruit and others as an added sugar.

Sources include: USDA MyPyramid Equivalents Database (version 2.0); USDA Database for the Added Sugar Content of Selected Foods, 2006; US Dietary Guidelines for Americans, 2005.

commonly consumed foods and beverages high in naturally occurring and added sugars[22] is presented in **Table 2**.

CONSUMPTION PATTERNS AND TRENDS

National survey data indicate that, from 1977 to 1978 to 1994 to 1996, the consumption of added sugars among Americans ages 2 years and older increased from 13.1% to 16.0% of total energy intake.[3] More recently, consumption has decreased. Between 1999 to 2000 and 2007 to 2008, the mean consumption of total added sugar in the United States is estimated to have decreased by almost one-fifth, from 18.1% to 14.6% of total energy intake,[2] with decreases observed among all race/ethnic, income, and age groups. During this period, the percent of total energy intake from added sugar consumption decreased among adolescents (ages 12–17 years) from 22.3% to 17.3%; among elementary school children (ages 6–11 years) from 20.6% to 17.0%; and among preschool children (ages 2–5 years) from 17.0% to 13.4%.[2] These trends are also reflected in USDA loss-adjusted food disappearance data, which, although known to overestimate intake, are useful for measuring trends. Estimates obtained using disappearance data indicate that consumption of added sugars increased by 6.5% between 1995 and 2000 and decreased by 6.3% between 2000 and 2003.[23]

As SSBs are the largest source of added sugars in the American diet, trends in total added sugar consumption closely track trends in SSB consumption. Between the 1960s and 2000, the consumption of soft drinks and other SSBs increased dramatically. Adults in 1965 consumed only an estimated 50 kcal/d (2.5% of total energy) as SSBs, while by 2002 this consumption had increased to 230 kcal/d (9.3% of total energy).[24] Then, between 1999 to 2000 and 2007 to 2008, SSB consumption decreased from 9.3% to 6.6% of total energy intake among Americans 2 years of age and older. This decrease in sugar intake from SSBs represents two-thirds of the absolute decrease in total added sugars intake observed over this time period.[2]

Although added sugar consumption has decreased significantly, the relative importance of soft drinks and other large contributors of added sugar in the American diet have remained the same over the past decade. From 2007 to 2008,[2] as from 1994 to 1996,[25] soft drinks contributed the most added sugars, followed by sugars and candies, cakes and cookies, fruit drinks (including sports drinks), and dairy desserts. Consumption of added sugars begins early, well before the age of 2 years. In 2002, almost 30% of 12- to 14-month-old children, 37% of 15- to 18-month-old children, and 44% of 19- to 24-month-old children consumed fruit drinks and/or carbonated soft drinks at least once in a day.[26] Among preschool and elementary school children, added sugars are a substantial component of calories consumed; from 2007 to 2008, 13.4% of total calories consumed by 2 to 5-year-olds and 17.0% of total calories consumed by 6 to 11-year-olds came from sugars added to the foods and beverages they consumed.[2]

POSSIBLE ROLE OF ADDED SUGARS IN CHILD OBESITY

Several studies have shown an association between the consumption of added sugars and higher calorie intake, weight gain, or obesity in adults as well as children, but others have not. Early findings, based primarily on the results of cross-sectional studies, were inconsistent, but multiple studies, including meta-analyses, randomized controlled trials, and long-term prospective studies published in recent years strengthen the evidence of this association.

While there has been little study of the health effects of total added sugar intake, the results of a meta-analysis and a systematic review published in 2006 report that the

Table 2
Sugar and other nutrient content of commonly consumed sources of added and naturally occurring sugars

	Unit Size	Total Calorie (kcals)	Total Sugars (g)	Fructose (g)	Glucose (g)	Sucrose[a] (g)	Lactose (g)	Fiber (g)	Calcium (mg)	Protein (g)
Sources of added sugar										
Cola drink	12 oz	151	38.9	22.5	16.5	0	0	0	0	0
Source of naturally occurring sugar										
Apple juice	12 oz	168	35.8	21.4	9.8	4.7	0	0.8	30	0.4
Apple whole	Medium[b]	95	18.9	10.7	4.4	3.8	0	4.4	11	0.5
Orange juice	12 oz	176	32.7	9.1	8.5	15.2	0	1.1	37.5	2.6
Orange whole	Medium[c]	69	11.9	3.2	2.8	6.0	0	3.1	60	1.3
Reduced-fat plain milk	12 oz	183	18.5	0.03	0.03	0.03	19.1	0	448	12.3
Source of added and naturally occurring sugars										
Reduced-fat chocolate milk	12 oz	285	35.9	1.5	2.0	18.0	14.4	2.7	408	11.3

[a] Disaccharide composed of and metabolized as 50% fructose and 50% glucose.
[b] 3" diameter.
[c] 2–7/8" diameter.
Data from United States Department of Agriculture, Economic Research Service. National Agricultural Library National Nutrient Database for Standard Reference. Available at: http://www.nal.usda.gov/fnic/foodcomp/cgi-bin/measure.pl. Accessed June 15, 2011.

consumption of SSBs is associated with increased risk of weight gain and obesity among adults as well as children.[7,27] The meta-analysis done by Vartanian and colleagues[7] included cross-sectional, short-term, and long-term experimental studies and found that consumption of SSBs was associated with an increase in total calorie consumption and a small but significant increase in body weight among adults and children. Similar findings were reported in a review done by Malik and colleagues.[27] A third meta-analysis published in 2008 analyzed the results from studies in children and adolescents and found no significant association between the consumption of SSBs and weight status,[28] although a follow-up reanalysis of the same data reported a positive association.[29]

Several other studies in children have been published recently. A prospective study of 2.5- to 4.5-year-olds (n = 1944) demonstrated that those who consumed more SSBs between meals (4–6 times/wk or more) were more likely to be overweight at 4.5 years of age.[30] A longitudinal study following children from preschool to school ages reported that high consumption of SSBs (>2 servings/d) at age 5 years was associated with a higher percentage of body fat and higher waist circumference and body weight through age 15 years.[31] A longitudinal study of low-income African American children aged 3 to 5 years (n = 365) showed that the intake of SSBs predicted development of overweight and obesity.[32] A randomized controlled pilot study among teens showed the home delivery of no-calorie beverages for 25 weeks decreased SSB intake among high consumers and reduced obesity risk among children in the highest body mass index (BMI) tertile at baseline. BMI change differed significantly between the intervention (-0.63 $\pm$ 0.23 kg/m^2) and control (+0.12 $\pm$ 0.26 kg/m^2) groups, a net effect of -0.75 plus or minus 0.34 kg/m^2.[33] Another large prospective study among preschool-aged children (n = 10,904) determined that low-income overweight children who consumed at least 1 sweet drink daily (sodas, fruit drinks, and fruit juice) were twice as likely to become obese at follow-up 1 year later as those who consumed less.[34]

OTHER ASSOCIATED HEALTH OUTCOMES

Several other chronic disease risk factors and conditions have been associated with high consumption of added sugars, including insulin resistance and diabetes,[8,12,35] cardiovascular disease (CVD),[36,37] elevated lipid levels,[12,35,38] nonalcoholic fatty liver disease,[39] hypertension,[35] elevated uric acid levels,[40,41] gout,[42] decreased diet quality,[10] and dental caries.[43] Most of these studies were in adults, but there is also increasing evidence of adverse health outcomes in adolescents and children, as will be briefly summarized.

Insulin Resistance and CVD Risk

A cross-sectional study using national data on adolescents showed that the intake of added sugars in the diet was positively associated with lipid measures known to increase cardiovascular disease risk among adolescents, independent of weight status, and with insulin resistance among those overweight.[12] In a study of overweight Latino youth 10 to 17 years of age (n = 120), total sugar intake was associated with lower insulin sensitivity.[44]

Diet Quality

A review of the association between SSBs consumption and diet quality demonstrated that SSB intake was inversely correlated with milk consumption and with calcium intake.[7] In a national survey of children and adolescents, consumption of SSBs, sugars and sweets, and sweetened grains was associated with a lower likelihood of meeting the Dietary Reference Intakes (DRI) for calcium, folate, and iron while consumption of presweetened cereals was associated with a higher likelihood of meeting the DRI for these nutrients. In this study, the consumption of sweetened dairy products increased the likelihood of meeting the requirement for calcium.[10]

Dental Caries

Associations between sugar consumption and dental caries have been mixed. A recent review identified 10 observational studies among children; 1 study showed a positive association, 4 showed mixed results, and 5 reported no association. Several factors, including the presence or absence of bacteria (related to differences in dental care), availability of fluoride, and the length of dental exposure to sugar confounded the relationship between sugar intake and dental health.[45]

SUGAR METABOLISM AND HYPOTHESIZED MECHANISMS FOR INCREASED OBESITY RISK

The primary role of sugars is to provide energy to cells in the body. All forms of carbohydrates are digested, absorbed, and transported through the body as monosaccharides (simple sugars), including glucose (most common), fructose, and some galactose.[46] Various mechanisms have been hypothesized to explain the association between the intake of sugars, specifically fructose and glucose (alone or in combination), and obesity risk.

One hypothesized mechanism relates to the fact that a large proportion of added sugars is consumed as liquids in SSBs. The compensation at later meals for calories consumed as liquids may be incomplete,[47] thereby leading to an excess in energy intake, weight gain, and obesity. Incomplete compensation may result from liquid's poor stimulation of satiety signals, taste appeal of sweetened beverages, perception that energy in beverages does not count, and their low cost.[48]

Other possible mechanisms are specific to the types of sugar commonly consumed. Consumption of foods high in glucose promotes a spike in insulin levels (glycemic response). This results in a rapid drop in blood glucose levels, which can lead to hunger and increased energy intake. Over the long term, diets high in such glucose-rich foods could contribute to weight gain or inability to lose excess weight.[49] The metabolism of fructose, which differs substantially from that of glucose, may contribute to weight gain through other mechanisms. Fructose has little effect on serum glucose concentrations; therefore, its consumption does not elicit an insulin response.[46] Without an insulin response, the satiety hormone leptin is not activated, nor is ghrelin, the hunger-promoting hormone, suppressed. This has been hypothesized to lead to a dysregulation in energy balance, resulting in excess consumption and weight gain.[50] Further study is needed to fully understand the metabolic impact of these sugars when they are consumed together in approximately equal amounts, as is the case with most added sugars.

CONSUMPTION GUIDELINES

US Dietary Guidelines for Americans, which form the basis of national nutrition policy, have been advising Americans to limit their consumption of sugars for years. The 1977 Dietary Goals for the United States recommended that total sugar consumption be limited to 15% of total energy,[51] while more recent versions of the dietary guidelines have not specified an upper limit. In 2000, Americans were advised to "choose beverages and foods to moderate" their intake of sugars[52] and, in 2005, to "choose prepared food and beverages with little added sugars or caloric sweeteners.[1] In the

2005 dietary guidelines, added sugars were grouped together with solid fats and alcohol in a category referred to as "discretionary calories," or calories to be consumed within the limits of total energy needs once nutrient requirements have been met. The discretionary calories allowable to an individual are calculated as the difference between the total calories needed based on body size, level of physical activity, and the number of calories consumed in meeting daily nutrient requirements. In the 2010 dietary guidelines, a limit for total discretionary calorie intake of 5% to 15% of total energy, depending on energy needs, was advised.[4] In line with these guidelines, the American Heart Association recommends that added sugar intake be limited to one-half of the allowable discretionary calories.[5]

STRATEGIES FOR REDUCING CHILDREN'S ADDED SUGAR CONSUMPTION

Pediatricians and other primary health care providers are uniquely positioned to identify children whose intake of added sugars exceeds the recommended limit and to promote positive behavior change as a part of well-child visits.[53] Following are examples of strategies that health care providers can discuss with children and their families as part of efforts to define a behavior change approach that can effectively reduce added sugar consumption. A brief summary of some of the research evidence in support of these strategies is also provided.

Limit Family Intake of SSBs

The Advisory Committee for the 2010 Dietary Guidelines for Americans recommended that avoiding SSBs should be one of the strategies for reducing obesity risk.[54] As consumption of SSBs among children has been shown to be positively correlated with that of their parents,[55] it may be necessary for parents to change their own intake to facilitate changes for their children.

Minimize Availability of SSB and Other Foods High in Added Sugars in the Home

Most added sugars in the US diet are consumed in the home.[3,6] Access is an important determinant of consumption among children; children with greater access to SSBs at home are more likely to consume such beverages,[56] while those with greater home access to milk have been shown to consume more milk.[57]

Replace SSBs with Water or with Nutrient-Rich Beverages

Low-fat milk[58] or water[59,60] in place of SSBs has been associated with lower calorie intake and lower body weight. The evidence regarding the benefits of fruit juice intake is mixed, as some studies have shown associations between fruit juice consumption and overweight or obesity, and others have not.[34,61,62] While they are also high in sugars, fruit juices may be a healthier alternative to SSBs, because they are associated with better diet quality,[63] lipid measures,[64,65] and insulin sensitivity.[66] While artificially sweetened beverages present another alternative for replacing SSBs, the limited available evidence examining the association between artificial sweetener intake and weight gain in children[67] and adults[68] has provided mixed results. Further research is needed to determine how the consumption of artificially sweetened beverages impacts diet, weight status, and health of children.

Avoid Offering Foods and Beverages Containing High Amounts of Added Sugars to Infants and Young Children

Consumption of added sugars begins for many children well before the age of 2 years.[26] High added sugar consumption at early ages raises concerns for immediate as well as long-term diet quality and health of children. Research suggests that eating patterns established in early childhood influence long-term dietary habits and weight status.[69]

Eat Family Meals Together

Children who eat dinner with their families have healthier intake, better calorie control, and more nutrient-dense diets[70] and may be at lower risk of obesity.[71,72]

Minimize Fast Food Consumption

The consumption of fast foods has been associated with greater intake of SSBs[73] and obesity.[74]

Avoid the Use of Sugary Foods and Beverages as Rewards

Research has suggested that using food as a reward increases a child's preference for that food, whereas pressuring or prompting a child to eat to obtain a reward tends to decrease a child's preference for the promoted food.[75]

Use Food Labels to Select Lower-Sugar (More Nutrient Dense) Foods and Beverages

Use of food labels has been shown to be associated with consuming a higher-quality diet.[76] Therefore, it is important that parents (and to the extent possible, children) know how to identify added sugars on the ingredients lists provided on packaged foods and to use the Nutrition Facts Panel to compare similar products to identify those with the least amount of added sugars (and best overall nutritional quality). In addition to educating and advising families, health care providers may also play a role in advocating to the FDA for a change in food labels that requires added sugars to be specifically listed.

SUMMARY: PRACTICAL ADVICE FOR PATIENTS/BOTTOM LINE

Results of recent high-quality studies have strengthened the body of evidence demonstrating that high intake of added sugars, particularly in SSBs, is associated with greater risk of obesity in children. This evidence, together with that which links added sugar consumption to increased risk of chronic disease and decreased diet quality, provides strong support for efforts to minimize children's consumption, which, despite recent decreases, continues to exceed recommended limits. Pediatricians and other health care providers can play a valuable role in guiding parents of young children in the importance of establishing healthy beverage consumption patterns (ie, low-fat milk and water) among their infants and toddlers and maintaining them throughout childhood. Providers are also uniquely positioned to identify children who consume high levels of added sugar, to counsel them and their parents in the importance of reducing this intake, and to guide them in the selection and implementation of strategies that can help them reduce this intake and achieve their diet and health goals.

REFERENCES

1. Dietary guidelines for Americans. 6th edition. US Department of Health and Human Services and US Department of Agriculture; 2005. Available at: www.healthierus.gov/dietaryguidelines. Accessed June 16, 2011.
2. Welsh JA, Sharma AJ, Grellinger L, et al. Consumption of added sugars is decreasing in the United States. Am J Clin Nutr 2011;94(3):726–34.
3. Popkin BM, Nielsen SJ. The sweetening of the world's diet. Obes Res 2003;11: 1325–32.

4. Dietary Guidelines for Americans. 7th edition. US Department of Health and Human Services and US Department of Agriculture; 2010. Available at: www.healthierus.gov/dietaryguidelines. Accessed July 17, 2011.

5. Johnson RK, Appel LJ, Brands M, et al. Dietary sugars intake and cardiovascular health: a scientific statement from the American Heart Association. Circulation 2009;120:1011–20.

6. Wang YC, Bleich SN, Gortmaker SL. Increasing caloric contribution from sugar-sweetened beverages and 100% fruit juices among us children and adolescents, 1988-2004. Pediatrics 2008;121:e1604–14.

7. Vartanian LR, Schwartz MB, Brownell KD. Effects of soft drink consumption on nutrition and health: a systematic review and meta-analysis. Am J Public Health 2007;97:667–75.

8. Schulze MB, Manson JE, Ludwig DS, et al. Sugar-sweetened beverages, weight gain, and incidence of type 2 diabetes in young and middle-aged women. JAMA 2004;292:927–34.

9. Marshall TA, Eichenberger Gilmore JM, et al. Diet quality in young children is influenced by beverage consumption. J Am Coll Nutr 2005;24:65–75.

10. Frary CD, Johnson RK, Wang MQ. Children and adolescents' choices of foods and beverages high in added sugars are associated with intakes of key nutrients and food groups. J Adolesc Health 2004;34:56–63.

11. Stanhope KL, Griffen SC, Bair BR, et al. Twenty-four hour endocrine and metabolic profiles following consumption of high-fructose corn syrup-, sucrose-, fructose-, and glucose-sweetened beverages with meals. Am J Clin Nutr 2008;87:1194–203.

12. Welsh JA, Sharma AS, Cunningham SA, et al. Consumption of added sugars and indicators of cardiovascular disease risk among US adolescents. Circulation 2011;123:249–57.

13. Aeberli I, Gerber PA, Hochuli M, et al. Low-to-moderate sugar-sweetened beverage consumption impairs glucose and lipid metabolism and promotes inflammation in healthy young men: a randomized controlled trial. Am J Clin Nutr 2011;94:479–85.

14. Ballinger RA. A history of sugar marketing through 1974. US Department of Agriculture. Agricultural Economic Report No. 382. Available at: http://www.ers.usda.gov/publications/aer382/aer382.pdf. Accessed July 6, 2011.

15. Sigman-Grant M, Morita J. Defining and interpreting intakes of sugars. Am J Clin Nutr 2003;78:815S–26S.

16. Institute of Medicine, Food and Nutrition Board. Dietary Reference Intakes for Energy, Carbohydrates, Fiber, Fat, Fatty Acids, Cholesterol, Protein, and Amino Acids. Washington, DC: The National Academies Press; 2005.

17. Hanover LM, White JS. Manufacturing, composition, and applications of fructose. Am J Clin Nutr 1993;58(5):724S–32S.

18. Bray GA. Soft drink consumption and obesity: it is all about fructose. Curr Opin Lipidol 2010;21:51–7.

19. Van Horn L, Johnson RK, Flickinger BD, et al. Translation and implementation of added sugars consumption recommendations. Circulation 2010;122:2470–90.

20. USDA Database for the Added Sugars Content of Selected Foods, Release 1. US Department of Agriculture, Agricultural Research Service. Available at: http://www.ars.usda.gov/SP2UserFiles/Place/12354500/Data/Add_Sug/addsug01.pdf. Accessed September 30, 2011.

21. Bowman S, Friday J, Moshfegh A. Mypyramid Equivalents Database 2.0 for USDA survey food codes, 2003-2004: Documentation and User Guide. 2006.

Available at: http://www.ars.usda.gov/ba/bhnrc/fsrg. Accessed September 1, 2010.

22. United States Department of Agriculture, Economic Research Service. National Agricultural Library National Nutrient Database for Standard Reference. Available at: http://www.nal.usda.gov/fnic/foodcomp/cgi-bin/measure.pl. Accessed June 15, 2011.

23. Sugars and sweetener situation and outlook yearbook. SSS-2004. Economic Research Service, US Department of Agriculture; 2004. Available at: http://usda.mannlib.cornell.edu/usda/ers/SSS-yearbook/2000s/2004/SSS-yearbook-08-31-2004.pdf. Accessed July 8, 2011.

24. Duffey KJ, Popkin BM. Shifts in patterns and consumption of beverages between 1965 and 2002. Obesity 2007;15:2739–47.

25. Guthrie JF, Morton JF. Food sources of added sweeteners in the diets of Americans. J Am Diet Assoc 2000;100:43–51.

26. Fox MK, Pac S, Devaney B, et al. Feeding infants and toddlers study: What foods are infants and toddlers eating? J Am Diet Assoc 2004;104:22–30.

27. Malik VS, Schulze MB, Hu FB. Intake of sugar-sweetened beverages and weight gain: a systematic review. Am J Clin Nutr 2006;84:274–88.

28. Forshee RA, Anderson PA, Storey ML. Sugar-sweetened beverages and body mass index in children and adolescents: a meta-analysis. Am J Clin Nutr 2008; 87:1662–71.

29. Malik VS, Willett WC, Hu FB. Sugar-sweetened beverages and BMI in children and adolescents: reanalyses of a meta-analysis. Am J Clin Nutr 2009;89: 438–9.

30. Dubois L, Farmer A, Girard M, et al. Regular sugar-sweetened beverage consumption between meals increases risk of overweight among preschool-aged children. J Am Diet Assoc 2007;107:924–34.

31. Fiorito LM, Marini M, Francis LA, et al. Beverage intake of girls at age 5 y predicts adiposity and weight status in childhood and adolescence. Am J Clin Nutr 2009; 90:935–42.

32. Lim S, Zoellner JM, Lee JM, et al. Obesity and sugar-sweetened beverages in African-American preschool children: a longitudinal study. Obesity 2009;17: 1262–8.

33. Ebbeling CB, Feldman HA, Osganian SK, et al. Effects of decreasing sugar-sweetened beverage consumption on body weight in adolescents: a randomized, controlled pilot study. Pediatrics 2006;117:673–80.

34. Welsh JA, Cogswell ME, Rogers S, et al. Overweight among low-income preschool children associated with the consumption of sweet drinks: Missouri, 1999–2002. Pediatrics 2005;115:e223–9.

35. Dhingra R, Sullivan L, Jacques PF, et al. Soft drink consumption and risk of developing cardiometabolic risk factors and the metabolic syndrome in middle-aged adults in the community. Circulation 2007;116:480–8.

36. Chen L, Appel LJ, Loria C, et al. Reduction in consumption of sugar-sweetened beverages is associated with weight loss: the premier trial. Am J Clin Nutr 2009; 89:1299–306.

37. Fung TT, Malik V, Rexrode KM, et al. Sweetened beverage consumption and risk of coronary heart disease in women. Am J Clin Nutr 2009;89:1037–42.

38. Welsh JA, Sharma A, Abramson JL, et al. Caloric sweetener consumption and dyslipidemia among US adults. JAMA 2010;303:1490–7.

39. Assy N, Nasser G, Kamayse I, et al. Soft drink consumption linked with fatty liver in the absence of traditional risk factors. Can J Gastroenterol 2008;22:811–6.

40. Nguyen S, Choi HK, Lustig RH, et al. Sugar-sweetened beverages, serum uric acid, and blood pressure in adolescents. J Pediatr 2009;154:807–13.

41. Gao X, Qi L, Qiao N, et al. Intake of added sugar and sugar-sweetened drink and serum uric acid concentration in US men and women. Hypertension 2007;50: 306–12.

42. Choi HK, Willett W, Curhan G. Fructose-rich beverages and risk of gout in women. JAMA 2010;304:2270–8.

43. Marshall TA, Eichenberger-Gilmore JM, Larson MA, et al. Comparison of the intakes of sugars by young children with and without dental caries experience. J Am Dent Assoc 2007;138:39–46.

44. Davis JN, Alexander KE, Ventura EE, et al. Associations of dietary sugar and glycemic index with adiposity and insulin dynamics in overweight Latino youth. Am J Clin Nutr 2007;86:1331–8.

45. Ruxton CH, Gardner EJ, McNulty HM. Is sugar consumption detrimental to health? A review of the evidence 1995-2006. Crit Rev Food Sci Nutr 2010; 50(1):1–19.

46. Stipanuk MH. Biochemical, physiological, molecular aspects of human nutrition. 2nd edition. Philadelphia: Saunders; 2006.

47. DiMeglio D, Mattes R. Liquid versus solid carbohydrate: effects on food intake and body weight. Int J Obes 2000;24:794–800.

48. Crawford PB, Woodward-Lopez G, Ritchie L, et al. How discretionary can we be with sweetened beverages for children? J Am Diet Assoc 2008;108:1440–4.

49. Hu FB. Obesity epidemiology. New York: Oxford University Press; 2008.

50. Elliott SS, Keim NL, Stern JS, et al. Fructose, weight gain, and the insulin resistance syndrome. Am J Clin Nutr 2002;76:911–22.

51. Dietary Goals for the United States. Senate Select Committee on Nutrition and Human Needs. Washington DC: US Government Printing Office; 1977. Available at: http://zerodisease.com/archive/Dietary_Goals_For_The_United_States.pdf. Accessed August 21, 2011.

52. US Department of Agriculture and US Department of Health and Human Services. Nutrition and your health: Dietary Guidelines for Americans. 5th edition. Washington, DC: US Government Printing Office; 2000. Home and Garden Bulletin No. 232.

53. Barlow SE, Expert Committee. Expert committee recommendations regarding the prevention, assessment, and treatment of child and adolescent overweight and obesity: summary report. Pediatrics 2007;120:S164–92.

54. Report of the Dietary Guidelines Advisory Committee on the Dietary Guidelines for Americans, 2010. Available at: http://www.Cnpp.Usda.Gov/dgas2010-dgacreport.htm. Accessed July 3, 2011.

55. Vereecken C, Legiest E, De Bourdeaudhuij I, et al. Associations between general parenting styles and specific food-related parenting practices and children's food consumption. Am J Health Promot 2009;23:233–40.

56. Haerens L, Craeynest M, Deforche B, et al. The contribution of psychosocial and home environmental factors in explaining eating behaviours in adolescents. Eur J Clin Nutr 2008;62:51–9.

57. Albala C, Ebbeling CB, Cifuentes M, et al. Effects of replacing the habitual consumption of sugar-sweetened beverages with milk in Chilean children. Am J Clin Nutr 2008;88:605–11.

58. Dougkas A, Reynolds CK, Givens ID, et al. Associations between dairy consumption and body weight: a review of the evidence and underlying mechanisms. Nutr Res Rev 2011;24:72–95.

59. Stookey J, Constant F, Popkin B, et al. Drinking water is associated with weight loss in overweight dieting women independent of diet and activity. Obesity 2008;16:2481–8.

60. Daniels MC, Popkin BM. Impact of water intake on energy intake and weight status: a systematic review. Nutr Rev 2010;68:505–21.

61. Faith MS, Dennison BA, Edmunds LS, et al. Fruit juice intake predicts increased adiposity gain in children from low-income families: Weight status-by-environment interaction. Pediatrics 2006;118:2066–75.

62. Dennison BA, Baker SL. Excess fruit juice consumption by preschool-aged children is associated with short stature and obesity. Pediatrics 1997;99(1):15–22.

63. O'Neil CE, Nicklas TA, Zanovec M, et al. Diet quality is positively associated with 100% fruit juice consumption in children and adults in the United States: NHANES 2003–2006. Nutr J 2011;10:17.

64. Hyson D, Studebaker-Hallman D, Davis PA, et al. Apple juice consumption reduces plasma low-density lipoprotein oxidation in healthy men and women. J Med Food 2000;3:159–66.

65. Kurowska EM, Spence JD, Jordan J, et al. HDL cholesterol-raising effect of orange juice in subjects with hypercholesterolemia. Am J Clin Nutr 2000;72:1095–100.

66. Ghanim H, Mohanty P, Pathak R, et al. Orange juice or fructose intake does not induce oxidative and inflammatory response. Diabetes Care 2007;30:1406–11.

67. Brown RJ, de Banate MA, Rother KI. Artificial sweeteners: a systematic review of metabolic effects in youth. Int J Pediatr Obes 2010;5(4):305–12.

68. Bellisle F, Drewnowski A. Intense sweeteners, energy intake and the control of body weight. European Journal of Clinical Nutrition 2007;61:691–700.

69. Skinner JD, Bounds W, Carruth BR, et al. Predictors of children's body mass index: a longitudinal study of diet and growth in children aged 2–8. Int J Obes Relat Metab Disord 2004;28:476–82.

70. Rovner AJ, Mehta SN, Haynie DL, et al. Perceived benefits, barriers, and strategies of family meals among children with type 1 diabetes mellitus and their parents: Focus-group findings. J Am Diet Assoc 2010;110:1302–6.

71. Gillman MW, Rifas-Shiman SL, Frazier AL, et al. Family dinner and diet quality among older children and adolescents. Arch Fam Med 2000;9:235–40.

72. Patrick H, Nicklas TA. A review of family and social determinants of children's eating patterns and diet quality. J Am Coll Nutr 2005;24:83–92.

73. French SA, Story M, Neumark-Sztainer D, et al. Fast food restaurant use among adolescents: Associations with nutrient intake, food choices and behavioral and psychosocial variables. Int J Obes 2001;25:1823–33.

74. MacFarlane A, Cleland V, Crawford D, et al. Longitudinal examination of the family food environment and weight status among children. Int J Pediatr Obes 2009;4(4):343–52.

75. Birch LL. Development of food preferences. Annu Rev Nutr 1999;19:41–62.

76. Campos S, Doxey J, Hammond D. Nutrition labels on pre-packaged foods: a systematic review. Public Health Nutr 2011;14(8):1496–506.

Artificial Sweetener Use Among Children: Epidemiology, Recommendations, Metabolic Outcomes, and Future Directions

Allison Sylvetsky, BA[a],*, Kristina I. Rother, MD, MHSc[b], Rebecca Brown, MD, MHSc[c]

KEYWORDS

- Artificial sweeteners • Non-nutritive sweeteners
- Noncaloric sweeteners • Low-calorie sweeteners
- Sugar substitutes • Obesity • Overweight

ARTIFICIAL SWEETENERS AND OBESITY

Childhood obesity is associated with many unfavorable consequences, including type 2 diabetes mellitus, nonalcoholic fatty liver disease, hypertension, and psychosocial problems, and often results in obesity during adulthood.[1] Consumption of added sugars is positively associated with higher energy intakes and is thought to be a significant contributor to the rapid rise in obesity worldwide.[2] Because the majority of added sugars are obtained from consumption of soft drinks,[3] artificially sweetened beverages have emerged as an alternative, providing the desired sweetness and palatability without contributing to caloric intake.[4] In addition to their use in "diet" and "light" beverages, artificial sweeteners are often used to replace added sugars in various foods, including yogurts, puddings, baked goods, and ice cream, among many other

This work was supported, in part, by the Intramural Research Program of the National Institutes of Health, and the National Institute of Diabetes, Digestive, and Kidney Diseases.
The authors have nothing to disclose.
[a] Graduate Division of Biological and Biomedical Sciences, Emory University, 1462 Clifton Road, Suite 314, Atlanta, GA 30322, USA
[b] Diabetes, Endocrinology and Obesity Branch, National Institute of Diabetes, Digestive and Kidney Diseases, Building 10, Room 8C-432A, 9000 Rockville Pike, Bethesda, MD 20892, USA
[c] Diabetes, Endocrinology and Obesity Branch, National Institute of Diabetes, Digestive and Kidney Diseases, Building 10, Room 7C-432A, 9000 Rockville Pike, Bethesda, MD 20892, USA
* Corresponding author.
E-mail address: asylvet@emory.edu

items frequently consumed by children and adolescents.[5] Despite their widespread and increasing use,[6] the effects of artificial sweeteners in children have not been well studied.

The purpose of this review is to summarize the existing literature pertaining to the epidemiology and current recommendations for artificial sweetener use in children and to present the results of studies investigating metabolic responses to artificial sweeteners among children. In addition, this review touches on the growing body of literature about taste, craving, and addiction to sweet taste. Artificial sweeteners have also been studied in relation to dental cavities, fetal outcomes, and carcinogenesis, but these issues are not addressed in this review. In presenting and analyzing the current scientific evidence on the metabolic safety of artificial sweeteners and their potential effectiveness in promoting weight loss and weight management, this review aims to provide clinicians with a comprehensive understanding of current knowledge about artificial sweetener usage in children.

REGULATORY STATUS OF ARTIFICIAL SWEETENERS

There are currently 5 artificial sweeteners approved by the Food and Drug Administration (FDA) for use in the United States (**Table 1**). These include aspartame, acesulfame potassium, saccharin, sucralose, and neotame.[7] In addition, stevia, a natural sweetener made from extracts of the intensely sweet *Stevia rebaudiana* Bertoni plant has been approved for limited use.[8] For each sweetener, the FDA establishes an acceptable daily intake (ADI),[9] in mg per kg body weight, which is the amount of sweetener thought to be safe to consume every day for a lifetime. The ADI is typically 100 times lower than the dose of the sweetener that caused toxicity in animal studies. To determine if a sweetener should be approved for use, the FDA then must establish that typical human intake of the sweetener (estimated daily intake [EDI]) is below the ADI. If the EDI is below the ADI, then the sweetener is considered safe for human use. Aspartame, saccharin, sucralose, and neotame are classified as food additives by the FDA, whereas stevia is classified as generally recognized as safe (GRAS), meaning that similar data consistent with its safety exist as for food additives.

Key Points

- There are 5 artificial sweeteners currently approved for use in the United States as well as stevia, a natural noncaloric sweetener.
- For each sweetener, the FDA establishes an ADI, which is the amount of sweetener thought to be safe to consume every day for a lifetime.

ARTIFICIAL SWEETENER CONSUMPTION AMONG CHILDREN

Apparent consumption of artificial sweeteners (based on servings of foods and beverages containing these sweeteners) has increased with time across all age groups.[10] Because the FDA does not require manufacturers to report the actual amounts of sweeteners contained in foods and beverages,[11] quantification of the precise amount of sweeteners present in the food supply is difficult. Hence, information about the total quantity of sweeteners in use is extracted from intake information for the various foods that contain them, using food composition tables and validated food databases.[12] The sweetening power of the artificial sweeteners (listed previously) is hundreds of times

Table 1
FDA-approved artificial sweeteners

Sweetener	FDA Status	ADI	Sweetness Relative to Sucrose
Acesulfame potassium	NNS, REG	15 mg/kg (~30 cans of diet soda)	200×
Aspartame	NUTRS, REG, GMP	50 mg/kg (~18 cans of diet soda)	160–220×
Neotame	NNS, REG, GMP	2 mg/kg	7000×–13,000×
Saccharin	NNS, REG/ITEM	5 mg/kg	300×
Stevia	GRAS	5 mg/kg	300×
Sucralose	NNS, REG, GMP	5 mg/kg (~6 cans of diet soda)	600×

The 6 sweeteners currently approved by the FDA are described in terms of the approval status by the FDA and the ADI and EDI levels for adults and children. If ADI is greater than or equal to the EDI, the sweetener is approved for use. Aspartame has caloric value, hence is defined as a nutritive sweetener; however, because it is so much sweeter than sucrose, its caloric value is negligible in the quantities typically consumed.

Abbreviations: GMP, good manufacturing practices, NNS, non-nutritive sweetener; NUTRS, nutritive sweetener; REG, food additives for which a petition has been filed and a regulation issued.

greater than that of sucrose (see **Table 1**).[13] Therefore, it takes a much smaller amount of an artificial sweetener relative to caloric sugars to produce the same level of sweetness in a product.

Because of their smaller size and high intake of beverages, children consume the highest amount of artificial sweeteners relative to their body weight per day.[5] A recent systematic review estimated that between 4% and 18% of total carbonated beverage intake among children is from artificially sweetened beverages.[14] A second review determined that approximately 15% of the total US population above the age of 2 years uses artificial sweeteners.[10] A third study, comparing NHANES data from 1999–2000 to 2007–2008,[15] and a recent study (Jean Welsh, PhD, unpublished data, 2011) showed that consumption of artificially sweetened beverages has increased in the general population and doubled among children during those years. Artificial sweetener consumption in foods has increased to a greater extent than in beverages. Furthermore, of those who already consume artificially sweetened products, the amount of these products being consumed has increased.[10] Given the extent to which consumption of artificially sweetened products is rising, it is important that more intervention studies testing the effects are conducted, to develop evidence-based recommendations for artificial sweetener usage in the prevention and treatment of childhood obesity.

Key Points

- Artificial sweetener consumption is increasing in all age groups, particularly in children.
- Because the FDA does not require manufacturers to report the actual amounts of sweeteners contained in foods and beverages,[11] quantification of the precise amount of sweeteners in food is difficult.

CURRENT RECOMMENDATIONS

There are few explicit recommendations regarding consumption of artificially sweetened foods and beverages in children; however, the American Dietetic Association (ADA) states that both nutritive and artificial sweeteners may comprise part of a diet that follows the Dietary Guidelines for Americans.[5] Specifically, a position statement from the ADA stated that artificial sweeteners can allow consumers to enjoy sweetness while continuing to manage weight, diabetes, and other chronic illnesses. With regard to children specifically, the ADA stated that artificial sweeteners are safe to use within the range of the ADI, which varies for each of the 5 FDA-approved artificial sweeteners. Current intake levels of artificial sweeteners among children are believed well below the ADI but range from approximately 10% of the ADI for current levels of aspartame consumption to as high as 60% of the ADI for acesulfame potassium.[5] In contrast, the Institute of Medicine does not support artificial sweetener use in children because artificially sweetened beverages have been shown to displace milk and 100% juice at mealtimes. In addition, the Institute of Medicine stated that more research is needed on the effectiveness of artificial sweeteners for weight management and that more studies are needed on safety effects when artificial sweeteners are consumed for many years starting in childhood or adolescence. Similarly, the American Academy for Pediatrics stated that artificial sweeteners have been inadequately studied for use in children and that they should not form a significant part of a child's diet. Other medical societies have stated their positions on the use of artificial sweeteners, which are outlined in **Table 2**. These statements are not sweetener specific, however, and many do not make recommendations for the use of these sweeteners in a pediatric population.

Key Points

- There are few explicit recommendations for artificial sweetener consumption in children.
- Recommendations from medical societies are conflicting.

ARTIFICIAL SWEETENERS AND THE CONTROL OF BODY WEIGHT

Although artificial sweeteners do not contribute significantly to energy intake, their effectiveness in promoting weight loss and weight control has been questioned.[16] To date, 8 observational studies have explored the relationship between consumption of artificial sweeteners and weight in children.[17–22] Of the 3 cross-sectional studies, including between 385 and 3311 children, the 2 conducted in school-age and adolescent children showed positive associations between artificial sweetener consumption and body mass index (BMI),[19,21] whereas the study in 2-year-old to 5-year-old children did not find an association.[20] Similarly, 4 of the 5 longitudinal cohort studies, including between 166 and 11,654 children, showed positive associations between artificially sweetened beverage consumption and weight related outcomes, including BMI change (in boys but not girls),[23] BMI z score,[17] energy intake (but not BMI),[24] and fat mass (no longer significant after adjustment for covariates).[25] A single study showed no association between artificially sweetened beverage intake and BMI but an inverse correlation with incident obesity, meaning that children who consumed fewer artificially sweetened beverages were less likely to become obese.[26] Given the observational nature of these studies, these data cannot establish that

Table 2
Position statements for use of sweeteners from various scientific organizations

Scientific Organization	Year	Position Statement	Population Considered
American Dietetic Association	2004, 2009	Consumers can safely use artificial sweeteners when consumed in a diet guided by current federal nutrition recommendations. The wide range of artificial sweeteners available in food supply should keep artificial sweetener intake in children well below the acceptable daily intakes	Children and adults
American Academy of Pediatrics	2010	The use of artificial sweeteners to provide health benefits for children and adolescents has been inadequately studied. As such, they should not form a significant part of a child's diet	Specific to children
American Heart Association	2010	People with diabetes can use artificial sweeteners, as can people on a weight loss diet	General population
American Diabetes Association	2010	Foods and drinks that contain artificial sweeteners are an option for those with diabetes to consume fewer calories and carbohydrates when replaced for a food or drink containing sugar	General population
Institute of Medicine	2007	No recommendations are made regarding foods containing artificial sweeteners because (1) artificially sweetened beverages have been shown to displace milk and 100% juice at mealtimes, (2) more research is needed on the effectiveness of artificial sweeteners in foods for weight management, and (3) more studies are needed on safety effects when artificial sweeteners are consumed for many years starting in childhood or adolescence	Specific to children

consumption of artificially sweetened beverages was the cause of increased body weight or food intake. There are likely to be many differences, both genetic and cultural, between families that do or do not offer their children artificially sweetened beverages. Children consuming artificial sweeteners may be those who are at risk of weight gain, thus reversing the direction of the causal relationship.

One proposed explanation for the association between artificial sweetener consumption and weight gain in epidemiologic studies is that knowledge of consuming a substance lower in energy could drive people to eat more[10]; this phenomenon has been best described in the context of low-fat foods, in which people overeat foods after receiving a food labeled as low fat.[27] In addition, studies in animals (who have no cognitive awareness of the energy content of foods) have shown that the disconnect between sweetness and caloric content from use of artificial sweeteners may impair energy regulation and lead to positive energy balance.[28,29] It has also been suggested that the observed paradoxic relationship between artificial sweetener intake and body weight may be due to alteration of gut microbiota.[30] Although these hypotheses are intriguing, few data exist to support them, especially in children, and future human studies are greatly needed.

Although it is expected that substituting artificially sweetened beverages for sugar-sweetened beverages would lead to weight loss due the lower caloric intake, experimental studies have shown that the assumed calorie deficit is not maintained.[31–34] One reason for this is that people tend to compensate for the "missing calories" in an artificially sweetened food or drink by subsequently eating more. Compensation involves the ability to account for excess calorie consumption by reducing intake later or, in the case of an artificially sweetened beverage, to account for the missing calories, by subsequently consuming more. Seven studies have evaluated how children compensate for changes in calorie density due to use of caloric versus artificial sweeteners. These studies involved between 14 and 262 participants, ages 2 to 14 years.[32,35–40] The results of these studies are complex and vary significantly based on study design. In general, younger children seemed to compensate better for missing calories in artificially sweetened foods and drinks by increasing subsequent food intake, thus raising questions about the efficacy of these products for weight control in young children. This study design, however, only provides insight into effects that occur within hours, whereas changes in body weight occur over much longer time frames.[41] In addition, these studies generally take place in laboratory settings and it may not be accurate to generalize their findings to "real life." It is, therefore, of great interest to evaluate changes in food intake and body weight that occur with chronic consumption of artificial sweeteners over the course of weeks, months, or years.

There are few randomized controlled trials evaluating the effects of artificial sweeteners on weight change in children. One study randomized 103 adolescents of varying BMI to either consume only noncaloric beverages (including both water and artificially sweetened beverages) or to maintain their normal beverage consumption habits. At the end of the 25-week intervention, no difference in BMI was found between groups; however, a post hoc subgroup analysis including only overweight participants did show lower BMI in the treatment group.[42] The effect of increased water versus artificially sweetened beverages, however, cannot be determined. A confirmatory study enrolling only overweight adolescents is currently in progress.[43] A second trial randomized overweight adolescent girls to a restricted, 1500 kcal per day diet that either permitted sugar-sweetened soda (within the 1500-kcal limit), or permitted only water or artificially sweetened beverages.[44] Both diets led to a modest amount of weight loss, but there were no significant differences between groups in this small pilot study. In a third study designed to prevent excess weight gain, children in the intervention group were assigned to replace sugar with artificial sweeteners and increase physical activity. As in other studies, the primary outcome of change in BMI z score was not different between groups, but fewer children in the intervention group increased their BMI z score. The effect of the artificial sweetener and the physical activity intervention, however, cannot be separated.[45] Finally, a study conducted shortly after the approval of aspartame randomized 55 children and young adults to consume an aspartame capsule 3 times daily or a placebo while on a calorie-restricted diet. No significant difference in weight loss was observed at the end of the 13-week intervention.[46]

Key Points

- The majority of observational studies show a positive association between artificial sweetener consumption and body weight.

- The results of short-term satiety studies are complex and vary significantly based on study design. In general, younger children seem to compensate better for lower calories in artificially sweetened drinks by increasing subsequent food intake.

- Unlike observational studies, randomized controlled trials of artificial sweeteners in children have not shown that artificial sweeteners cause weight gain. The current studies are not sufficient, however, to show that these sweeteners aid in weight loss, either.

EFFECTS ARTIFICIAL SWEETENERS ON GLYCEMIA AND GLUCOREGULATORY HORMONES

Because artificial sweeteners are frequently recommended for use by patients with diabetes, it is critical to understand their effects on glycemia. Early studies in adults with diabetes did not show acute or chronic effects artificial sweeteners on blood glucose or insulin levels.[47,48] This topic has recently been readdressed, however, as a result of new evidence that artificial sweeteners may be biologically active in the gastrointestinal tract, via binding to sweet taste receptors located on enteroendocrine L cells.[49,50] The biologic relevance of intestinal sweet taste receptors on gut hormone secretion in humans has been demonstrated in two recent studies. In both experiments, blockade of these receptors using the sweet taste antagonist, lactisole, reduced glucose-stimulated secretion of glucagon-like peptide 1 (GLP-1) and peptide YY (PYY), both of which are made by L cells. The effects of artificial sweeteners binding to intestinal sweet taste receptors are still being elucidated. In vitro studies demonstrated that artificial sweetener binding to intestinal sweet taste receptors increased secretion of the incretin hormones GLP-1 and gastric inhibitory peptide, and, in rodents in vivo, increased the rate of intestinal glucose absorption by up-regulating the apical glucose transporter, GLUT2.[51] The relevance of these findings in humans is under active investigation, and this review focuses on studies conducted in humans.

In contrast to in vitro data, human studies do not support an effect of artificial sweeteners in isolation on gut hormone secretion. When artificial sweeteners were delivered in 240-mL solutions by intragastric infusion to adults, none had an effect on ghrelin, PYY, glucose, GLP-1, or insulin.[52] In a similar study, no changes in insulin, glucose, GLP-1, or gastric emptying were observed after intragastric infusions of sucralose solutions.[53] A third study provided adults with equisweet solutions of glucose, fructose, saccharin, or aspartame via intragastric infusion.[54] The artificial sweeteners alone did not slow gastric emptying to a greater extent than water, although the caloric glucose and fructose solutions did. In another study, 8 healthy adults orally ingested

50 mL of sucralose solution versus water, and no differences in PYY, insulin, or GLP-1 were observed.[55] Finally, when aspartame was provided in a tablet form, no insulin or glucose response was observed.[56]

A recent study conducted by Brown and colleagues[57] suggests that artificial sweeteners might affect gut hormone secretion when given in combination with caloric sugars. In this study, healthy adolescents and young adults drank 240 mL of diet soda, containing acesulfame potassium and sucralose, before a 75-g glucose load. No significant changes in glucose or insulin were observed, but the diet soda led to a higher GLP-1 response when compared with carbonated water. This study suggests that artificial sweeteners do not affect glucoregulatory hormones when delivered alone but might have an effect when administered in conjunction with an energy-containing food item. In contrast, however, in a human study where intraduodenal infusion of glucose was accompanied by an intraduodenal infusion of sucralose or a saline control, sucralose had no effect on either GLP-1 secretion or the absorption of glucose from the small intestine.[58]

The conflicting data from available studies might be related to differences in sweetener dose, content (acesulfame potassium plus sucralose vs sucralose alone), mode of delivery (oral vs intraduodenal), or infusion rates. Artificial sweeteners each have a different chemical structure and may affect metabolic response differently. Similarly, the physiologic response to a sweetener ingested orally may be different from a sweetener infused intragastrically due to interactions with taste and reward pathways and with cephalic phase responses, in which small insulin responses are observed in response to gustatory stimulation, before the absorption of nutrients.[59] Cephalic phase insulin response has been observed before swallowing nonsweet nutritive substances and artificially sweetened energy-containing substances in humans. Sweet noncaloric stimuli alone, however, have not been sufficient to generate an expectatory, cephalic phase response in humans.[59] Further studies are needed to determine whether artificial sweeteners can reliably elicit a gut hormone response in humans.

Key Points

- Human studies do not support an effect of artificial sweeteners in isolation on gut hormone secretion.
- Recent studies suggest that artificial sweeteners might affect gut hormone secretion when given in combination with caloric sugars.

ARTIFICIAL SWEETENERS AND THEIR POTENTIAL EFFECTS ON TASTE, REWARD, AND ADDICTION PATHWAYS

In an effort to further understand and explain the etiology behind the rising epidemic of obesity, a new research area exploring potentially addictive properties of sugar has emerged. The concept of addiction is hard to define but is commonly characterized by compulsive and uncontrollable behaviors that are driven by cravings. Although most addiction research examines more common drugs of abuse, such as alcohol, cocaine, morphine, and nicotine, various studies have drawn parallels between drug-seeking behavior and food-seeking behavior. This has led some to believe that sugar and other sweet substances could become physiologically addictive.[60]

Both feeding patterns and drug use involve learned habits, intense reinforcement, and reward pathways, which persist despite the likelihood of negative consequences.[61] The neurobiologic pathways that underlie drug addiction and proposed sugar addiction share the same neurotransmitters and the same receptors and activate many of the same brain regions.[62] A recent study in children demonstrated that familial alcoholism and depressive symptoms were associated with a preference for more concentrated sucrose solutions and a greater liking of sweet foods.[63] Specifically, sugar has been shown to cause release of endogenous opioids, endorphins, and dopamine from the brain in an analogous manner to addictive drugs.[64] Furthermore, artificially sweetened solutions have, like sugar, been shown to be effective for pain reduction in infants, providing solid evidence that perception of sweet taste alters central responses.[65] In rats, gene expression for dopamine receptors and opioids is altered in sugar-dependent rats in a similar manner to morphine-dependent rats.[66] Sugar dependence, defined by indices of bingeing, withdrawal, and increased intake after deprivation, arises when rats are maintained on a schedule of intermittent access to a sugar and chow, which leads to behavioral and neurologic changes.[64,66] Although animals can be conditioned to follow particular eating patterns, which may evoke a drug-like response, this cannot be replicated in humans, and the observed reaction may result from the specific feeding pattern rather than a physical addiction.[67]

Limited data from humans and animal models suggest that some, but not all, effects of caloric sugars on brain reward systems are recapitulated by artificial sweeteners. Although sweet taste from either caloric or artificial sweeteners produces activation of dopaminergic reward systems in wild-type mice, rodents with an inability to sense sweet-taste only increase dopamine in response to caloric sugars, not artificial sweeteners.[68] In addition, in humans, drinking a calorically versus artificially sweetened beverage led to greater activation of the amygdala in functional MRI studies.[69] Both of these studies suggest that although artificial sweeteners can stimulate reward pathways, the nutritive value of sweet foods and drinks plays a role in brain reward signaling, independent of their sweetness.

It has also been proposed that frequent exposure to highly sweet items alters food preferences rather than promoting tolerance; hence, humans develop an expectation that foods and beverages ingested will be sweet and increase their intake of sweet items in accordingly.[67] Recent animal data suggest that artificial sweeteners can be ingested during infancy through breast milk and prenatally through amniotic fluid, exerting changes in sweetness preferences of exposed offspring.[70] Further supporting this view, experimental studies in young children have shown that early and repeated exposure to sweet taste can shape preferences for sugar-rich food items.[71] The idea of habituation to consume a palatable, low-energy substance leading to inability to compensate for higher-energy variants with similar flavor was tested by randomizing healthy adults to consume a yogurt drink of low or high energy and then reversing the energy content after a 9-week habituation period.[72] Participants who switched from the low-energy yogurt drink to the identically flavored high-energy yogurt drink were unable to compensate for the additional calories and overate at the subsequent ad libitum meal. Meanwhile, those who were habituated to the high-energy variant did not alter their energy intake when they were provided with the lower-energy yogurt.[72] Similar findings were observed in 3-year-old to 5-year-old children habituated to aspartame-sweetened versus maltodextrin-sweetened pudding.[38] This inability for both children and adults to adequately alter their energy intake after repeated experience with a specific pairing of flavor and calories supports the idea that regular consumption of artificial sweeteners, which provide sweetness without calories, might lead to overconsumption when presented with a sweet energy-containing food or beverage.

Key Points

- Sugar has been shown to cause release of endogenous opioids, endorphins, and dopamine from the brain in an analogous manner to addictive drugs.

- More research is needed to further examine if consumption of artificial sweeteners can evoke similar brain responses that may lead to increased craving for sweet taste.

SUMMARY

This review aims to provide clinicians with current and comprehensive information regarding the effects of artificial sweeteners on food intake, body weight, glycemic control, and sweet liking, craving, and addiction in children. Understanding and critically evaluating past research will assist clinicians in making informed recommendations for use of artificial sweeteners as a means of combating pediatric obesity. Taking into consideration the evidence that exists, the authors cautiously conclude that there are no benefits of artificial sweetener use in young children, although it is possible that consumption of artificial sweeteners may be beneficial in limiting weight gain in overweight adolescents. To recommend consuming or avoiding artificially sweetened products as a weight control strategy, more studies evaluating the effect of artificial sweeteners on hormonal and metabolic response and on sweet craving must be conducted in children. It is also imperative that longer-term studies be performed in children, because metabolic and behavioral alterations that occur in response to artificial sweeteners introduced and conditioned during childhood may accumulate throughout adolescence and adulthood. Continued research about the various mechanisms that underlie energy compensation, satiety, sweet craving, food intake, and weight control will contribute to the growing body of literature examining the role of artificial sweeteners in combating childhood obesity.

REFERENCES

1. Biro FM, Wien M. Childhood obesity and adult morbidites. Am J Clin Nutr 2010; 91:1499S–505S.
2. Drewnowski A, Bellisle F. Liquid calories, sugar, and body weight. Am J Clin Nutr 2007;85(3):651–61.
3. Malik VS, Schulze MB, Hu FB. Intake of sugar-sweetened beverages and weight gain: a systematic review. Am J Clin Nutr 2006;84(2):274–88.
4. Blackburn GL, Kanders BS, Lavin PT, et al. The effect of aspartame as part of a multidisciplinary weight-control program on short- and long-term control of body weight. Am J Clin Nutr 1997;65(2):409–18.
5. American Dietetic Association. Position of the American dietetic association: use of nutritive and nonnutritive sweeteners. J Am Diet Assoc 2004;104:255–75.
6. Fowler SP, Williams K, Resendez RG, et al. Fueling the obesity epidemic? Artificially sweetened beverage use and long-term weight gain. Obesity (Silver Spring) 2008;16(8):1894–900.
7. Artificial sweeteners: no calories…sweet! FDA Consum 2006;40(4):27–8.
8. Gardana C, Scaglianti M, Simonetti P. Evaluation of steviol and its glycosides in Stevia rebaudiana leaves and commercial sweetener by ultra-high-performance liquid chromatography-mass spectrometry. J Chromatogr A 2010;1217(9): 1463–70.
9. Food and Drug Administration, U.S. Department of Health and Human Services. Guidance for industry and other stakeholders: toxicological

principles for the safety assessment of food ingredients. College Park (MD): Office of Food Additive Safety, Center for Food Safety and Applied Nutrition; 2000, revised July 2007.

10. Mattes RD, Popkin BM. Nonnutritive sweetener consumption in humans: effects on appetite and food intake and their putative mechanisms. Am J Clin Nutr 2009;89(1):1–14.

11. International Food Information Council. Food ingredients and colors. Washington, DC: Food and Drug Administration, U.S. Department of Health and Human Services; 2004, revised April 2010.

12. Magnuson BA, Burdock GA, Doull J, et al. Aspartame: a safety evaluation based on current use levels, regulations, and toxicological and epidemiological studies. Crit Rev Toxicol 2007;37(8):629–727.

13. Renwick AG, Molinary SV. Sweet-taste receptors, low-energy sweeteners, glucose absorption and insulin release. Br J Nutr 2010;104(10):1415–20.

14. Brown RJ, de Banate MA, Rother KI. Artificial sweeteners: a systematic review of metabolic effects in youth. Int J Pediatr Obes 2010;5(4):305–12.

15. Welsh JA, Sharma AJ, Grellinger L, et al. Consumption of added sugars is decreasing in the United States. Am J Clin Nutr 2011;94(3):726–34.

16. Blundell JH, Hill AJ. Paradoxical effects of an intense sweetener (aspartame) on appetite. Lancet 1986;1:1092–3.

17. Blum JW, Jacobsen DJ, Donnelly JE. Beverage consumption patterns in elementary school aged children across a two-year period. J Am Coll Nutr 2005;24(2): 93–8.

18. Ludwig DS, Peterson KE, Gortmaker SL. Relation between consumption of sugar-sweetened drinks and childhood obesity: a prospective, observational analysis. Lancet 2001;357(9255):505–8.

19. Forshee RA, Storey ML. Total beverage consumption and beverage choices among children and adolescents. Int J Food Sci Nutr 2003;54(4):297–307.

20. O'Connor TM, Yang SJ, Nicklas TA. Beverage intake among preschool children and its effect on weight status. Pediatrics 2006;118(4):e1010–8.

21. Giammattei J, Blix G, Marshak HH, et al. Television watching and soft drink consumption: associations with obesity in 11- to 13-year-old schoolchildren. Arch Pediatr Adolesc Med 2003;157(9):882–6.

22. Kral TV, Stunkard AJ, Berkowitz RI, et al. Beverage consumption patterns of children born at different risk of obesity. Obesity (Silver Spring) 2008;16(8):1802–8.

23. Berkey CS, Rockett HR, Field AE, et al. Sugar-added beverages and adolescent weight change. Obes Res 2004;12(5):778–88.

24. Striegel-Moore RH, Thompson D, Affenito SG, et al. Correlates of beverage intake in adolescent girls: the National Heart, Lung, and Blood Institute Growth and Health Study. J Pediatr 2006;148(2):183–7.

25. Johnson L, Mander AP, Jones LR, et al. Is sugar-sweetened beverage consumption associated with increased fatness in children? Nutrition 2007;23(7–8): 557–63.

26. Ludwig DS. Relation between consumption of sugar sweetened drinks and childhood obesity: a prospective, observational analysis. Lancet 2001;357(9255): 505–8.

27. Shide DJ, Rolls BJ. Information about the fat content of preloads influences energy intake in healthy women. J Am Diet Assoc 1995;95(9):993–8.

28. Swithers SE, Baker CR, Davidson TL. General and persistent effects of high-intensity sweeteners on body weight gain and caloric compensation in rats. Behav Neurosci 2009;123(4):772–80.

29. Swithers SE, Doerflinger A, Davidson TL. Consistent relationships between sensory properties of savory snack foods and calories influence food intake in rats. Int J Obes (Lond) 2006;30(11):1685–92.

30. Pepino MY, Bourne C. Non-nutritive sweeteners, energy balance, and glucose homeostasis. Curr Opin Clin Nutr Metab Care 2011;14(4):391–5.

31. Rogers PJ, Blundell JE. Separating the actions of sweetness and calories: effects of saccharin and carbohydrates on hunger and food intake in human subjects. Physiol Behav 1989;45(6):1093–9.

32. Birch LL, McPhee L, Sullivan S. Children's food intake following drinks sweetened with sucrose or aspartame: time course effects. Physiol Behav 1989;45(2): 387–95.

33. Kim JY, Kissileff HR. The effect of social setting on response to a preloading manipulation in non-obese women and men. Appetite 1996;27(1):25–40.

34. Drewnowski A, Massien C, Louis-Sylvestre J, et al. Comparing the effects of aspartame and sucrose on motivational ratings, taste preferences, and energy intakes in humans. Am J Clin Nutr 1994;59(2):338–45.

35. Anderson GH, Saravis S, Schacher R, et al. Aspartame: effect on lunch-time food intake, appetite and hedonic response in children. Appetite 1989;13(2): 93–103.

36. Bellissimo N, Pencharz PB, Thomas SG, et al. Effect of television viewing at mealtime on food intake after a glucose preload in boys. Pediatr Res 2007;61(6): 745–9.

37. Bellissimo N, Thomas SG, Goode RC, et al. Effect of short-duration physical activity and ventilation threshold on subjective appetite and short-term energy intake in boys. Appetite 2007;49(3):644–51.

38. Birch LL, Deysher M. Conditioned and unconditioned caloric compensation: evidence for self-regulation of food intake in young children. Learn Motiv 1985; 16:341–55.

39. Birch LL, Deysher M. Caloric compensation and sensory specific satiety: evidence for self regulation of food intake by young children. Appetite 1986; 7(4):323–31.

40. Johnson SL, Taylor-Holloway LA. Non-Hispanic white and Hispanic elementary school children's self-regulation of energy intake. Am J Clin Nutr 2006;83(6): 1276–82.

41. Swinburn BA, Sacks G, Lo SK, et al. Estimating the changes in energy flux that characterize the rise in obesity prevalence. Am J Clin Nutr 2009;89(6):1723–8.

42. Ebbeling CB, Feldman HA, Osganian SK, et al. Effects of decreasing sugar-sweetened beverage consumption on body weight in adolescents: a randomized, controlled pilot study. Pediatrics 2006;117(3):673–80.

43. Reducing sugar-sweetened beverage consumption in overweight adolescents (BASH). Available at: http://www.clinicaltrials.gov/ct2/show/NCT00381160. Accessed February 2, 2011.

44. Williams CL, Strobino BA, Brotanek J. Weight control among obese adolescents: a pilot study. Int J Food Sci Nutr 2007;58(3):217–30.

45. Rodearmel SJ, Wyatt HR, Stroebele N, et al. Small changes in dietary sugar and physical activity as an approach to preventing excessive weight gain: the America on the Move family study. Pediatrics 2007;120(4):e869–79.

46. Knopp RH, Brandt K, Arky RA. Effects of aspartame in young persons during weight reduction. J Toxicol Environ Health 1976;2(2):417–28.

47. Grotz VL, Henry RR, McGill JB, et al. Lack of effect of sucralose on glucose homeostasis in subjects with type 2 diabetes. J Am Diet Assoc 2003;103(12):1607–12.

48. Shigeta H, Yoshida T, Nakai M, et al. Effects of aspartame on diabetic rats and diabetic patients. J Nutr Sci Vitaminol (Tokyo) 1985;31(5):533–40.

49. Margolskee RF, Dyer J, Kokrashvili Z, et al. T1R3 and gustducin in gut sense sugars to regulate expression of Na+-glucose cotransporter 1. Proc Natl Acad Sci U S A 2007;104(38):15075–80.

50. Jang HJ, Kokrashvili Z, Theodorakis MJ, et al. Gut-expressed gustducin and taste receptors regulate secretion of glucagon-like peptide-1. Proc Natl Acad Sci U S A 2007;104(38):15069–74.

51. Mace OJ, Affleck J, Patel N, et al. Sweet taste receptors in rat small intestine stimulate glucose absorption through apical GLUT2. J Physiol 2007;582(Pt 1):379–92.

52. Steinert RE, Frey F, Topfer A, et al. Effects of carbohydrate sugars and artificial sweeteners on appetite and the secretion of gastrointestinal satiety peptides. Br J Nutr 2011;105(9):1320–8.

53. Ma J, Bellon M, Wishart JM, et al. Effect of the artificial sweetener, sucralose, on gastric emptying and incretin hormone release in healthy subjects. Am J Physiol Gastrointest Liver Physiol 2009;296(4):G735–9.

54. Little TJ, Gupta N, Case RM, et al. Sweetness and bitterness taste of meals per se does not mediate gastric emptying in humans. Am J Physiol Regul Integr Comp Physiol 2009;297(3):R632–9.

55. Ford HE, Peters V, Martin NM, et al. Effects of oral ingestion of sucralose on gut hormone response and appetite in healthy normal-weight subjects. Eur J Clin Nutr 2011;65(4):508–13.

56. Abdallah L, Chabert M, Louis-Sylvestre J. Cephalic phase responses to sweet taste. Am J Clin Nutr 1997;65(3):737–43.

57. Brown RJ, Walter M, Rother KI. Ingestion of diet soda before a glucose load augments glucagon-like peptide-1 secretion. Diabetes Care 2009;32(12):2184–6.

58. Ma J, Chang J, Checklin HL, et al. Effect of the artificial sweetener, sucralose, on small intestinal glucose absorption in healthy human subjects. Br J Nutr 2010; 104(6):803–6.

59. Teff KL, Devine J, Engelman K. Sweet taste: effect on cephalic phase insulin release in men. Physiol Behav 1995;57(6):1089–95.

60. Avena NM, Rada P, Hoebel BG. Evidence for sugar addiction: behavioral and neurochemical effects of intermittent, excessive sugar intake. Neurosci Biobehav Rev 2008;32(1):20–39.

61. Volkow ND, Wise RA. How can drug addiction help us understand obesity? Nat Neurosci 2005;8(5):555–60.

62. Fortuna JL. Sweet preference, sugar addiction and the familial history of alcohol dependence: shared neural pathways and genes. J Psychoactive Drugs 2010; 42(2):147–51.

63. Mennella JA, Pepino MY, Lehmann-Castor SM, et al. Sweet preferences and analgesia during childhood: effects of family history of alcoholism and depression. Addiction 2010;105(4):666–75.

64. Rada P, Avena NM, Hoebel BG. Daily bingeing on sugar repeatedly releases dopamine in the accumbens shell. Neuroscience 2005;134(3):737–44.

65. Bucher HU, Baumgartner R, Bucher N, et al. Artificial sweetener reduces nociceptive reaction in term newborn infants. Early Hum Dev 2000;59(1):51–60.

66. Spangler R, Wittkowski KM, Goddard NL, et al. Opiate-like effects of sugar on gene expression in reward areas of the rat brain. Brain Res Mol Brain Res 2004;124(2):134–42.

67. Benton D. The plausibility of sugar addiction and its role in obesity and eating disorders. Clin Nutr 2010;29(3):288–303.

68. de Araujo IE, Oliveira-Maia AJ, Sotnikova TD, et al. Food reward in the absence of taste receptor signaling. Neuron 2008;57(6):930–41.
69. Smeets PA, Weijzen P, de Graaf C, et al. Consumption of caloric and non-caloric versions of a soft drink differentially affects brain activation during tasting. Neuroimage 2011;54(2):1367–74.
70. Zhang GH, Chen ML, Liu SS, et al. Effects of Mother's dietary exposure to acesulfame-k in pregnancy or lactation on the adult offspring's sweet preference. Chem Senses 2011. [Epub ahead of print].
71. Liem DG, Mars M, De Graaf C. Sweet preferences and sugar consumption of 4- and 5-year-old children: role of parents. Appetite 2004;43(3):235–45.
72. Zandstra EH, Stubenitsky K, De Graaf C, et al. Effects of learned flavour cues on short-term regulation of food intake in a realistic setting. Physiol Behav 2002; 75(1–2):83–90.

The Role of Physical Activity in Pediatric Obesity

Kate Lambourne, PhD*, Joseph E. Donnelly, EdD

KEYWORDS

• Exercise • Youth • Health • Development • Intervention
• Academic achievement • Cognition

BENEFITS OF PHYSICAL ACTIVITY IN CHILDREN AND ADOLESCENTS

Decreased physical activity in today's youth is a contributing factor to the obesity epidemic in the United States. Obesity has a negative impact on physical health and quality of life in children and adolescents. Chronic diseases such as type 2 diabetes and metabolic syndrome that were once only seen in adults are becoming increasingly common in children. Obesity in children is also linked to poor academic performance, poor self-esteem, and negative social consequences, such as teasing by peers and discrimination.

Children and adolescents experience multiple physical and mental health benefits when they participate in regular physical activity. The benefits of physical activity in youth are typically considered in terms of future health status, although other considerations exist. For instance, movement plays a critical role in development as the child learns to integrate sensation, perception, action, and the external environment. Physical activity has a role in the critical developmental window during which the foundation is laid for future cognitive abilities. Recent evidence also links physical activity to improvements in academic achievement and cognitive functioning. Promotion of physical activity is imperative as an obesity prevention measure and to improve the physical and mental well-being of children and adolescents. Recommendations to promote physical activity in children center on increasing play time, outdoor time, and active transportation; reducing sedentary time; and promoting physical education and physical activity throughout the day.

Effects of Physical Activity on Obesity

Recent estimates indicate that 25% of children in the United States are overweight and 11% are obese.[1] Obesity in children is a risk factor for several diseases (eg, diabetes,

Disclosures: None.
Department of Internal Medicine, University of Kansas Medical Center, 3901 Rainbow Boulevard, Kansas City, KS 66045, USA
* Corresponding author.
E-mail address: katel@ku.edu

hypertension, elevated blood cholesterol). When diagnosed at an early age, the overall impact of the disease is more deleterious than adult-onset diseases because of the likelihood of complications over the course of a lifetime. Obesity has a negative impact on longevity, and the current population of children may live less-healthy and potentially shorter lives than their parents.[2] Adults who were obese as children have increased morbidity and mortality irrespective of their adult weight.[3] Comorbidities are discussed in more detail by other authors elsewhere in this issue.

Obesity also has been linked to poorer cognitive performance[4–6] and academic achievement.[7,8] One potential factor contributing to poor academic performance is discrimination of obese students by teachers and peers.[9] Obesity is highly stigmatized and has social consequences, such as weight bias and weight-based teasing.[10] Evidence also shows long-term consequences, such as social and economic discrimination.[10,11] The role of weight bias in the lives of children and adults is receiving more attention by researchers and the media, but much needs to be done to increase public awareness and examine stigma-reducing strategies.

Physical inactivity is strongly related to the increased prevalence of childhood obesity in the United States.[12] Physical activity plays a role in obesity because it alters the balance between caloric intake and expenditure. Energy intake in excess of energy expenditure results in a positive energy balance and weight gain, whereas expenditure in excess of intake results in weight loss. Physical activity is the largest modifiable component of energy expenditure, accounting for 15% to 30% of total daily energy expenditure. The mechanisms leading to the increased prevalence of overweight and obesity in children and adolescents are not well understood, but lifestyle changes leading to increased sedentary time and decreased physical activity undoubtedly play a role.

Obesity is a complex issue, with contributions from biologic, social, behavioral, environmental, and economic factors. Interventions designed to reduce obesity in children are most effective when they are part of a comprehensive strategy to address dietary and physical activity change, including social support and environmental change.[13] Effective prevention programs likely involve strategies that affect multiple settings and address both energy intake and expenditure.[14] A meta-analysis of obesity prevention studies for children and adolescents showed that the most successful programs for preventing weight gain targeted a variety of health behaviors rather than only weight control.[15] However, current prevention programs are only minimally effective, highlighting the need for more research to identify components of successful interventions for preventing and treating overweight and obesity.

Prevention may be a more critical target in the obesity epidemic because the effects of behavioral interventions for weight loss in overweight and obese children and adolescents are small to moderate.[16] Behavioral family-based physical activity and diet interventions have been successful in achieving weight loss,[15] as have combined dietary, behavioral, and physical activity interventions.[17] Children may benefit from early interventions to diminish obesity, because lifestyle behaviors are learned at an early age and children may have a greater capacity to change their behavior than adults.[12] However, much research is needed to examine interactions between determinants of weight management and how interventions might target these complex behaviors.

Health Benefits

The level of evidence supporting the benefits of physical activity on musculoskeletal health, components of cardiovascular health, and adiposity in overweight youth is strong.[18] Exercise has been shown to reduce triglyceride and insulin levels in overweight children.[19,20] Furthermore, adequate evidence suggests that physical activity benefits lipid and lipoprotein level, blood pressure, and adiposity in normal-weight youth.[18] Increasing physical activity during childhood has been associated with an increased life expectancy and decreased risk of cardiovascular disease.[21] Developing chronic diseases as a child is problematic because the diseases persist into adulthood, making promotion of physical activity an important disease prevention strategy.

Physical activity is positively associated with aerobic fitness in children,[22–24] and aerobic fitness has been linked to the risk for chronic diseases and metabolic syndrome. Metabolic syndrome is a group of risk factors that occur concurrently and increase the odds of coronary artery disease, stroke, and type 2 diabetes. In children, these factors include abdominal obesity and the presence of two or more other health risks: elevated triglycerides, low high-density lipoprotein cholesterol, high blood pressure, and increased plasma glucose.[25] In a cross-sectional analysis of fitness and metabolic syndrome,[26] the number of metabolic syndrome risk factors in elementary school children increased across body mass index groups, with the normal-weight, high-fit group possessing the lowest number of risk factors, and the overweight, unfit group possessing the highest number of risk factors. A high fitness level was associated with a lower number of metabolic syndrome risk factors in overweight children than in low-fit, overweight children. Increasing a child's fitness level could be a viable approach to reducing the risk of obesity-related comorbidities.[27]

An increase in sedentary, indoor activities has contributed to the rise in childhood chronic diseases and obesity. These lifestyle changes have led to concern in the public health community because this "nature-deficit disorder"[28] is depriving children of opportunities to experience the outdoors and engage in physical activity.[29] Time spent outdoors is related to increased physical activity. A longitudinal study of 10- to 12-year-old children showed that each additional hour spent outdoors was associated with an increase in physical activity of 27 minutes a week, and the prevalence of overweight at follow-up was 27% to 41% lower among those spending more time outdoors at baseline.[30] Outdoor activity not only promotes increases in physical activity but also is associated with prevention of other pediatric health issues, such as asthma, myopia, vitamin D deficiency, stress, and attention-deficit hyperactivity disorder.[29] The Child and Nature Initiative was launched to encourage pediatric health care providers to promote time spent outdoors to children and their families. Pediatricians write "prescriptions" for the amount of physical activity recommended by health organizations; however, the physical activity is to be taken outdoors. The prescription includes ideas such as going to a park or playground, riding a bike, and going bird watching.

The Role of Physical Activity in Cognitive Development

Movement itself is a critical component of cognitive development. As a child moves, the interaction between sensorimotor integration and the environment plays an important role in the development of cognitive abilities.[31] The child's actions become coupled with perceptions of the environmental consequences, which influences further actions. Small variations in how children practice these actions may influence how they learn associations between physical actions and their effects. For this reason, physical activity games that are unpredictable and require problem solving may provide conditions that foster the emergence and development of cognitive abilities.[32]

This action-perception coupling that occurs during movement plays a role in the development of children's motor skills. Children with greater motor proficiency may find it easier to engage in physical activity. Positive associations between motor proficiency in preschoolers and time spent in moderate-to-vigorous physical activity (MVPA),[33,34] and inverse associations between motor proficiency and sedentary time have been observed.[34] Similar associations between motor skills and physical activity level have been shown in older children (aged 8–10 years).[35] Targeting improvement in motor skills could be an important way to increase physical activity in children with poor motor skills.

Encouraging unstructured play is another way to increase physical activity levels in children, and could be a strategy to reduce the obesity epidemic.[36] Currently, a trend has been seen away from free play to more structured activities in schools and at home because of family structure and increased focus on academics and enrichment activities. Unstructured play is important for healthy brain development; children learn to engage and interact with the world through play. During play, children gain experience in working in groups, negotiating, conflict resolution, and self-advocacy.[37] It is important for teachers and parents to promote free play because it contributes to the cognitive, physical, social, and emotional development of a child and provides an opportunity for physical activity.

A considerable amount of research has examined the role of physical activity in cognitive function during childhood and adolescent development. A meta-analysis conducted by Sibley and Etnier[38] suggested that physical activity is related to cognitive function during development. A positive association was found between physical activity and cognitive function, including perceptual skills, intelligence quotient, academic achievement, verbal tests, mathematics tests, developmental level, and academic readiness in school-aged children (aged 4–18 years). The results of this meta-analysis highlighted the importance of promoting physical activity in children and adolescents for the purpose of optimizing cognitive development.

The Impact of Physical Activity on Academic and Cognitive Performance

Increasing evidence supports the notion that children who engage in more physical activity have better academic performance. Several large-scale correlational studies have shown associations among measures of physical activity,[39] fitness,[39–43] and academic achievement. Experimental studies have also supported the role of physical activity in improving standardized achievement scores,[44] reading scores,[45] and grades.[46] Other experimental and correlational studies have shown no effect of physical activity on school achievement.[47–49] However, the results of some of these studies must be interpreted cautiously because of lack of random assignment and potentially biased measures of achievement.[50]

Recent studies have also shown the positive relation between cardiovascular fitness and cognition in preadolescent children using several measures, such as reaction time and response accuracy,[51] brain function,[52] and brain structure.[53] Evidence from a randomized controlled trial also shows that sedentary children who become physically active experience enhanced cognitive abilities.[54,55] Children who were randomized to a 13-week exercise program performed better on the "planning" scale of the Cognitive Assessment System, a standardized assessment of cognitive processes. The results suggest that physical activity interventions may have selective effects on children's cognition. Increasing physical activity in children may produce the greatest improvements in complex mental processing, known as *executive function*, which includes the ability to achieve goal-directed behavior, self-monitoring, and self-control.

Schools provide a unique opportunity for young people to engage in physical activity, because most children in the United States spend most of their day there. Unfortunately, many school districts have removed physical activity opportunities from the school day despite increasing literature showing the impact of physical activity on cognitive and academic performance.[41] Studies that examined physical activity during physical education classes, at recess, and in the classroom were recently reviewed in a publication by the Centers for Disease Control and Prevention

(CDC).[56] Much of the research in this area has examined the influence of physical education classes on academic achievement. Of the 14 studies of physical education interventions, 11 reported one or more positive associations between physical education and academic performance; the remaining 3 showed no significant associations.

Other studies that were included in the CDC review examined the effects of classroom-based physical activity in the form of physically active academic lessons or short activity breaks between regular academic lessons. Eight of the nine reviewed studies reported a positive significant association between classroom-based physical activity and indicators of academic achievement. The results of a 3-year randomized control trial by Donnelly and colleagues[26] were not included in the CDC review. This study examined the impact of physically active academic lessons on academic achievement and BMI. Physically active academic lessons of moderate intensity improved performance on a standardized test of academic achievement and slowed the rate of BMI gains in students with the greatest exposure to the intervention. Physically active academic instruction does not compete for time allocated for academic instruction and provides an inexpensive, easily implemented, and sustainable approach that may allow elementary schools to meet the competing demands of improving student health while also improving academic achievement.

CURRENT LEVELS OF PHYSICAL ACTIVITY IN CHILDREN AND ADOLESCENTS

It is recommended that children get at least 60 minutes of physical activity of sufficient intensity to increase their heart rate each day (see next section for specific recommendations by various public health organizations). Many children are not meeting this recommendation, and physical activity declines as children get older.[57] According to the Youth Risk Behavior Surveillance Survey (YRBSS), 18.4% of youth in grades 9 through 12 participated in 60 minutes of physical activity per day on each of the 7 days before the survey.[58] The percentage of students meeting this recommendation was higher among boys than girls (24.8% and 11.4%, respectively). The percentages of students meeting the guideline of 60 min/d of activity and participating in daily physical education classes by age and race are shown in **Table 1**.

Table 1
Data (percentages) from youth risk behavior surveillance survey

	Meeting Recommendation to Engage in 60 min of PA Every Day		Participated in Physical Education Classes on a Daily Basis	
	Boys	Girls	Boys	Girls
Race/Ethnicity				
White	26.2	12.4	31.4	29.7
Black	24.2	10.0	40.1	34.0
Hispanic	20.7	10.5	41.5	39.5
Grade				
9th	28.0	13.6	45.5	48.2
10th	25.3	12.7	34.9	32.3
11th	23.3	10.3	29.7	25.5
12th	21.9	8.6	25.2	19.6

Data from Centers for Disease Control. Youth risk behavior surveillance - United States, 2009. MMWR Surveill Summ 2009;59(SS-5):1–142.

With a rise in sedentary activities, physical education classes are the only place that some children and adolescents engage in physical activity. Requirements for physical education class attendance vary among states, and only a handful of states require daily physical education for all grades from kindergarten through 12th grade.[59] The YRBSS reported that 56.4% of students attended physical education classes on one or more days in an average week when they were in school. The discrepancy in state mandates for physical education are reflected in the wide range in percentages of youth attending physical education classes, from 29.1% to 92.0% (median, 43.8%) across state surveys.

RECOMMENDATIONS FOR PHYSICAL ACTIVITY IN CHILDREN AND ADOLESCENTS

Recommendations for amounts of physical activity for children have been made by several organizations, including the CDC,[60] the American Heart Association (AHA),[59] and the National Association for Sport and Physical Education (NASPE).[59] Very young children (toddlers to 5 years of age) should have up to 120 minutes of moderate-to-vigorous physical activity (MVPA) per day, with 60 minutes of it as structured activity and 60 minutes as unstructured or free play.[61] Older children and adolescents should perform 60 minutes or more of physical activity each day,[60] and MVPA that is aerobic in nature should make up most of the 60 or more minutes of physical activity. Muscle and bone strengthening activities, such as gymnastics, calisthenics (ie, push-ups, jumping jacks), jumping rope, and running, should be included at least 3 days per week as part of the 60 minutes.

A recent joint publication by NASPE and the AHA recommends that schools provide 150 minutes per week of instructional physical education for elementary school children, and 225 minutes per week for middle and high-school students. NASPE also recommends limiting sedentary behavior in children and adolescents, and discouraging extended periods of inactivity (2 hours or more) for children.[62]

Practical Recommendations

Based on the current knowledge in the area of physical activity and childhood obesity, the following recommendations can be made to parents, educators, and health care providers. These recommendations target reduction of sedentary time, emphasis of free play, and use of existing evidence-based programs.

Children spend more time using media (eg, television, video games, and Internet) than any other activity besides sleeping.[63] The American Academy of Pediatrics recommends that children and adolescents limit their screen time to 1 to 2 hours per day[64]; however, children spend an average of 5.5 hours per day in front of a screen.[65] Potential linkages between screen time and obesity are the displacement of physically active behaviors, increased energy intake during TV viewing (often triggered by advertising), and decreased metabolic rate while seated. Television in particular is associated with a greater level of stillness than other sedentary activities, such as reading or drawing.[66] Targeting sedentary time has been shown to be as effective in reducing body fat in obese children as trying to increase physical activity[67] Interventions that aim to reduce sedentary behaviors are associated with improved BMI, which provides a proxy for body fat.[68]

Outdoor play is a recommended strategy to reduce obesity.[37] Play has a critical role in physical, cognitive, social, and emotional development. Play is so important to the well-being of children that it is recognized as a right by the United Nations High Commission for Human Rights.[69] Self-directed play is a part of the optimal developmental environment along with academic and social enrichment activities, and a healthy balance between these must be achieved. Targeting free play in children, particularly outdoor play, is associated with increased physical activity and could have a role in reducing the burden of childhood obesity in the United States.

The safety of the neighborhood must be taken into account when advising parents to encourage children to play outdoors. Several studies have shown that parental concerns about neighborhood safety are associated with limiting of children's outdoor activities in underserved, inner-city populations.[70] Negative perceptions of neighborhood safety disproportionately affect those living in poor communities, who also have higher prevalence of overweight and obesity.[71] For this reason, improved options for physical activity should be advocated for children living in impoverished areas. Parental concerns about safety are also associated with decreases in active transportation to school by children and adolescents. Nevertheless, the "walking school bus" has become popular and circumvents some of the safety concerns because the children are supervised by adults during their walk to school.

The child or adolescent's attitude toward sports and exercise affects the level of participation in physical activity. In a longitudinal study of 1902 adolescents participating in Project Eating and Activity in Teens (EAT), positive attitudes toward sports, exercise, and fitness were associated with activity levels 5 and 10 years later.[72] It is important to introduce children and adolescents to a variety of sport and exercise options and encourage them to pursue activities that they enjoy. Being forced to exercise has negative repercussions on activity levels later in life.[73,74] Parents can foster the development of positive attitudes toward physical activity through modeling positive attitudes and behaviors to their children.

In summary, childhood obesity has become a major concern in the United States partly because of the associated health issues and its negative impact on children's psychosocial development. Discrimination based on weight bias can have long-term psychological, social, and economic consequences. Physical inactivity is one factor contributing to the obesity epidemic, and intervening to change patterns of inactivity is critical in childhood because a sedentary lifestyle often becomes a lifelong habit. Physical activity has an important role in childhood and adolescence because it enhances fitness, fosters cognitive development, and provides an opportunity to learn about the world. Physical activity also diminishes chronic disease and provides health benefits for children who are already overweight or obese. Many interventional approaches can be considered, but more comprehensive approaches are necessary because of the pervasiveness of sedentary activities in a child's environment and the complexity of factors contributing to obesity. Comprehensive interventions that saturate the environment with opportunities for physical activity will be critical in stopping and reversing the obesity epidemic. Valid targets for behavioral intervention include promoting play time, outdoor activity, active transportation, and physical activity in

---

Box 1
Internet Resources

Walking School Bus: http://www.walkingschoolbus.org/

We Can!: http://www.nhlbi.nih.gov/health/public/heart/obesity/wecan/

VERB: http://www.cdc.gov/youthcampaign/

Fuel up to Play 60; http://school.fueluptoplay60.com/welcome/

Let's Move: http://www.letsmove.gov/programs

the classroom. Furthermore, several evidence-based programs developed by various health organizations can be incorporated by parents and educators to increase physical activity in children and adolescents. A list of these programs is provided in **Box 1**.

REFERENCES

1. Dehghan M. Childhood obesity, prevalence and prevention. Nutr J 2005;4(1): 24–32.
2. Olshansky SJ, Passaro DJ, Hershow RC, et al. A potential decline in life expectancy in the United States in the 21st century. N Engl J Med 2005;352(11): 1138–45.
3. Must A, Strauss RS. Risks and consequences of childhood and adolescent obesity. Int J Obes Relat Metab Disord 1999;23(Suppl 2):S2–11.
4. Li Y, Dai Q, Jackson JC, et al. Overweight is associated with decreased cognitive functioning among school-age children and adolescents. Obesity (Silver Spring) 2008;16(8):1809–15.
5. Roberts CK. Low aerobic fitness and obesity are associated with lower standardized test scores in children. J Pediatr 2010;156(5):711–8.
6. Yu ZB. Intelligence in relation to obesity: a systematic review and meta-analysis. Obes Rev 2010;11:656–70.
7. Datar A, Sturm R, Magnabosco JL. Childhood overweight and academic performance: national study of kindergartners and first-graders. Obes Res 2004;12(1): 58–68.
8. Shore SM, Sachs ML, Lidicker JR, et al. Decreased scholastic achievement in overweight middle school students. Obesity (Silver Spring) 2008;16(7):1535–8.
9. Puhl R, Brownell KD. Bias, discrimination, and obesity. Obes Res 2001;9(12): 788–805.
10. Puhl RM, Heuer CA. The stigma of obesity: a review and update. Obesity (Silver Spring) 2009;17(5):941–64.
11. Boreham C, Riddoch C. The physical activity, fitness and health of children. J Sports Sci 2001;19(12):915–29.
12. Steinbeck KS. The importance of physical activity in the prevention of overweight and obesity in childhood: a review and an opinion. Obes Rev 2001;2:117–30.
13. Summerbell CD, Waters E, Edmunds L, et al. Interventions for preventing obesity in children. Cochrane Database Syst Rev 2005;3:CD001871.
14. Dietz WH, Gortmaker SL. Preventing obesity in children and adolescents. Annu Rev Public Health 2001;22:337–53.
15. Stice E, Shaw H, Marti CN. A meta-analytic review of obesity prevention programs for children and adolescents: the skinny on interventions that work. Psychol Bull 2006;132(5):667–91.
16. Whitlock EP, O'Connor EA, Williams SB, et al. Effectiveness of weight management interventions in children: a targeted systematic review for the USPSTF. Pediatrics 2010;25:e396–418.
17. Nemet D, Barkan S, Epstein Y, et al. Short- and long-term beneficial effects of a combined dietary–behavioral–physical activity intervention for the treatment of childhood obesity. Pediatrics 2005;115(4):e443–9.
18. Strong WB, Malina RM, Blimkie CJ, et al. Evidence based physical activity for school-age youth. J Pediatr 2005;146(6):732–7.
19. Ferguson MA, Gutin B, Le N, et al. Effects of exercise training and its cessation on components of the insulin resistance syndrome in obese children. Int J Obes 1999;22:889–95.

20. Hardin DS, Hebert JD, Bayden T, et al. Treatment of childhood syndrome X. Pediatrics 1997;100(2):E5.
21. Williams CL, Hayman LL, Daniels SR, et al. Cardiovascular health in childhood. Circulation 2002;106(1):143–60.
22. Burgi F, Meyer U, Granacher U, et al. Relationship of physical activity with motor skills, aerobic fitness and body fat in preschool children: a cross-sectional and longitudinal study (Ballabeina). Int J Obes 2011;35(7):937–44.
23. Dencker M, Bugge A, Hermansen B, et al. Objectively measured daily physical activity related to aerobic fitness in young children. J Sports Sci 2010;28(2):139–45.
24. Ruiz JR, Rizzo NS, Hurtig-Wennlof A, et al. Relations of total physical activity and intensity to fitness and fatness in children: the European Youth Heart Study. Am J Clin Nutr 2006;84(2):299–303.
25. Zimmet P, Alberti KG, Kaufman F, et al. The metabolic syndrome in children and adolescents—an IDF consensus report. Pediatr Diabetes 2007;8(5):299–306.
26. Donnelly JE, Greene JL, Gibson CA, et al. Physical Activity Across the Curriculum (PAAC): a randomized controlled trial to promote physical activity and diminish overweight and obesity in elementary school children. Prev Med 2009;49:336–41.
27. DuBose KD, Eisenmann JC, Donnelly JE. Aerobic fitness attenuates the metabolic syndrome score in normal-weight, at-risk-for-overweight, and overweight children. Pediatrics 2007;120(5):1262–8.
28. Louv R. Last child in the woods: saving our children from nature deficit disorder. Chapel Hill (NC): Algonquin Books; 2006.
29. McCurdy LE, Winterbottom KE, Mehta SS, et al. Using nature and outdoor activity to improve children's health. Curr Probl Pediatr Adolesc Health Care 2010;40(5):102–17.
30. Cleland V, Crawford D, Baur LA, et al. A prospective examination of children's time spent outdoors, objectively measured physical activity and overweight. Int J Obes 2008;32(11):1685–93.
31. Spencer JP, Clearfield M, Corbetta D, et al. Moving toward a grand theory of development: in memory of Esther Thelen. Child Dev 2006;77(6):1521–38.
32. Tomporowski PD, Lambourne K, Okumura MS. Physical activity interventions and children's mental function: an introduction and overview. Prev Med 2011;52(Suppl 1):S3–9.
33. Fisher A, Reilly JJ, Kelly LA, et al. Fundamental movement skills and habitual physical activity in young children. Med Sci Sports Exerc 2005;37(4):684–8.
34. Williams HG, Pfeiffer KA, O'Neill JR, et al. Motor skill performance and physical activity in preschool children. Obesity (Silver Spring) 2008;16(6):1421–6.
35. Wrotniak BH, Epstein LH, Dorn JM, et al. The relationship between motor proficiency and physical activity in children. Pediatrics 2006;118(6):e1758–65.
36. Council on Sports Medicine and Fitness, Council on School Health. Active healthy living: prevention of childhood obesity through increased physical activity. Pediatrics 2006;117(5):1834–42.
37. Ginsburg KR. The importance of play in promoting healthy child development and maintaining strong parent-child bonds. Pediatrics 2007;119(1):182–91.
38. Sibley BA, Etnier JL. The relationship between physical activity and cognition in children: a meta-analysis. Pediatr Exerc Sci 2003;15(3):243–56.
39. Dwyer T, Sallis JF, Blizzard L, et al. Relation of academic performance to physical activity and fitness in children. Pediatr Exerc Sci 2001;13:225–37.
40. California Department of Education. California physical fitness test: a study of the relationship between physical fitness and academic achievement in California

using 2004 test results. Available at: http://www.fmschools.org/webpages/twiniecki/files/California%20Study%202004.pdf. Accessed September 15, 2011.

41. Castelli DM, Hillman CH, Buck SM, et al. Physical fitness and academic achievement in third- and fifth-grade students. J Sport Exerc Psychol 2007;29(2):239–52.

42. Welk G. The association of health-related fitness with indicators of academic performance in Texas schools. Res Q Exerc Sport 2010;81(3):S16–23.

43. Grissom JB. Physical fitness and academic achievement. J Exerc Physiol Online 2005;8:11–25.

44. Ismail AH. The effects of a well-organized physical education program on intellectual performance. Res Phys Educ 1968;1:31–8.

45. McCormick CC, Schnobrich JN, Footlik SW, et al. Improvement in reading achievement through perceptual-motor training. Res Q Exerc Sport 1968;39(3):627–33.

46. Coe DP, Pivarnik JM, Womack CJ, et al. Effect of physical education and activity levels on academic achievement in children. Med Sci Sports Exerc 2006;38(8):1515–9.

47. Ahamed Y, Macdonald H, Reed K, et al. School-based physical activity does not compromise children's academic performance. Med Sci Sports Exerc 2007;39(2):371–6.

48. Sallis JF, McKenzie TL, Kolody B, et al. Effects of health-related physical education on academic achievement: project SPARK. Res Q Exerc Sport 1999;70(2):127–34.

49. Tremblay MS, Inman JW, Willms JD. The relationship between physical activity, self-esteem, and academic achievement in 12-year-old children. Pediatr Exerc Sci 2000;12:312–23.

50. Tomporowski PD, Davis CL, Miller PH, et al. Exercise and children's intelligence, cognition, and academic achievement. Educ Psychol Rev 2008;20(2):111–31.

51. Hillman CH, Kramer AF, Belopolsky AV, et al. A cross-sectional examination of age and physical activity on performance and event-related brain potentials in a task switching paradigm. Int J Psychophysiol 2006;59(1):30–9.

52. Pontifex MB, Raine LB, Johnson CR, et al. Cardiorespiratory fitness and the flexible modulation of cognitive control in preadolescent children. J Cogn Neurosci 2011;23(6):1332–45.

53. Chaddock L, Erickson KI, Prakash RS, et al. Basal ganglia volume is associated with aerobic fitness in preadolescent children. Dev Neurosci 2010;32(3):249–56.

54. Davis CL, Tomporowski PD, Boyle CA, et al. Effects of aerobic exercise on overweight children's cognitive functioning: a randomized controlled trial. Res Q Exerc Sport 2007;78(5):510–9.

55. Davis CL, Tomporowski PD, McDowell JE, et al. Exercise improves executive function and achievement and alters brain activation in overweight children: a randomized controlled trial. Health Psychol 2011;30(1):91–8.

56. Centers for Disease Control and Prevention. The association between school-based physical activity, including physical education, and academic performance. Atlanta (GA): Centers for Disease Control and Prevention; 2010.

57. Pate RR, Freedson PS, Sallis JF, et al. Compliance with physical activity guidelines: prevalence in a population of children and youth. Ann Epidemiol 2002;12(5):303–8.

58. Centers for Disease Control. Youth risk behavior surveillance - United States, 2009. MMWR Surveill Summ 2009;59(SS-5):1–142.

59. National Association for Sport and Physical Education & American Heart Association. 2010 Shape of the nation report: Status of physical education in the USA. Reston (VA): National Association for Sport and Physical Education; 2010.

60. Office of Disease Prevention & Health Promotion. 2008 Physical Activity Guidelines for Americans. US Department of Health and Human Services Web site. Available at: http://www.health.gov/paguidelines. Accessed August 23, 2011.

61. National Association for Sport and Physical Education. Moving into the future: National standards for physical education. 2nd edition. Reston (VA): National Association for Sport and Physical Education; 2004.

62. National Association for Sport and Physical Education. Physical Activity for Children: A Statement of Guidelines for Children Ages 5-12. Reston (VA): National Association for Sport and Physical Education; 2004.

63. Robinson TN. Reducing children's television viewing to prevent obesity. JAMA 1999;282(16):1561–7.

64. American Academy of Pediatrics. Committee on Public Education. American Academy of pediatrics: children, adolescents, and television. Pediatrics 2001; 107(2):423–6.

65. Roberts DF, Foehr UG. Kids and media in America. Cambridge (UK): Cambridge University Press; 2004.

66. Dietz WH, Bandini LG, Morelli JA, et al. Effect of sedentary activities on resting metabolic rate. Am J Clin Nutr 1994;59:556–9.

67. Epstein LH, Paluch RA, Gordy CC, et al. Decreasing sedentary behaviors in treating pediatric obesity. Arch Pediatr Adolesc Med 2000;154(3):220–6.

68. DeMattia L, Lemont L, Meurer L. Do interventions to limit sedentary behaviours change behaviour and reduce childhood obesity? A critical review of the literature. Obes Rev 2007;8(1):69–81.

69. Office of the United Nations High Commissioner for Human Rights. Convention on the Rights of the Child. Available at: http://www2.ohchr.org/english/law/crc.htm. Accessed September 15, 2011.

70. Weir LA, Etelson D, Brand DA. Parents' perceptions of neighborhood safety and children's physical activity. Prev Med 2006;43(3):212–7.

71. Wang Y, Beydoun MA. The obesity epidemic in the United States–gender, age, socioeconomic, racial/ethnic, and geographic characteristics: a systematic review and meta-regression analysis. Epidemiol Rev 2007;29:6–28.

72. Graham DJ, Sirard JR, Neumark-Sztainer D. Adolescents' attitudes toward sports, exercise, and fitness predict physical activity 5 and 10 years later. Prev Med 2011;52(2):130–2.

73. Janz KF, Witt J, Mahoney LT. The stability of children's physical activity as measured by accelerometry and self-report. Med Sci Sports Exerc 1995;27(9): 1326–32.

74. Taylor WC, Blair SN, Cummings SS, et al. Childhood and adolescent physical activity patterns and adult physical activity. Med Sci Sports Exerc 1999;31: 118–23.

The Fault, Dear Viewer, Lies Not in the Screens, But in Ourselves: Relationships Between Screen Media and Childhood Overweight/Obesity

Sarah McKetta, A.B[a], Michael Rich, MD, MPH[b],*

KEYWORDS
- Child obesity • Child overweight • Television • Media
- Advertising • Video games • Cell phones • Computers

SCREEN TIME AND PEDIATRIC OVERWEIGHT/OBESITY: CURRENT KNOWLEDGE

Over the past 25 years, cross-sectional epidemiologic studies have demonstrated a significant and consistent relationship between time spent watching television (TV) and risk of childhood overweight/obesity.[1] A 2008 meta-analysis of exposure to screen media and weight status found a dose-response relationship with the prevalence of overweight/obesity with increasing longer average screen-viewing durations, quantifying this relationship as equivalent to taking in an extra 100 calories per hour of TV watched.[1,2] Prospective studies have shown that TV viewing is a risk factor for subsequent weight gain,[3] and a randomized controlled trial has demonstrated that body mass index (BMI, calculated as the weight in kilograms divided by height in meters squared) can be reduced by decreasing TV viewing.[4] Although the relationship between screen time and overweight/obesity was first described in the United States,

The authors have no relationship with commercial companies with direct financial interest in the subject matter or materials discussed.

[a] Department of Society, Human Development, and Health, Harvard School of Public Health, 677 Huntington Avenue, Boston, MA 02115, USA
[b] Center on Media and Child Health, Children's Hospital Boston, 300 Longwood Avenue, Boston, MA 02115, USA
* Corresponding author.
E-mail address: michael.rich@childrens.harvard.edu

Pediatr Clin N Am 58 (2011) 1493–1508
doi:10.1016/j.pcl.2011.09.010
0031-3955/11/$ – see front matter © 2011 Elsevier Inc. All rights reserved.

pediatric.theclinics.com

it has been found around the world.[5–8] However, the relationship is not always as robust nor as reliable in other countries, suggesting that there may be factors that make TV viewing more "fattening" in certain cultures than in others.[9,10]

A SCREEN-RICH ENVIRONMENT

Several studies examining the effects of media on childhood weight status have investigated TV as the primary medium of concern and measured screen time, the duration of TV viewing, as the key independent variable. TV was the first widely used electronic screen medium and is still the medium used for the greatest number of hours by most American children, so the effects of TV screen time have been the longest and best studied. However, the past decade has seen the development of a wide variety of screen media technologies that are used to communicate a plethora of messages in many different ways. Because media devices have evolved, researchers have become increasingly interested in the relationships between uses of emerging media types and childhood overweight/obesity. Studies of relationships between video games and overweight/obesity have provided an opportunity to examine the pros and cons of screen time with different content, compare more active engagement with and contexts of using screen media, and investigate how the effects of exposure to different content can interact with childhood overweight/obesity. For example, a 2009 study on video game use found that the length of game play time in a single sitting, frequency of video game playing, and years of video game playing were each correlated with less exercise and higher BMI,[11] which was consistent with previous findings about the relationship between video game use and childhood overweight/obesity.[12] However, these results are not always consistent, with some studies finding no relationship between video game play and increased BMI.[6,13] The 2008 meta-analysis of screen time and overweight found that there was no relationship between video game use and BMI but that video game use nevertheless was associated with an increased energy intake, equivalent to 92 calories per hour played, that exceeded energy output.[2] Other research shows that the type of game played is much more predictive than exposure to video games per se.[14] Exergames, interactive video games that require players to be highly active during game play, have very different content and elicit very different metabolic processes than passive games. Exergames have been proposed as a potential alternative to reducing screen time for increasing children's physical activity.[15–18] Several studies have shown that exergaming can increase metabolic rate and expend more energy than watching TV or playing a hand-controlled video game but still falls short of the energy expenditure required to actually play the sports that exergaming emulate.[19–22]

Associations between computer screen time and childhood overweight/obesity have been found but are neither as robust nor as consistent as TV screen time.[6,13] Similar to TV, computers target children with advertising, both through banner advertisements on child-oriented sites and through dedicated Web sites offering advergaming,[23,24] engaging electronic games branded for sugared cereals, candy, or other calorie-dense nutrition-poor foods. Uniquely, computer capabilities of operating multiple programs in separate windows simultaneously make media multitasking with a single device not only possible but also a routine for young people, who can simultaneously do homework, download music, interact via social media, play games, surf the web, and use traditional media such as listening to music and watching TV programs. For the most part, researchers are yet to catch up with the capabilities of computers. When investigating computer use, children are very rarely asked about the actual activities in which they are engaged while using the computer and are only asked about the total hours of computer use.[6] It is likely that the reason results vary among studies of computer screen time and overweight/obesity because the content and activities to which one child is exposed can differ dramatically from the exposures of another child with the same cumulative computer screen time.

Because smartphone technology is evolving rapidly and can be used for a variety of different tasks, there is little research so far on associations between cell phone screen time and overweight or obesity. One study linked cell phone use to poor sleep habits,[25] an established risk factor for childhood overweight/obesity. Another study found that playing electronic games, but no other activities, on cell phones was associated with increased BMI, demonstrating that, as with other screens, the content to which users are exposed is heterogeneous and of variable risk for overweight/obesity.[26] Most of the research on cell phones and overweight/obesity has been focused on developing interventions, such as using cell phone gaming or social networking to reduce BMI.[27]

Current research on screen media is indicating that as technology evolves and media content converges, device-based research is becoming increasingly obsolete. Mixed research findings, particularly on devices such as computers and cell phones, which can present a variety of content and formats, emphasize the need to measure contexts of use and exposure to content, rather than simply estimating the time one is in front of specific types of electronic screens. As screen media technologies emerge and new applications are developed, with programming and advertising becoming available on cell phones, computers, video games, and even uninvestigated screens such as global positioning system devices, it is increasingly clear that screens are most important as delivery mechanisms for content. Caloric intake, activity levels, and eating behaviors have been found to vary across content used and the ways in which that content is used.[28] It is not the duration of exposure to screen media that increases risk but the nature of exposure. It is how one uses screen media, the content to which one is exposed, and the contexts in which those exposures occur that drive the relationships between screen media and overweight/obesity. As an example of context rather than duration being critical to overweight/obesity outcomes, children who have TVs in their bedroom are more likely to be overweight than those who watch the same amount of TV but do not have a set in their bedroom.[29] Investigating the mechanisms underlying relationships between screen time and childhood overweight/obesity is critical to understanding and responding to risk in a constantly changing media environment.

PROPOSED MECHANISMS

Although the significant dose-response relationship between TV screen time and childhood overweight/obesity has been demonstrated at a population level, associations are less consistent with other electronic screen media use or at an individual level. For exposure to electronic screen media to be a risk factor for overweight/obesity, effects of screen-viewing experience on human physiology, of screen content on human psychology, or of screen use contexts on human behavior must create conditions in which the child's energy intake exceeds energy expenditure. For screen time to increase risk of overweight/obesity, evidence must indicate that features of screen media use contribute to decreased activity, increased consumption, or both.

Decreased Energy Expenditure

Because it seems as if the only time that children sit still is when they are in front of a screen, the first and most extensively investigated proposed mechanism for screen time's promoting overweight/obesity is decreased energy expenditure due to the sedentary nature of screen viewing. Findings of one early study indicated that basal metabolic rate might be lower while watching TV than during rest or even sleep, suggesting that TV uniquely slowed human metabolism.[30] Although this mechanism has face validity for anyone who has spent too many sedentary hours in front of a TV, none of the several follow-up studies have been able to replicate the original findings; energy expenditure while watching TV was found to be 18% higher than during rest, similar to that of other sedentary activities.[31–33]

Although energy expenditure while watching TV is not less than when resting, it is less than when engaged in strenuous physical activity. The most commonly accepted mechanism, that sedentary screen time displaces strenuous physical activity, is based on the assumption that if children were not watching TV, they would be running around and playing outside.[34] However, studies have shown that this assumption is not accurate; children whose TV watching is curtailed replace it with other sedentary behaviors rather than strenuous physical activities.[35] Although they are not more active, the weight status of children does improve.[36] Research into communication media, such as texting and social networking Web sites, has shown that children are as sedentary when using these media as when they are watching TV,[37] despite media devices becoming increasingly mobile.

Neither screen time nor other sedentary behaviors have a clear relationship with physical activity. Research has demonstrated that, when comparing people who viewed TV for a long time with those who viewed for a short time, there is no significant difference in physical activity.[38] Other sedentary behaviors, such as reading, have been associated with higher levels of physical activity among children; others had no relationship with weight status at all.[39] This lack of supportive evidence for sedentary behavior as the mechanism of increased risk for overweight/obesity has also been demonstrated indirectly through inconclusive research on screen time using video games, computers, and other media platforms. A methodological problem with some of the studies that have linked screen time and overweight/obesity is that they use screen time (usually TV, sometimes computer use as well) as a proxy for sedentary behavior without examining other types of inactivity.[40,41] Using screen time as an independent variable does not demonstrate that sedentary behavior is the mechanism of action but simply reaffirms the relationship between exposure to screen and childhood overweight/obesity.

Increased Consumption of Calories

Research has also examined whether watching TV and using other screen media influence children to eat more or eat differently than they might without screen media use. Increased screen time has been associated with more energy-rich nutrition-poor diets in children.[42–45] The relationship between obesogenic diets and screen media has been explained by 2 different, but complementary, pathways: eating while watching TV and exposure to food advertising.

Eating in front of a screen

A systematic review has shown increased consumption of snack foods, sugar-sweetened beverages, and food that lacks proper nutrients while watching TV and decreased consumption of fruits and vegetables with increases in TV viewing.[46] Children have been found to snack more in proportion to how much TV they watch.[47] A 2004 randomized controlled trial investigated whether eating habits while watching TV varied from eating habits while listening to a book on tape or with no media use.[48] Researchers found that people who ate while watching TV or listening to a recorded story ate larger meals but did not report more satiety, more palatable food, or reduced feelings of hunger compared with eating without any stimulus.[49] Laboratory research found that participants ate more while watching TV than in the absence of a TV screen.[50] A 2005 study in which obese adolescents were given camcorders to document their day-to-day experiences revealed what investigators termed unconscious eating when eating in front of a screen. Children consumed "high-sensation" foods and salt-, sugar-, and fat-containing choices that stimulated their taste buds because their eyes and ears were stimulated by the media they were using.[51] Children took whole bags of snacks, containers of ice cream, or serving bowls of pasta and ate until the containers were empty, completely focused on screens. These observations, coupled with laboratory findings on consumption and auditory/visual stimulation,[50,52] showed that eating while in the presence of an engaging stimulus such as screen media may lead to a disconnect from physiologic cues of hunger and satiety, leading to unconscious consumption of supraphysiologic calories.

These results are consistent with other research showing that children's eating while watching TV is more affected by different types of screen stimuli than by hunger.[53] A recent study on computer use found that when children were distracted by a computer game, they ate more and felt less full after eating than children who did not play a game.[51,54] Although children have shown signs of unconscious eating in controlled trials involving video games, the type of game played affected this behavior. In one trial of game play, boys ate more while playing only fighting games but not puzzle games, and girls ate less when playing video games than when just sitting around in a control environment.[14] Children do not eat consistently in front of every screen type, and the results of comparable studies have not been consistent from country to country, which provides further evidence that sedentary behavior is not the only, or even the predominant, mechanism by which screen time promotes overweight/obesity but that the contexts of media use and content of the media used may be more important than the duration of use.[9]

Food advertising and product placement

Food is advertised very aggressively to children, despite the fact that children themselves do not actually make household food purchases. The food advertised is most frequently energy-dense nutrition-poor sugared cereals, snack foods, and candy.[55] TV advertising directed toward children is very effective. Children exposed to advertising show clear preferences for the advertised foods[56] and choose branded food products over identical but nonbranded products whether or not it is a known or recognizable brand.[57] Parents want their children to eat better and often buy food items that children request so that they will eat something; thus food sales often parallel effective commercial campaigns.[58] In young children, even an exposure as short as 30 seconds has been shown to significantly influence food preferences.[59] Food advertisements, when compared with advertisements for nonfood produces, have an immediate effect, increasing food consumption at the time of exposure,[60–62] and there is some evidence that the unconscious eating in front of the screen may be motivated by advertising.[61]

Advertising is ubiquitous on TV and Internet. Successful advertising requires only brief exposure and a low level of comprehension to be effective. One study found that even when viewers fast-forward through advertisements on digital video recorders (DVRs), they absorb advertising messages as if they were watching them at their normal speed.[63] Children younger than about 7 years do not yet have the neurodevelopment to discern persuasive intent[64]; often they do not perceive any difference between programming and commercials, viewing advertising for candy from the same perspective as a lesson about dinosaurs: more information about something interesting. However, even a child who is media literate, able to deconstruct the persuasive messages of advertising, is not immunized against finding advertised food products desirable.[65] Obese children have proven to be better able to recognize food cues in advertising than nonobese children, suggesting that increased education and heightened awareness about food advertising is not an effective technique for decreasing the impact of advertising on food consumption among children.[66,67] Increasing children's media literacy and ability to discern persuasive intent has been shown not to protect them against advertising influence but may actually have a boomerang effect in which they believe that if advertisers have gone through so much trouble and expense to let them know about a product, it must be really good (Chervin A. The relationship between children's knowledge of persuasive intent and persuasion: the case of televised food marketing. Unpublished doctoral dissertation, University of Pennsylvania. 2007: Paper AAI3292015).[67]

Content analyses of food advertising consistently show that the food advertised on TV, in some research, specifically food advertisements directed toward children, is unhealthy, often high in sugar and fat, and does not represent the necessary parts of a balanced diet, such as sufficient amounts of fruits and vegetables.[68–71] The amount of food advertising on TV has been highly correlated with rates of childhood overweight/obesity in international comparisons.[72] Advertising is so highly related to overweight/obesity so that 1 analysis predicted that, had their exposure to TV advertising been limited, as many as 1 in 3 obese children in the United States would have a healthy weight.[73]

Because commercials are often skipped by leaving the room or fast-forwarding a DVR, an increasingly prevalent variation on food advertising is product placement, the insertion of specific products or advertising for those products into the programming itself. Although the Federal Communications Commission has set limitations on the amount of advertising that can occur during breaks in children's TV programming, it does not have any restrictions for advertising products within program content or any restrictions for advertising on primetime TV, which many children watch.[74] A review of the most-watched TV shows in 2005 found that product placement is extremely common; in 2005, the number 1 show American Idol had more than 3000 counts of product placement.[75] Product placement is also common in movies, with nearly 70% of the movies in the box office top 20 from 1996 to 2005 containing product placement for food, beverage, or food retail establishments.[76] The Internet was built on commerce, with products being featured and sold on many sites, banner advertisements for products supporting even unrelated Web sites, and products deeply embedded in the content of seemingly noncommercial sites. The most overt example of this is the relatively recent phenomenon of advergaming.[24] Cereal, candy, and other companies have created Web destinations for children, which feature engaging games that are branded with the company's products and logos, offer discounts or other deals, and provide the opportunity for young consumers to share these games with their friends. However, to date there is little research on the effects of advergaming and product placement on eating behaviors and weight outcomes in children.

What distinguishes food advertising and product placement from other possible mechanisms influencing childhood overweight/obesity is that the hypothesized obesogenic effects are driven by *exposure to screen content* rather than *energy imbalance while using screen media*. Screen media content, in the forms of food advertising and product placement, has been shown to be a robust predictor of BMI. Longitudinal research has shown that educational programming, with no commercials, does not have the positive relationship with childhood overweight/obesity that commercial programming has.[77] Distinctly different relationships between screen time and childhood overweight/obesity observed in different countries may be the result of different regulations and practices regarding broadcast of food advertising and product placement.[78]

ENVIRONMENTAL AND CULTURAL MODERATORS

Childhood overweight and obesity, an epidemic in the United States and other developed countries, is clearly multifactorial in origin and varies among individuals and across cultures, developing and continuing because of an array of lifestyle expectations and choices (of which screen media use is one). To date, there have been no studies investigating the relative contributions of different mechanisms by which exposure to screen media may influence risk of overweight/obesity. Empirically, it is most likely that there are multiple mechanisms by which screen media use affects risk of overweight or obesity in each individual. Sedentary screen-viewing behavior combined with exposure to obesogenic content and unconscious eating may cumulatively contribute to overweight/obesity in individuals or groups for whom each mechanism alone may not predict risk. Although the dose-response relationship between TV viewing and childhood overweight/obesity has been consistently demonstrated at the population level, insufficient power of each mechanism combined with individual and cultural moderators may explain variations among individuals and subgroups.

Relationships between screen time and childhood overweight/obesity vary around the world, modified by socioeconomic status (SES), local broadcast standards, and cultural customs of media use, eating, and activity. A 2003 study in China, in which household TV was not common before 1997, children's screen time was about one-fourth of that of American children, and statutory guidelines regulate advertising to children,[60] failed to find any significant relationship between screen time and weight status.[9] Subgroups within countries can also show variation; a 2009 multivariate analysis of health behaviors among children in US racial and ethnic subgroups found screen time not to be related to overweight/obesity among black and Hispanic children, suggesting that reducing screen time among these subgroups does not affect their weight status.[79] A recent study showed that although Hispanic and black adolescent women had significantly higher BMIs than their white counterparts, a relationship between TV screen time and BMI was found only among whites.[80]

Within-group differences can sometimes be attributed to factors such as family environment or SES. Eating dinner routinely with one's family has been shown to be a protective moderator between overall exposure to screen media and childhood overweight/obesity[81]; eating family meals while the TV is on erases this protective effect.[82] An Australian study associated children's weight and screen time with their mothers' employment status; children of mothers who worked part-time watched less TV and were not as overweight as those whose mothers worked full-time or were unemployed, indicating nonlinear modification by lifestyle or SES of the screen time–overweight/obesity relationship.[83] Children whose parents perceived their neighborhoods to be unsafe played outside less, watched TV more, and had higher BMIs.[84] Because lower SES predicts both perception of neighborhood safety[82] and length of parental work days,[85,86] it seems to be an important moderator of the findings that children of families with low SES watch more TV and have higher BMIs.[87]

Children who have TVs in their bedrooms have been consistently found at greater risk for overweight/obesity than those who do not,[29,88] an association that led one Centers for Disease Control and Prevention expert panel to make removing TVs from bedrooms a leading recommendation for combating childhood overweight/obesity.[89] Children with TVs in their bedroom watch more TV overall, and their viewing is less supervised; so they are likely exposed to greater amounts of food advertising and product placement as well as content that might contribute to nightmares or other sleep disturbance. A randomized controlled trial has shown that both evening TV viewing and exposure to violent programming disrupt children's sleep patterns but nonviolent daytime TV does not.[90] Sleep may be an important moderator of the screen media–overweight/obesity relationship. TV viewing has repeatedly been associated with getting less or poorer-quality sleep,[29,88] and getting sufficient sleep has been associated with healthier weight. A longitudinal study of young children who were controlled for initial BMI and a variety of sociodemographic risk factors (but not screen media) found a dose-response relationship between hours of sleep and risk of overweight/obesity, with each additional hour of sleep per night coming to an associated 0.56 decrease in BMI.[91] Another study found that preschool children who had screen media limits, got adequate sleep, and ate meals as a family had approximately 40% lower risk of obesity than those who had none of these routines.[81]

Because individuals filter media messages through their own experiences and perspectives,[92] children's gender can influence the effects of exposure to screen media on their risk of overweight/obesity. However, in the limited research that has been stratified by gender, the direction of gender-specific influences is mixed. Among US high school students, boys and girls who watched TV for less than 1 h/d had no increased risk of overweight/obesity, and boys only had increased risk when they watched more than 4 h/d combined with low levels of moderate physical activity.[93] For girls, moderate physical activity for 3 to 5 d/wk combined with less than 1 h/d TV viewing seemed to be protective, but more than 4 h/d TV viewing increased risk of overweight/obesity in an inverse dose-response relationship to their level of physical activity.[93] Similarly, a study in France found screen time to be associated with overweight among girls but not among boys.[7] Conversely, a US study found that a TV in a child's bedroom, often used as a proxy for increased screen time, was associated with overweight among boys but not girls.[29]

Because of cultural ideals and gender-related expectations, exposure to food-related screen media content can affect girls in different ways than it affects boys. When 8- to 12-year-old boys and girls watched movies with food commercials or nonfood commercials, boys who watched food commercials ate more than those who watched nonfood commercials, but girls who watched food commercials ate less than those who watched nonfood commercials.[60] A Dutch study of emotional eaters found that boys snacked while watching TV, whereas girls did not.[53] Screen media, even for young children, have portrayed and promoted a thin body ideal for women that can become internalized[94,95] and lead to girls' dissatisfaction with their bodies and subsequent weight loss behaviors.[92,96–99] The difference between how TV sitcoms criticize overweight female characters and have fun with overweight male characters is one example of how different media portrayals may contribute to different eating habits between the genders.[100,101] Although gender clearly plays a moderating role in how children receive and respond to media messages, the directions of children's weight-related responses and mechanism of influence require more extensive research to clarify.

RECOMMENDATIONS
For Parents

1. Take the TV and computer out of the child's bedroom. Screen media in a child's bedroom has consistently been shown to increase risk of the child being

overweight.[29,88,102] Moving children's screen media use into public areas of the home is an easy effective way to make a big impact.

2. Have household TV rules, and make sure children know the rules and both parents enforce them. Limiting screen time is straightforward, especially when parents make their expectations clear and model healthy screen media use themselves.[48,103] The American Academy of Pediatrics recommends a limit of 1 to 2 hours of educational screen time per day for children older than 2 years, but every household is different. Children of different ages have different academic and social demands, so it is most important to make household rules that work for one's family and then adhere to them. For example, school-aged children are increasingly being asked to do homework online. It is more important for them to clearly distinguish online work from entertainment and get their work done without simultaneously texting, downloading music, and using social media than it is to limit their overall screen time. A good rule of thumb is to establish a routine in which all essential activities, that is, homework, exercise (preferably outdoors), a family meal, and adequate sleep, are taken care of before entertainment.

3. Dissociate screen media use from food consumption. Eat at least one family meal together every day. During these meals, do not turn the TV on (even in the background), respond to texts, or read a tablet. If possible, avoid temptation by even having screens viewable from eating areas removed. Given the research showing that advertised foods tend to be energy dense and nutrient poor, avoiding them is a good general rule, and, when children ask for foods they have seen advertised on TV or online, take the opportunity to talk about the nutritional value (or lack thereof) of these food items rather than succumbing to their commercial-motivated requests. Because snacking in front of the TV is particularly obesogenic, it should be avoided. If the dining room or kitchen does not have screen media, prohibiting unconscious snacking in front of a screen can be as simple as implementing a "no eating in the living room" rule.

4. Pay attention to content. If possible, watch TV with your children or have them watch in an area where you can monitor programming and advertising to which they are being exposed. Use a DVR to capture educational and entertainment programs they watch, so that children can view them when their essential activities are done and they can skip (rather than fast-forward) through commercials. If their total screen time is limited, teach them to do this to optimize their entertainment in the limited time available. When watching broadcast media, mute the sound during commercials.

5. Use the capabilities of new media technologies to use media in healthier ways. Control content with content filters offered by many cable and satellite companies and with DVR. If children are computer or video gamers, invest in their health with a console that uses active controllers and purchase physically active games.

For Pediatricians

Consistent with recommendations from the American Academy of Pediatricians, doctors ought to take a history of media use and incorporate anticipatory guidance about media usage in their annual health maintenance visits, much the way they ask questions about nutrition and injury prevention.[104]

DISCUSSION

Children's exposure to electronic screen media can influence their risk of overweight/obesity, but the evidence indicates that it is how they use media and what media they use that matters rather than simply the amount of time they are in front of a screen. The complicated relationships between screen media and childhood overweight/obesity speak to a deeper truth about these technologies: electronic screen media have children's attention and are very effective communication tools. If children are exposed to messages about eating energy-dense nutrition-poor foods, they are more likely to eat those foods. If children have access to engaging and fun active video games, they will be more active. Using electronic screen media as interventions for childhood overweight/obesity has shown real promise, although few interventions use TV, the best communicator in history and still the screen medium that more children use for longer durations than any other.

Although there is little evidence that use of screen media places young people at increased risk for overweight/obesity by displacing strenuous physical activity at the moment, contemporary lifestyles are more sedentary than those of earlier generations. Technology has made both work and leisure more efficient and less physically demanding. The attractions of electronic screen media over other activities is a major contributor to a cultural shift toward more sedentary lifestyles overall. Thus, when children decrease their total TV viewing, they simply substitute another sedentary behavior. However, increasing use of mobile media devices may herald a paradigm shift. Historically, viewers needed to sit in one place to watch TV or even talk on the telephone. Now young people can run on a treadmill and watch video on a tablet or interact on social media while walking to school. With intermittent multitasking uses of increasing mobile devices, duration of exposure to screen media has become an obsolete and clinically irrelevant measure. What affects young people's overweight/obesity risk and overall physical, mental, and social health is the media content to which they are exposed; when and how these media are consumed; and the contexts, that is, where, with whom, and what else is happening, in which the media are used. Improving media messages accessible to children can be very effective in health promotion and obesity prevention at a population level, but media production and regulation are in the hands of entertainment industries and policymakers[105–108] who are motivated by concerns other than child health, so their feasibility is uncertain. However, those who receive and respond to the media messages are we ourselves, dear viewer. We can reduce risk of overweight/obesity for ourselves and for the children for whom we care by using screen media wisely, focusing on prohealth media content and using contexts that promote physical and mental health, and turning off these powerful tools when we are done.

SUMMARY/POINTS FOR RECALL

- Exposure to electronic screen media can powerfully influence the risk of childhood overweight/obesity.
- The mechanisms of increased overweight/obesity are primarily increased food consumption due to both altered eating behaviors and exposure to advertising; sedentary screen viewing behaviors may contribute but not as predominantly as originally believed.
- Moderators of the relationship between screen media use and overweight/obesity include context of use, family culture and SES, gender of viewer, and sleep.
- Informed and focused screen media use has real potential for improving risk of overweight/obesity.

REFERENCES

1. Dietz W, Gortmaker SL. Do we fatten our children at the television set? Obesity and television viewing in children and adolescents. Pediatrics 1985;75(5):807–12.

2. Sonneville KR, Gortmaker SL. Total energy intake, adolescent discretionary behaviors, and the energy gap. Int J Obes 2008;32(Suppl 6):S19–27.

3. Hancox RJ, Poulton R. Watching television is associated with childhood obesity: but is it clinically important? Int J Obes 2006;30(1):171–5.

4. Epstein LH, Paluch RA, Gordy CC, et al. Decreasing sedentary behaviors in treating pediatric obesity. Arch Pediatr Adolesc Med 2000;154(3):220–6.

5. Jones RA, Okely AD, Caputi P, et al. Relationships between child, parent and community characteristics and weight status among young children. Int J Pediatr Obes 2010;5(3):256–64.

6. Kautiainen S, Koivusilta L, Lintonen T, et al. Use of information and communication technology and prevalence of overweight and obesity among adolescents. Int J Obes 2005;29(8):925–33.

7. Dupuy M, Godeau E, Vignes C, et al. Socio-demographic and lifestyle factors associated with overweight in a representative sample of 11–15 year olds in France: results from the WHO-Collaborative Health Behaviour in School-aged Children (HBSC) cross-sectional study. BMC Public Health 2011;11:442.

8. Ozmert EN, Ozdemir R, Pektas A, et al. Effect of activity and television viewing on BMI z-score in early adolescents in Turkey. World J Pediatr 2011;7(1):37–40.

9. Waller CE, Du S, Popkin BM. Patterns of overweight, inactivity, and snacking in Chinese children. Obes Res 2003;11(8):957–61.

10. Manios Y, Kourlaba G, Kondaki K, et al. Obesity and television watching in preschoolers in Greece: the genesis study. Obesity (Silver Spring) 2009; 17(11):2047–53.

11. Ballard M, Gray M, Reilly J, et al. Correlates of video game screen time among males: body mass, physical activity, and other media use. Eat Behav 2009; 10(3):161–7.

12. Vicente-Rodriguez G, Rey-Lopez JP, Martin-Matillas M, et al. Television watching, videogames, and excess of body fat in Spanish adolescents: the AVENA study. Nutrition 2008;24(7–8):654–62.

13. Vandewater EA, Shim MS, Caplovitz AG. Linking obesity and activity level with children's television and video game use [special issue on video games and youth]. J Adolesc 2004;27(1):71–85.

14. Cessna T, Raudenbush B, Reed A, et al. Effects of video game play on snacking behavior. Appetite 2007;49(1):282.

15. Daley AJ. Can exergaming contribute to improving physical activity levels and health outcomes in children? Pediatrics 2009;124(2):763–71.

16. Maddison R, Foley L, Ni Mhurchu C, et al. Feasibility, design and conduct of a pragmatic randomized controlled trial to reduce overweight and obesity in children: The electronic games to aid motivation to exercise (eGAME) study. BMC Public Health 2009;9(1):146.

17. Papastergiou M. Exploring the potential of computer and video games for health and physical education: a literature review. Comput Educ 2009;53(3): 603–22.

18. Murphy EC, Carson L, Neal W, et al. Effects of an exercise intervention using Dance Dance Revolution on endothelial function and other risk factors in overweight children. Int J Pediatr Obes 2009;4(4):205–14.

19. Graf DL, Pratt LV, Hester CN, et al. Playing active video games increases energy expenditure in children. Pediatrics 2009;124(2):534–40.

20. Graves L, Stratton G, Ridgers ND, et al. Comparison of energy expenditure in adolescents when playing new generation and sedentary computer games: cross sectional study. BMJ 2007;335(7633):1282–4.

21. Graves LE, Ridgers ND, Stratton G. The contribution of upper limb and total body movement to adolescents' energy expenditure whilst playing Nintendo Wii. Eur J Appl Physiol 2008;104(4):617–23.

22. Lanningham-Foster L, Foster RC, McCrady SK, et al. Activity-promoting video games and increased energy expenditure. J Pediatr 2009;154(6):819–23.

23. Rideout VJ. It's child's play: advergaming and the online marketing of food to children. Washington, DC: Kaiser Family Foundation; 2006.

24. Jain A. Temptations in cyberspace: new battlefields in childhood obesity. Health Aff (Millwood) 2010;29(3):425–9.

25. Brunborg GS, Mentzoni RA, Molde H, et al. The relationship between media use in the bedroom, sleep habits and symptoms of insomnia. J Sleep Res 2011; 20(3).

26. Yen CF, Hsiao RC, Ko CH, et al. The relationships between body mass index and television viewing, internet use and cellular phone use: the moderating effects of socio-demographic characteristics and exercise. Int J Eat Disord 2010;43(6): 565–71.

27. Woolford SJ, Clark SJ, Strecher VJ, et al. Tailored mobile phone text messages as an adjunct to obesity treatment for adolescents. J Telemed Telecare 2010; 16(8):458–61.

28. Chaput JP, Klingenberg L, Astrup A, et al. Modern sedentary activities promote overconsumption of food in our current obesogenic environment. Obes Rev 2011;12(5):e12–20.

29. Delmas C, Platat C, Schweitzer B, et al. Association between television in bedroom and adiposity throughout adolescence. Obesity (Silver Spring) 2007; 15(10):2495–503.

30. Klesges RC, Shelton ML, Klesges LM. Effects of television on metabolic rate: potential implications for childhood obesity. Pediatrics 1993;91(2):281–6.

31. Buchowski MS, Sun M. Energy expenditure, television viewing and obesity. Int J Obes Relat Metab Disord 1996;20(3):236–44.

32. Lanningham-Foster L, Jensen TB, Foster RC, et al. Energy expenditure of sedentary screen time compared with active screen time for children. Pediatrics 2006;118(6):e1831–5.

33. Conway JM, Irwin ML, Ainsworth BE. Estimating energy expenditure from the Minnesota Leisure Time Physical Activity and Tecumseh Occupational Activity questionnaires—a doubly labeled water validation. J Clin Epidemiol 2002; 55(4):392–9.

34. Dietz W, Gortmaker SL. TV or not TV: fat is the question. Pediatrics 1993;91(2): 499–501.

35. Biddle S, Gorely T, Marshall S. Is television viewing a suitable marker of sedentary behavior in young people? Ann Behav Med 2009;38(2):147–53.

36. Goldfield GS, Mallory R, Parker T, et al. Effects of open-loop feedback on physical activity and television viewing in overweight and obese children: a randomized, controlled trial. Pediatrics 2006;118(1):e157–66.

37. Leatherdale ST. Factors associated with communication-based sedentary behaviors among youth: are talking on the phone, texting, and instant messaging new sedentary behaviors to be concerned about? J Adolesc Health 2010;47:315–8.

38. Biddle SJ, Gorely T, Stensel DJ. Health-enhancing physical activity and sedentary behavior in children and adolescents. J Sports Sci Med 2004;22(8):679–701.

39. Koezuka N, Koo M, Allison KR, et al. The relationship between sedentary activities and physical inactivity among adolescents: results from the Canadian Community Health Survey. J Adolesc Health 2006;39(4):515–22.

40. Thibault H, Contrand B, Saubusse E, et al. Risk factors for overweight and obesity in French adolescents: physical activity, sedentary behavior and parental characteristics. Nutrition 2010;26(2):192–200.

41. Sisson SB, Church TS, Martin CK, et al. Profiles of sedentary behavior in children and adolescents: the US National Health and Nutrition Examination Survey, 2001–2006. Int J Pediatr Obes 2009;4(4):353–9.

42. Vader AM, Walters ST, Harris TR, et al. Television viewing and snacking behaviors of fourth- and eighth-grade schoolchildren in Texas. Prev Chronic Dis 2009; 6(3):A88.

43. Ranjit N, Evans MH, Byrd-Williams C, et al. Dietary and activity correlates of sugar-sweetened beverage consumption among adolescents. Pediatrics 2010;126(4):e754–61: peds.2010-1229.

44. Miller SA, Taveras EM, Rifas-Shiman SL, et al. Association between television viewing and poor diet quality in young children. Int J Pediatr Obes 2008;3(3): 168–76.

45. Taveras EM, Sandora TJ, Shih MC, et al. The association of television and video viewing with fast food intake by preschool-age children. Obesity (Silver Spring) 2006;14(11):2034–41.

46. Pearson N, Biddle SJ. Sedentary behavior and dietary intake in children, adolescents, and adults a systematic review. Am J Prev Med 2011;41(2):178–88.

47. Pearson P, Ball K, Crawford D. Mediators of longitudinal associations between television viewing and eating behaviours in adolescents. Int J Behav Nutr Phys Activ 2011;30(8):23.

48. Springer AE, Kelder SH, Barroso CS, et al. Parental influences on television watching among children living on the Texas-Mexico border. Prev Med 2010; 51(2):112–7.

49. Bellisle F, Dalix AM, Slama G. Non food-related environmental stimuli induce increased meal intake in healthy women: comparison of television viewing versus listening to a recorded story in laboratory settings. Appetite 2004;43(2):175–80.

50. Higgs S, Woodward M. Television watching during lunch increases afternoon snack intake of young women. Appetite 2009;52(1):39–42.

51. Rich M, Patashnick J, Huecker D, et al. Living with obesity: visual narratives of overweight adolescents. J Adolesc Health 2002;30(2):100.

52. Chaput JP, Visby T, Nyby S, et al. Video game play increases food intake in adolescents: a randomized crossover study. Am J Clin Nutr 2011;93(6):1196–203.

53. Snoek HM, Van Strien T, Janssens JMAM, et al. The effect of television viewing on adolescents' snacking: individual differences explained by external, restrained and emotional eating. J Adolesc Health 2006;39:448–51.

54. Oldham-Cooper RE, Hardman CA, Nicoll CE, et al. Playing a computer game during lunch affects fullness, memory for lunch, and later snack intake. Am J Clin Nutr 2011;93:308–13.

55. Batada A, Seitz MD, Wootan MG, et al. Nine out of 10 food advertisements shown during Saturday morning children's television programming are for foods high in fat, sodium, or added sugars, or low in nutrients. J Am Diet Assoc 2009; 108(4):673–8.

56. Koordeman R, Anschutz DJ, van Baaren RB, et al. Exposure to soda commercials affects sugar-sweetened soda consumption in young women. An observational experimental study. Appetite 2010;54(3):619–22.

57. Robinson TN, Borzekowski DL, Matheson DM, et al. Effects of fast food branding on young children's taste preferences. Arch Pediatr Adolesc Med 2007;161(8): 792–7.

58. Hawkes C. Sales promotions and food consumption. Nutr Rev 2009;67(6): 333–42.

59. Borzekowski DL, Robinson TN. The 30-second effect: an experiment revealing the impact of television commercials on food preferences of preschoolers. J Am Diet Assoc 2001;101(1):42–6.

60. Anschutz DJ, Engels RC, Van Strien T. Side effects of television food commercials on concurrent nonadvertised sweet snack food intakes in young children. Am J Clin Nutr 2009;89(5):1328–33.

61. Harris JL, Bargh JA, Brownell KD. Priming effects of television food advertising on eating behavior. Health Psychol 2009;28(4):404–13.

62. Buijzen M, Schuurman J, Bomhof E. Associations between children's television advertising exposure and their food consumption patterns: a household diary-survey study. Appetite 2008;50(2–3):231–9.

63. Armbruster A. Don't give up on TV ads just yet. Television Week 2007;26(30):16.

64. Carter OB, Patterson LJ, Donovan RJ, et al. Children's understanding of the selling versus persuasive intent of junk food advertising: Implications for regulation. Soc Sci Med 2011;72(6):962–8.

65. Mehta K, Coveney J, Ward P, et al. Australian children's views about food advertising on television. Appetite 2010;55(1):49–55.

66. Halford JCG, Gillespie J, Brown V, et al. Effect of television advertisements for foods on food consumption in children. Appetite 2004;42(2):221–5.

67. Parvanta SA, Brown JD, Du S, et al. Television use and snacking behaviors among children and adolescents in China. J Adolesc Health 2010;46(4):339–45.

68. Bell RA, Cassady D, Culp J, et al. Frequency and types of foods advertised on Saturday morning and weekday afternoon English- and Spanish-language American television programs. J Nutr Educ Behav 2009;41(6):406–13.

69. Adams J, Hennessy-Priest K, Ingimarsdottir S, et al. Food advertising during children's television in Canada and the UK. Arch Dis Child 2009;94(9):658–62: adc.2008.151019.

70. Harris J, Pomeranz J, Lobstein T, et al. A crisis in the marketplace: how food marketing contributes to childhood obesity and what can be done. Annu Rev Public Health 2009;30(1):211–25.

71. Mink M, Evans A, Moore CG, et al. Nutritional imbalance endorsed by televised food advertisements. J Am Diet Assoc 2010;110(6):904–10.

72. Goris JM, Petersen S, Stamatakis E, et al. Television food advertising and the prevalence of childhood overweight and obesity: a multicountry comparison. Public Health Nutr 2009;13(7):1–10.

73. Veerman JL, Van Beeck EF, Barendregt JJ, et al. By how much would limiting TV food advertising reduce childhood obesity? Eur J Public Health 2009;19(4): 365–9.

74. Jordan AB. Children's media policy. Future Child 2008;18(1):235–53.

75. Edwards J. On TV, kids and placements often show up together. Brandweek 2006;47(11):43–5.

76. Sutherland LA, MacKenzie T, Purvis LA, et al. Prevalence of food and beverage brands in movies: 1996–2005. Pediatrics 2010;125(3):468–74.

77. Zimmerman FJ, Bell JF. Associations of television content type and obesity in children. Am J Public Health 2010;100(2):334–40.

78. Hawkes C. Marketing food to children: the global regulatory environment. Geneva (Switzerland): WHO; 2004.

79. Russ SA, Larson K, Franke TM, et al. Associations between media use and health in US children. Acad Pediatr 2009;9(5):300–6.

80. Richmond TK, Walls CE, Gooding HC, et al. Television viewing is not predictive of BMI in black and Hispanic young adult females. Obesity (Silver Spring) 2010; 18(5):1015–20.
81. Anderson SE, Whitaker RC. Household routines and obesity in US preschool-aged children. Pediatrics 2010;125(3):420–8.
82. Fitzpatrick E, Edmunds LS, Dennison BA. Positive effects of family dinner are undone by television viewing. J Am Diet Assoc 2007;107(4):666–71.
83. Brown JE, Broom DH, Nicholson JM, et al. Do working mothers raise couch potato kids? Maternal employment and children's lifestyle behaviours and weight in early childhood. Soc Sci Med 2010;70(11):1816–24.
84. Cecil-Karb R, Grogan-Kaylor A. Childhood body mass index in community context: neighborhood safety, television viewing, and growth trajectories of BMI. Health Soc Work 2009;34(3):169–77.
85. Wilson DK, Kirtland KA, Ainsworth BE, et al. Socioeconomic status and perceptions of access and safety for physical activity. Ann Behav Med 2004;28(1): 20–8.
86. Warren R. Parental mediation of children's television viewing in low-income families. J Commun 2006;55(4):847–63.
87. Morgenstern M, Sargent JD, Hanewinkel R. Relation between socioeconomic status and body mass index: evidence of an indirect path via television use. Arch Pediatr Adolesc Med 2009;163(8):731–8.
88. Adachi-Mejia AM, Longacre MR, Gibson JJ, et al. Children with a TV in their bedroom at higher risk for being overweight. Int J Obes 2007;31(4):644–51.
89. Jordan AB, Robinson TN. Children, television viewing, and weight status: summary and recommendations from an expert panel meeting. Ann Am Acad Pol Soc Sci 2008;615(1):119–32.
90. Garrison MM, Liekweg K, Christakis DA. Media use and child sleep: the impact of content, timing, and environment. Pediatrics 2011;128(1):29–35.
91. Carter PJ, Taylor BJ, Williams SM, et al. Longitudinal analysis of sleep in relation to BMI and body fat in children: the FLAME study. BMJ 2011;342:d2712.
92. Moore ES, Lutz RJ. Children, advertising, and product experiences: a multimethod inquiry. J Consum Res 2000;27(1):31–48.
93. Eisenmann J, Bartee RT, Smith DT, et al. Combined influence of physical activity and television viewing on the risk of overweight in US youth. Int J Obes 2008; 32(4):613–8.
94. Herbozo S, Tantleff-Dunn S, Gokee-Larose J, et al. Beauty and thinness messages in children's media: a content analysis. Eat Disord 2004;12(1):21–34.
95. Tiggemann M. Television and adolescent body image: the role of program content and viewing motivation. J Soc Clin Psychol 2005;24:361–81.
96. Field AE, Camargo CAJ, Taylor CB, et al. Peer, parent, and media influences on the development of weight concerns and frequent dieting among preadolescent and adolescent girls and boys. Pediatrics 2001;107(1):54–60.
97. Field AE, Camargo CAJ, Taylor CB, et al. Relation of peer and media influences to the development of purging behaviors among preadolescent and adolescent girls. Arch Pediatr Adolesc Med 1999;153(11):1184–9.
98. Bissell K, Zhou P. Must-see TV or ESPN: entertainment and sports media exposure and body-image distortion in college women. J Commun 2006;54(1):5–21.
99. Carney T, Louw J. Eating disordered behaviors and media exposure. Soc Psychiatry Psychiatr Epidemiol 2006;41(12):957–66.
100. Fouts G, Burggraf K. Television situation comedies: female weight, male negative comments, and audience reactions. Sex Roles 2000;42:925–32.

101. Fouts G, Vaughan K. Television situation comedies: male weight, negative references, and audience reactions. Sex Roles 2000;46:439–42.

102. Rosenberg DE, Sallis JF, Kerr J, et al. Brief scales to assess physical activity and sedentary equipment in the home. Int J Behav Nutr Phys Activ 2010;7:10.

103. He M, Piche L, Beynon C, et al. Screen-related sedentary behaviors: children's and parents' attitudes, motivations, and practices. J Nutr Educ Behav 2010; 42(1):17–25.

104. American Academy of Pediatrics. Policy statement—children, adolescents, obesity, and the media. Pediatrics 2011;128(1):201–8.

105. King L, Hebden L, Grunseit A, et al. Industry self regulation of television food advertising: responsible or responsive? Int J Pediatr Obes 2011;6(2–2):e390–8.

106. Pomeranz J. Television food marketing to children revisited: the Federal Trade Commission has the constitutional and statutory authority to regulate. J Law Med Ethics 2010;38(1):98–116.

107. Robin AM, Orleans CT, Shiriki KK, et al. Considerations for an obesity policy research agenda. Am J Prev Med 2009;36(4):351–7.

108. Wilde P. Self-regulation and the response to concerns about food and beverage marketing to children in the United States. Nutr Rev 2009;67(3):155–66.

Media, Social Networking, and Pediatric Obesity

Elizabeth A. Vandewater, PhD*,
Laurence M. Denis, MD, MPH

KEYWORDS

- Media • Technology • Smartphones • Apps • Children
- Adolescents • Social Media • Health behavior • Obesity

MEDIA AND THE AMERICAN FAMILY

Since the advent of television in the early 1950s, its impact on American life, and especially its impact on children, has been the subject of great interest and great debate. The United States became a nation of television viewers between 1950 and 1960, and the popularity of television has continued unabated.[1] Consumer electronics are now requisite components of American family life. Ownership of televisions and other devices (eg, DVD players, video game system, computers) is nearly universal among families with children.[2] More telling is that, in 2009, American families reported owning an average of almost 4 (3.8) televisions, almost 3 (2.9) VCR/DVD players, and 2 computers. Eight-four percent had cable/satellite television as well as Internet access. Moreover, 71% of children between 8 and 18 years old had a television in their bedroom, 50% had cable/satellite channels, and a third had a computer with Internet access in their bedrooms.[2] American children are growing up with unprecedented levels of access to media, and this trend seems unlikely to decline.

The Digital Era and the New Media Landscape

During the first decade of the new millennium, the number of devices available for accessing media content (eg, televisions, DVDs, DVRs, computers, cell phones, tablets such as iPads, networked video game consoles such as the Wii or xBox360, or other devices whose sole purpose is to stream content to televisions or existing screens, such as AppleTV) increased rapidly. The current plethora of possibilities and platforms renders long-standing concerns of scholars and practitioners alike about the impact of television on children almost quaint. Although television remains

Michael & Susan Dell Center for Healthy Living, University of Texas School of Public Health, Austin Regional Campus, University of Texas Administration Building (UTA), 1616 Guadalupe Street, Suite 6.310, Austin, TX 78701, USA
* Corresponding author.
E-mail address: Elizabeth.Vandewater@tmc.uth.edu

Pediatr Clin N Am 58 (2011) 1509–1519
doi:10.1016/j.pcl.2011.09.012
0031-3955/11/$ – see front matter © 2011 Published by Elsevier Inc.

pediatric.theclinics.com

highly popular, technological advances have rendered the means of delivery of media content nearly irrelevant.

The large variety of consumer electronics and entertainment technology available to consumers has been greatly facilitated by the switch from analog to digital delivery technologies. Digital technology offers users the capability to use more media simultaneously, producing the phenomenon of media multitasking.[2,3] Computers, tablets (eg, iPads) and even cell phones can run multiple applications simultaneously, everything from streaming video to resident application programs. The combination of digital delivery with significant advances in component miniaturization, touch screens, and wireless technologies in recent years has forever changed the kinds of devices people rely on, the ways in which people use media, and how people access media content.

As an example, between 2004 and 2009, cell phone ownership among US youth has increased from about 48% to 84%.[4] Among youth aged 12 to 18 years, mobile-to-mobile texting has become the primary way they communicate with friends, surpassing face-to-face contact, email, instant messaging, and voice calling as the preferred mode of daily communication.[5] However, voice calling is still the preferred mode for reaching parents[5] (probably because of parental preferences rather than those of teens). Increasingly, even cell phones are morphing into smartphones, allowing Internet access and surfing, online game playing, video streaming, and all manner of activities far removed from the humble purpose of sending and receiving communications, either voice or text.

Facebook was launched in 2004, the same year that Google made its first public stock offering. Facebook now has 750 million active users (the youngest of whom are 13 years old), and Google has changed the lexicon: the verb to google can now be found in the Webster Collegiate and Oxford English Dictionaries, defined as "to use the Google search engine to obtain information on the Internet."[6,7] The first iPhone went on the market in June 2007, and Apple released the first iPad tablet computer in April 2010, selling 3 million of the devices in 80 days.[8]

These 3 products alone represent major conceptual and technological innovations that have altered the media landscape for current and future generations of children. In their own way, each has provided the foundation for ensuing paradigmatic shifts, altering the way people think about media, how people use it in their daily lives, what people expect from it, and the role people expect it to play in their lives and the lives of their children.

Regarding the impact of media, children and youth have always been a special audience, in part because they are developmentally vulnerable, and in part because they have always been among the earliest adopters and heaviest users of entertainment technology.[9] There is popular and scholarly consensus that today's adolescents, in particular, have widely adopted the use of digital media for daily life activities. An image of typical American teenagers is conjured up: these teenagers are in their rooms, doing homework on the computer, perhaps with a word-processing program open for text, surfing the Internet for information related to the topic of their particular paper. Although both writing and surfing, they are texting friends on their cell phones or about events at school, who likes whom, who dissed whom, or what a pain the assignment is. Alternatively, they are posting this same information in more public forums via updates on their own Facebook statuses, or posts on the walls of their Facebook friends. All this is happening with the television on in the background (or video content streamed via iPads, or networked game consoles), and/or while listening to music on their iPods. It is commonly thought that this image describes most adolescents in America today, and there is some evidence to support this notion.[2]

Influences of Media on Pediatric Obesity: the Good, the Bad, and the Equivocal

Youth of all ages spend a large proportion of their time using electronic media (eg, 3–5 hours a day watching television), more time than for any other single free-time activity except for sleep.[10] Partly because of this, the notion that media use is an important contributor to the increased prevalence of obesity in American youth is held by the lay public and scholars alike.[11–15] Moreover, this conviction has shaped prominent public health policies. The US Department of Health and Human Services listed the reduction of television viewing as a national health objective in both *Healthy People 2010* and *Healthy People 2020*. Likewise, the American Academy of Pediatrics (AAP) policy statement regarding the prevention of pediatric overweight and obesity identifies limiting television and videogame use to no more than 2 hours per day as an important strategy for preventing obesity among children and adolescents.[16]

However, empirical evidence for this belief is mixed. Despite high levels of media use[2,17] and a high incidence of obesity among youth, evidence that these concurrent trends are strongly related is poor.[18] In a recent meta-analysis, Marshall and colleagues[19] found that the associations between media use and obesity among youth, although consistently positive, are weak, and concluded that they are of little clinical relevance. Similarly, they reported average effect sizes (Pearson r) of -0.12 and -0.10 for the relationship between television viewing and video/computer game use, respectively, and physical activity. The investigators conclude that "…media-based inactivity may be unfairly implicated in recent epidemiologic trends of overweight and obesity among children and youth" (p. 1238).[19] They noted critical flaws with the current body of literature, including the general lack of attention to important contextual factors or confounders (including socioeconomic resources, parental weight status, and child pubertal status), a heavy reliance on cross-sectional correlations, and, because of a general lack of longitudinal studies, that temporal precedence has not been established.

These findings have important implications for the notion that electronic media use has contributed to the obesity epidemic in US youth via its impact on physical activity. There is ample evidence that American children are not active enough.[20] The question is whether electronic media use plays an important role in this problem. Generally, the assumption is that, if children were not using media, they would be outside running up and down a soccer field. However, the existing evidence suggests that this is not the case, and that media use mainly displaces other kinds of sedentary activities.[10,18,21] The current body of empirical evidence suggests that reduction of moderate to vigorous physical activity is not one of the major mechanisms by which media use contributes to childhood obesity.

If the role of media use in childhood obesity is not via its impact on physical activity, the other possible mechanism is caloric intake. Many hold advertising responsible for childhood obesity because of its abundant promotion of calorically dense food products with high proportions of fat, sugar, and salt.[22–24] Evidence for this hypothesis is more robust than for the sedentary lifestyle hypothesis. A large body of findings from diverse methods (eg, experimental, correlational, longitudinal) and samples (eg, community, convenience, population level) now exists. Taken together, it seems that (1) screen-based media viewing encourages indiscriminate eating and greater caloric intake[25,26]; (2) exposure to advertised food products increases children's choice of, and preference for, such products[27] and increases children's product purchase requests and parental product purchases,[27–29] with these purchase requests reflecting product advertising frequency[30]; and (3) media-based food advertising is related to both poor dietary habits[25,26,31] and increased caloric intake.[23,28]

Advertising works, and is likely to be a central mechanism linking screen media use to childhood obesity.

Effects of Social Networking, Friends, and Peers on Pediatric Obesity

For children and youth, literature in this area is scarce. Although researchers are aware of the popularity of social media, and the likelihood that friends and peers might influence behaviors, which might have implications for children's obesity and/or weight status, empirical evidence examining these issues is sparse to nonexistent. There is some literature examining implications of online social ties among youth.[32,33] However, this literature has focused almost exclusively on either the implications of online relationships for youth social competence and relationship development,[32,34,35] or on the dangers of online relationships and sexual predators.[36,37]

Friend Me: Implications of Social Media for Childhood Obesity

Social media is a term coined in the last few years, and generally refers to Web sites in which user members present information about themselves and connect with friends. As of 2011, Facebook and MySpace are the most prominent examples, and also the most popular among children, but other sites, typically with a more narrow purpose (LinkedIn, Twitter, and so forth) also exist. Because social media platforms are rapidly evolving, as companies try to develop the next big thing (eg, Google Plus), the importance of any particular social media site for youth is difficult to predict. Regardless, the commonality among all social media sites is that the fundamental purpose is to become part of a social network through linkages with other members.

The popularity of Facebook in terms of sheer numbers has resulted in some profound shifts in the ways people think about and use technology in their daily lives. As early adopters of virtually all new technology, this is particularly true of children and youth. In part because of the rapidity of changes in popularity and availability of social media, even simple descriptive information is scarce. Currently, one of the primary sources for information regarding teen use of social media is the Pew Internet & American Life Surveys. They report that, in 2009, 93% of youth aged 12 to 17 years went online, and use of social networking sites among online youth has increased steadily from 55% in 2006, to 65% in 2008, to 73% in 2009.[38]

If social networking sites continue in their popularity among youth, there may be the potential for using such sites to promote healthy behaviors and positive health behavior change. There is emerging evidence that support from peers, friends, and family can have important influences on youth weight-related behaviors, including physical activity and eating patterns.[35,39–41] There is evidence that family support is important for both youth physical activity and eating habits,[39,42] that youth are more motivated to be physically active in the presence of friends, and that the presence of peers can increase overweight youth's motivation to be physically active.[40]

Among adults, there is evidence that social contexts have important influences on eating behaviors,[43] and that social support (including online groups with shared goals, such as Weight Watchers) can facilitate individual success of desired behavior change.[44] At present, the power or potential of social media as sites of prevention and intervention programs intended to influence youth behaviors related to obesity and weight status have not been fully investigated.

Yes, There's an App for That

The term app originated within the technology industry as an abbreviation of application. This meaning morphed into apps as additional functionalities, tools, and resources for smartphones. Today, apps are commonly understood as software applications designed for mobile technologies, including smartphones or tablet computers with specific operating systems (eg, iPhone, iPad, or Android apps).

In some sense, apps are the tweets of the programming world. Apps are characterized by small storage and memory demands, a concise and focused objective, and ease of use with little or no training required. Covering a wide variety of topics (eg, education, entertainment, business, social life, health, fitness, lifestyle), apps have rapidly become a mainstay of daily life. It is estimated that apps were downloaded more than 18.5 billion times by midyear 2011.[45,46] The number of apps to choose from is so vast (estimated at more than half a million among the different platforms[47]) that finding relevant apps, even if you know what you want, can be difficult. Despite, or because of, the constant influx of new apps, more than 70% of Android and iPhone users report downloading apps in the last 30 days,[48] and 60% and 68% of them, respectively, report using their apps multiple times daily.[49]

Apps for Nutrition, Physical Activity, and Weight Loss

Most apps relevant to weight-related behaviors, such as caloric intake, nutrition, physical activity, or fitness, are categorized as health care and fitness apps, at least by Apple. Of the 459,923 active apps available from Apple, just 2% are in this category. As of August 2011, there were 1504 paid and 629 free health care and fitness apps. Most of these apps are electronic versions of strategies known to be effective for weight loss, namely logging caloric intake and physical activity. Many of them are app versions of popular Web-based logging programs, such as My Fitness Pal, thus offering users more opportunities to log without having to sit down to a computer with an Internet connection. Despite the large number of apps promoting health and fitness now available, most target adults. Thus far, although there are some cooking and recipe apps (mainly designed for parents) related to cooking with healthy child-friendly recipes, apps specifically designed to appeal to children and youth with the goal of either healthy weight maintenance or weight loss are an untouched market. In addition, despite their popularity, the efficacy of apps related to nutrition, physical activity, or weight loss has not yet been empirically evaluated, although discussions of their potential have begun to emerge in the scientific literature.[50,51]

The Intersection of Apps and Biometric Sensors

Embedded sensors, particularly in smartphones, have proved essential to the development of mobile health programs. Microphones, cameras, gyroscopes, global positioning systems (GPS), digital compasses, pedometers, and accelerometers provide information regarding the user's activities and location that can be used to foster health. Data from body-worn sensors can also be combined with data collected from mobile device sensors to enhance the richness of the data and/or ease of data transmission. In an ongoing chronic disease management study (eCAALYX [Enhanced Complete Ambient Assisting Living Experiment]), data from physiologic sensors embedded in a smart garment worn by patients is combined with smartphone-based GPS data.[52]

Many available health and fitness apps use built-in features/characteristics of smartphones such as pedometers, accelerometers, or GPS readings, and/or link to such data provided by body-worn sensors. Wahoo Fitness apps rely on data collected via proprietary fitness sensors to track, record, and relay data on physical activity performance.[53] Research has indicated that a positive feedback loop based on behavior monitoring data could promote individuals to engage in healthy behavior.[54] For instance, it has been shown that Nike+ users who uploaded personal exercise data more than 5 times to the analytics portal are likely to be engaged in the data analytics feedback loop, which encourages them to continue exercising and data uploading.[55]

Depending on the app and the amount of data collected, data can be stored on the smartphone, a company Web site, or the cloud database, allowing either real-time analysis or analysis at any later time. Although currently of limited availability to the general public, mainly because of their high cost, health sensors measuring blood pressure, temperature, weight, and glucose are available using ANT technology. However, data collected from such sensors are continuously streaming from the moment of initiation to ending. Thus, there are potentially millions of data points per user, depending on the epoch or length of time between assessments. Efforts are underway to cope with the amount of such data and issues related to how to reduce these data in ways that are meaningful either at the individual or population level; this is now called the problem of big data.[56]

A Rare Opportunity: the Intersection of Social Media and Mobile Apps

Numerous apps invite users to track and/or share their geographic position while practicing a physical activity such as running, walking, or cycling through social media sites. Combining aspects of behavioral theories with technological advances, apps like Fit Friendzy rely on the power of social networks and connections to motivate exercise plans among youth patients; the app lets them connect with friends, share scores, and encourages them to join in multiple fitness challenges.

The intersection between social media and fitness apps providing data collected via the smartphone/linked device, or data reported by the user, provides a rich opportunity for both clinicians and scholars to understand the power and potential of various aspects common to health behavior change intervention and prevention programs. First, although most apps are designed to communicate and share data with real or virtual friends, relevant data collected by the app could also be shared with designated individuals, such as coaches or health care providers. The implications of the public aspect of information relayed via social media sites has yet to be examined. Unanswered, but possibly important, questions include whether keeping track of progress publically has some added benefit to keeping track of it privately. Does it matter who one's public is or who many of them are watching one's progress? What is the effect of reminders, likes, or cheers from family, friends, or strangers?

App Regulation

There is no current governmental regulation of apps, although this may change soon.[57] In July 2010, the US Food and Drug Administration (FDA), in collaboration with the Federal Communications Commission issued a joint statement in which they acknowledged the potential benefits of wireless medical technology advances for the US population but also the need for "clear regulatory pathways, processes, and standards to bring broadband and wireless-enabled medical devices to market."[57] Although some fear that the cost related to getting FDA approval might refrain innovation, others deplores the lack of regulation.[58] For the first time in February 2011, the FDA cleared a software application for use by physicians to view images and make medical diagnoses from their portable devices such as the iPhone or Android.[59] However, in the absence of federal guidelines, some in the industry have established their own criteria in which patient safety and privacy are not core concerns. For example, Apple decides whether apps will be offered to consumers in their App Store based on design, inoffensive content, and lack of technical flaws. Neither veracity of claims by the app developers nor evaluations of effectiveness/efficacy are considered.

SUMMARY AND IMPLICATIONS

In the last decade, the media landscape, and hence the role of media in the lives of children and youth, has undergone important changes. As the result of major technological and conceptual innovations, electronic media have become part of the fabric of daily life in previously unimagined ways. They are the backdrop against which people's lives are set. They are an endemic part of daily life, and, in many ways, they provide the foundation for a large number of daily activities. They are used for information, for entertainment, for relaxation, for stress relief, as a means of socializing, as a tool for household management, for shopping, for work, for communication, for scheduling. People turn to electronic media for company when they are alone. People turn to them when they are bored, when they are lonely, when they are tired, when they need solace, when they need information, when they need entertainment. People turn to them for a myriad of uses, and they use them without thinking much about it.

Although the popularity of these media, and the technologically and media-saturated world in which American children are growing up has fostered a great deal of debate, controversy, and general anguish among parents, practitioners, policy makers, and scholars,[60] they are here to stay. The huge popularity of social media and mobile technologies, especially among youth, may make them likely to provide a fruitful hub for treatment, intervention, and prevention efforts to address pediatric obesity. However, few have taken advantage of this possibility, and research on the feasibility and efficacy of doing so is almost nonexistent. Given the rapidity of their growth and popularity (against the backdrop of the slow and often protracted process of securing research funding), this is perhaps not surprising. However, we argue that at least some of the dearth of attention in this area is the result of other, more personal factors on the part of professionals, including ambivalence about the usefulness of such media,[60] and discomfort with new technologies (largely as a result of generational cohort). For most clinicians, practitioners, and scholars (including the authors), the technologies discussed in this article represent departures from those we grew up with. Many of us (until forced to by teenage children) have taken little advantage of even the capabilities of our cell phones. As a consequence, the use of these technologies as a tool for contact, treatment, practice, or research is often an afterthought for us; they simply do not come to mind. This omission is not shared by the children we are hoping to help in either primary or secondary intervention programs. Although surveys still clumsily ask how much children and youth use different kinds of devices, this will soon become irrelevant. In the near future, all televisions, computers, tablets, phones (and yet-to-be invented devices) will become touch-screen and Internet connected, and the choice of where to stream chosen content will simply be a matter of which device we are closest to at the moment.

Despite more than 30 years of both prevention and remediation, the prevalence of overweight and obesity among US youth has proved surprisingly intractable.[61,62] Although energy imbalance is often cited as the root cause for overweight and obesity, if equilibrium were easy to achieve, more children would have been helped to achieve it by now.[63] The reasons for this imbalance are complex and varied. Whatever the solution, because obesity in childhood tends to persist in adulthood,[64,65] the striking increase in the prevalence of childhood obesity since the 1980s will dramatically affect public health expenses, programs, and priorities well into the twenty-first century. Given the rate of technological innovation, it seems likely (even guaranteed) that previously unimagined media devices may change the future media landscape in unimagined ways many times over. Current and future generations of children will never know life without the Internet, Wi-Fi, computers, touch screens, tablets, or smartphones. They are technological natives, and we clinicians ignore (or reject) the possible power of these new media and technologies as a way for reaching them at our (and their) peril.

REFERENCES

1. Schmidt ME, Vandewater EA. Media and attention, cognition, and school achievement. Future Child 2008;18(1):63–85.
2. Rideout VJ, Foehr UG, Roberts DF. Generation M2: media in the lives of 8- to 18-year-olds. Menlo Park (CA): Kaiser Family Foundation; 2010.
3. Roberts DF, Foehr UG. Kids & media in America. New York: Cambridge University Press; 2004.
4. Teens and mobile phones over the past five years: Pew Internet looks back. Pew Internet & American Life Project. 2009. Available at: http://www.pewinternet.org/Reports/2009/14–Teens-and-Mobile-Phones-Data-Memo.aspx. Accessed August 11, 2011.
5. Teens and mobile phones. Pew Internet & American Life Project. Available at: http://www.pewinternet.org/Reports/2010/Teens-and-Mobile-Phones.aspx. Accessed August 11, 2011.
6. Krantz M. Do you "google"? Google, Inc; 2006. Available at: http://googleblog.blogspot.com/2006/10/do-you-google.html. Accessed February 17, 2010.
7. Bylund A. To google or not to google. MSNBC; 2006. Archived from the original on July 7, 2006. Available at: http://www.fool.com/investing/dividends-income/2006/07/05/to-google-or-not-to-google.aspx. Accessed February 17, 2010.
8. Apple Inc. Apple sells three million iPads in 80 days. 2010; Press release. Available at: http://www.apple.com/pr/library/2010/06/22Apple-Sells-Three-Million-iPads-in-80-Days.html. Accessed August 1, 2011.
9. Schmidt ME, Anderson DR. The impact of television on cognitive development and educational achievement. In: Pecora N, Murray JP, Wartella EA, editors. Children and television: fifty years of research. Mahaw (NJ): Lawrence Erlbaum Associates; 2006. p. 65–84.
10. Huston AC, Wright JC, Marquis J, et al. How young children spend their time: television and other activities. Dev Psychol 1999;35:912–25.
11. Chen JL, Kennedy CM. Television viewing and children's health. J Pediatr Nurs 2001;6:35–8.
12. Dietz WH. The obesity epidemic in young children: reduce television viewing and promote playing. BMJ 2001;322:313.
13. Gortmaker SL, Dietz WH, Sobol AM, et al. Increasing pediatric obesity in the United States. Am J Dis Child 1987;141:535–40.
14. Dietz WH, Gortmaker SL. Do we fatten our children at the television set? Obesity and television viewing in children and adolescents. Pediatrics 1985;75:807–12.
15. Gortmaker SL, Must A, Sobol AM, et al. Television viewing as a cause of increasing obesity among children in the United States, 1986-1990. Arch Pediatr Adolesc Med 1996;150:356.
16. American Academy of Pediatrics. Prevention of pediatric overweight and obesity. Pediatrics 2003;112:424–30.
17. Lee SJ, Bartolic S, Vandewater EA. Predicting children's media use in the US: differences in cross-sectional and longitudinal analyses. Br J Dev Psychol 2009;27:123–43.

18. Davison KK, Marshall SJ, Birch LL. Cross-sectional and longitudinal associations between TV viewing and girls' body mass index, overweight status, and percentage of body fat. J Pediatr 2006;149:32–7.

19. Marshall SJ, Biddle SJ, Gorley T, et al. Relationships between media use, body fatness and physical activity in children and youth: a meta-analysis. Int J Obes 2004;28:1238–46.

20. Pate RR, Freedson PS, Sallis JF, et al. Compliance with physical activity guidelines: prevalence in a population of children and youth. Ann Epidemiol 2002; 12(5):303–8.

21. Vandewater EA, Bickham DS, Lee JH. Time well spent? Relating media use to children's free-time activities. Pediatrics 2006;117:e181–5.

22. Hastings G, Stead M, McDermott L. From the billboard to the school canteen: how food promotion influences children. Education Review 2002;17:17–23.

23. Schor J. Born to buy: the commercialized child and the new consumer culture. New York: Scribner; 2005.

24. Institute of Medicine. Food marketing to children and youth: threat or opportunity? Washington, DC: National Academies Press; 2006.

25. Buijzen M, Schuurman J, Bomhof E. Associations between children's television advertising exposure and their food consumption patterns: a household diary-survey study. Appetite 2008;50(2–3):231–9.

26. Harris JL, Bargh JA, Brownell KD. Priming effects of television food advertising on eating behavior. Official Journal Of The Division Of Health Psychology, American Psychological Association. Health Psychol 2009;28(4):404–13.

27. Calvert SL. Children as consumers: advertising and marketing. Future Child 2008;18(1):205–34.

28. Borzekowski DL, Robinson TN. The 30 second effect: an experiment revealing the impact of television commercials on food preferences of preschoolers. J Am Diet Assoc 2001;101:42–6.

29. Taras H, Zive M, Nader P, et al. Television advertising and classes of food products consumed in a paediatric population. Int J Ad 2000;19:487–93.

30. Coon KA, Tucker K. Television and children's consumption patterns. A review of the literature. Minerva Pediatr 2002;54:423–36.

31. Barr-Anderson DJ, Larson NI, Nelson MC, et al. Does television viewing predict dietary intake five years later in high school students and young adults? Int J Behav Nutr Phys Act 2009;6:7.

32. Bryant JA, Sanders-Jackson A, Smallwood AM. IMing, text messaging, and adolescent social networks. J Comput Mediat Commun 2006;11(2):577–92.

33. Wolak J, Mitchell KJ, Finkelhor D. Close online relationships in a national sample of adolescents. Adolescence 2002;37:441–55.

34. Bargh JA, McKenna KY. The internet and social life. Annu Rev Clin Psychol 2004; 55:573–90.

35. McKenna KY, Bargh JA. Causes and consequences of social interaction on the internet: a conceptual framework. Media Psychol 1999;1:249–69.

36. Wolak J, Mitchell K, Finkelhor D. Unwanted and wanted exposure to online pornography in a national sample of youth internet users. Pedatrics 2007;119: 247–57.

37. Moreno MA, Vanderstoep A, Parks MR, et al. Reducing at-risk adolescents' display of risk behavior on a social networking web site: a randomized controlled pilot intervention trial. Arch Pediatr Adolesc Med 2009;163(1):35–41.

38. Lenhart A, Purcell K, Smith A, et al. Social media and mobile internet use among teens and young adults: Pew internet & American Life Project, Feb 3, 2010.

Available at: http://www.pewinternet.org/Reports/2010/Social-Media-and-Young-Adults.aspx. Accessed June 20, 2011.

39. Dowda M, Dishman RK, Pfeiffer KA, et al. Family support for physical activity in girls from 8th to 12th grade in South Carolina. Prev Med 2007;44(2):153–9.

40. Salvy S-J, Roemmich JN, Bowker JC, et al. Effect of peers and friends on youth physical activity and motivation to be physically active. J Pediatr Psychol 2009; 34(2):217–25.

41. Hume C, Timperio A, Salmon J, et al. Walking and cycling to school: predictors of increases among children and adolescents. Am J Prev Med 2009;36(3):195–200.

42. Rockett HR. Family dinner: more than just a meal. J Am Diet Assoc 2007;107(9): 1498–501.

43. French SA, Story M, Jeffery RW. Environmental influences on eating and physical activity. Annu Rev Public Health 2001;22:309–35.

44. Wright KB. Computer-mediated support groups: an examination of relationships among social support, perceived stress, and coping strategies. Comm Q 1999; 47:402–14.

45. Brodkin J. (2011). Network world. Google: 100 million android devices activated, 4.5 billion apps downloaded. Available at: http://www.networkworld.com/news/ 2011/051011-google-io.html. Accessed July 1, 2011.

46. Florin. (2011). Apple iOS stats: 200 million devices sold (25 million iPads), 14 billion apps downloaded, and more. Available at: Unwiredview.com; http:// www.unwiredview.com/2011/06/06/apple-ios-stats-200-million-devices-sold-25-million-ipads-14-billion-apps-downloaded-and-more. Accessed July 6, 2011.

47. Just how many Android tablet apps are there? Available at: http://pogue.blogs. nytimes.com/2011/07/01/mystery-how-many-android-tablet-apps/?scp=2&sq= 500,000appsforapple&st=cse. Accessed July 1, 2011.

48. NielsenWire. You have an app for that … now what? 2010. Available at: http:// blog.nielsen.com/nielsenwire/consumer/you-have-an-app-for-that-now-what. Accessed July 7, 2011.

49. NielsenWire. In US, smartphones now majority of new cellphone purchases. 2011. Available at: http://blog.nielsen.com/nielsenwire/online_mobile/in-us-smartphones-now-majority-of-new-cellphone-purchases. Accessed June 30, 2011.

50. Rao A, Hou P, Golnik T, et al. Evolution of data management tools for managing self-monitoring of blood glucose results: a survey of iPhone applications. J Diabetes Sci Technol 2010;4(4):949–57.

51. Atienza AA, Patrick K. Mobile health: the killer app for cyberinfrastructure and consumer health. Am J Prev Med 2011;40(5 Suppl 2):S151–3.

52. Boulos MN, Wheeler S, Tavares C, et al. How smartphones are changing the face of mobile and participatory healthcare: an overview, with example from eCAALYX. Biomed Eng Online 2011;10:24.

53. Wahoo Fitness. Available at: http://www.wahoofitness.com/Apps/Apps/Ready-for-Use-101-CL.aspx. Accessed June 20, 2011.

54. Webb TL, Sniehotta FF, Michie S. Using theories of behaviour change to inform interventions for addictive behaviours. Addiction (Abingdon, England) 2010; 105(11):1879–92.

55. McClusky M. The Nike experiment: how the shoe giant unleashed the power of personal metrics. Available at: http://www.wired.com/medtech/health/magazine/ 17-07/lbnp_nike?currentPage=all. Accessed October 25, 2010.

56. Forman MR, Greene SM, Avis NE, et al. Bioinformatics: tools to accelerate population science and disease control research. Am J Prev Med 2010;38(6): 646–51.

57. US Food and Drug Administration and Federal Communications Commission. 2010. Joint statement on wireless medical devices. Available at: http://hraunfoss. fcc.gov/edocs_public/attachmatch/DOC-300200A1.pdf.
58. Medical smartphone apps may need new federal regulation. (2010). Available at: e-week.com; http://www.eweek.com/c/a/Health-Care-IT/Medical-Smartphone-Apps-May-Need-New-Federal-Regulation-607844. Accessed July 3, 2011.
59. US Food and Drug Administration. Press release. FDA clears first diagnostic radiology application for mobile devices. 2011. Available at: http://www.fda.gov/NewsEvents/Newsroom/PressAnnouncements/ucm242295.htm. Accessed July 3, 2011.
60. Strasburger VC, Jordan AB, Donnerstein E. Health effects of media on children and adolescents. Pediatrics 2010;125(4):756–67.
61. Huang TT, Drewnosksi A, Kumanyika S, et al. A systems-oriented multilevel framework for addressing obesity in the 21st century. Prev Chronic Dis 2009;6(3):A82.
62. Glass TA, McAtee MJ. Behavioral science at the crossroads in public health: extending horizons, envisioning the future. Soc Sci Med 2006;62(7):1650–71.
63. Robinson TN. Treating pediatric obesity: generating the evidence. Arch Pediatr Adolesc Med 2008;162(12):1191–2.
64. Must A, Jacques PF, Dallal GE, et al. Long-term morbidity and mortality of overweight adolescents: a follow-up of the Harvard Growth Study 1922 to 1935. N Engl J Med 1992;327:1350–5.
65. Must A. Morbidity and mortality associated with elevated body weight in children and adolescents. Am Soc Clin Nutr 1996;63:445S.

Policies to Support Obesity Prevention for Children: A Focus on of Early Childhood Policies

Marianne E. McPherson, MS, PhD*, Charles J. Homer, MD, MPH

KEYWORDS

- Childhood obesity prevention • Healthy weight • Policy
- Early childhood • Advocacy • Health care professionals

The epidemic of childhood obesity is one of the most urgent health challenges facing our nation today. Obesity rates among the nation's children have tripled in the past 30 years.[1] As of 2008, more than 30% of children aged 2 to 19 years had a body mass index (BMI) at or above the 85th percentile for their age.[2] Individuals make choices that influence their weight (or that of their children, especially in the case of very young children), including what and how much they eat and their participation in physical activity. Interventions to influence those choices and thus promote healthy weight exist on two broad levels: individual-level strategies such as clinical counseling on healthy weight and population-level strategies to shape the environment in which people make choices that influence their weight status, for example, providing safe places for children to play outside or access to affordable fresh fruits and vegetables.

Promoting environments whereby the healthy choice is the easy choice for individuals is the realm of environmental systems change. Landmark national initiatives, both in the public and private sectors, have promoted and funded policy and environmental change strategies for obesity prevention. Examples include the Centers for Disease Control and Prevention's (CDC's) Communities Putting Prevention to Work Initiative funded by the American Reinvestment and Recovery Act and the childhood obesity initiatives of the Robert Wood Johnson Foundation.[3,4] Enacting and protecting policies that promote healthy environments and thus support individuals in making healthier choices are levers for positively altering the environment in which individuals make the choices influencing their weight.

The authors have nothing to disclose.
National Initiative for Children's Healthcare Quality, 30 Winter Street, 6th Floor, Boston, MA 02108, USA
* Corresponding author.
E-mail address: mmcpherson@nichq.org

Both the environment potentially affecting obesity and the policies potentially affecting the environment are expansive categories. Policies exist, and therefore policy change may happen on a variety of levels, from worksite, to community, state, national, and even international levels. The environment affecting obesity can mean myriad specific contexts, including but not limited to the following: food policy and farm support, the built environment (ie, how buildings, roads, and communities are physically designed and built, including sidewalks and bike paths for streets or accessible stairways for buildings), transportation, schools and early child care centers and worksites, and the environment in which clinical care takes place (eg, fast food in children's hospitals, formula samples in newborn nurseries).

Given the potential for policy change to promote healthy environments and the broad definition of the environment described earlier, this article focuses on the example of early childhood-related policies as a window on policies to support obesity prevention. We include a discussion of policy on more macro, public levels such as federal or state policy and legislation as well as more micro, often private levels such as institutional and worksite policies. To further structure our discussion of areas of environment, we incorporate elements of the pillars and framework set forth in the 2010 White House Task Force on Childhood Obesity Report to the President.[5] We include a discussion of (1) breastfeeding as an example of an early childhood-specific issue, (2) providing healthy affordable food and information about food in community and child care settings, and (3) increasing physical activity. We also include information on the role of the health care sector using the example of promoting body mass screening and monitoring and highlight recommendations from a recent Institute of Medicine (IOM) report on early childhood prevention policies.[6] We also make the case for pediatricians and other pediatric health care providers to take an active role in policy advocacy and feature resources for advocacy.

IMPORTANCE OF EARLY CHILDHOOD-RELATED POLICIES AND PROMOTING BREASTFEEDING

As of 2008, nearly 10% of infants and toddlers (birth through age 2 years) were at or above the 95th percentile of weight for length, and more than 20% of children aged 2 to 5 years were overweight or obese (BMI of 85% or more).[2] A variety of expert committees, including the IOM and the White House Task Force on Childhood Obesity, have emphasized the importance of early childhood as a unique opportunity for prevention of childhood obesity.[5,6]

Early childhood contrasts to other periods of childhood and adulthood in the potential to establish positive healthy weight behaviors rather than needing to reverse or alter existing negative behaviors. The environment in which children spend their first years of life as well as the individuals who care for them (parents and other primary caregivers such as day care providers and extended family) and the environmental choices available to those caregivers influence children's developing behaviors and habits related to physical activity and eating and may help to shape developmental pathways to positively (or negatively) affect long-term risk of obesity and associated chronic diseases.[6]

Overview of Policy Opportunities in Early Care and Education Settings

Nationally, nearly 6 million children younger than 5 years, representing nearly 30% of American children, are enrolled in child care (including home day care) facilities, and they spend an average of more than 30 hours per week in these facilities.[7] Child care environments and the caregivers and teachers who staff them may contribute significantly to shaping children's emerging patterns for eating and drinking, participating in physical activity, and having screen time. States vary widely in their regulations for nutrition and physical activity, presenting an opportunity for strengthening and unifying licensing requirements for requiring healthier food, more physical activity, and less screen time.[8,9]

Regarding screen time, the American Academy of Pediatrics (AAP) recommends no television viewing for children younger than 2 years and limiting total media time to no more than 1 to 2 hours per day of quality programming for children aged 2 years and older.[10] Taking this recommendation to the child care setting, the IOM has recommended that "adults working with children should limit screen time, including television, cell phone, or digital media, to less than two hours per day for children aged two to five."[6(Rec.5-1)] There is a policy opportunity for regulations affecting child care centers to align with these recommendations as well as for academic training curricula for providers (undergraduate, graduate, and continuing education) to be modified to include current guidelines.

In 2011, a consortium of leading clinical and governmental organizations, including the AAP, the American Public Health Association, and the Maternal and Child Health Bureau released a revised set of evidence-based and expert consensus national standards for nutrition, physical activity, and screen time in all early care settings. These standards include age-specific nutrition requirements for infants, toddlers, and preschoolers; standards on food brought from home, meal service and supervision, nutrition education, and nutrition policies; standards concerning opportunities for physical activity and playtime; and guidelines for limiting screen time. The investigators also included suggested uses of these standards for families, caregivers and teachers, healthcare professionals, regulators, early childhood systems, policymakers, and academic faculty of early childhood programs.[11] Connecting quality improvement to policy, if these standards around nutrition, physical activity, and screen time are prominently included in regulatory and/or quality rating systems for child care facilities, and if those ratings systems influence payment to or licensing of facilities, the standards take on increased policy import.

Promoting Breastfeeding

The White House Task Force highlighted concerns specific to early childhood as one of its pillars, including the example of breastfeeding promotion. Breastfeeding may be protective against subsequent obesity for the breastfed infant.[12–14] In 2010, 75% of US mothers initiated breastfeeding, but only 13% were exclusively breastfeeding their infants at six months (43% any breastfeeding). These rates also reveal substantial geographic and racial/ethnic disparities.[15,16] Healthy People 2020 established targets for 82% of infants to be breastfed, 61% breastfed through six months, and 26% exclusively breastfed through six months.[17] These goals are aligned with recommendations of the AAP, the World Health Organization, the American College of Obstetricians and Gynecologists, the US Preventive Services Task Force, and the IOM to encourage exclusive breastfeeding through 6 months of life.[6,18–20]

Environments that may have a key role in promoting breastfeeding include clinical settings (both regarding prenatal care and the facility at which a baby is born and spends his/her first days of life) for supporting breastfeeding initiation in the immediate postpartum. In addition, community environments such as worksites and child care centers may support exclusive breastfeeding through 6 months and breastfeeding continuing through at least 1 year of life.

Promoting baby-friendly hospitals

The environment in which mothers deliver their infants and where the infants spend their first few days of life exerts a disproportionately large influence on the likelihood that the mothers will initiate breastfeeding and continue to breastfeed their infants (at all and exclusively) for an extended period. The World Health Organization identified and codified a set of practices, the Ten Steps to Successful Breastfeeding, through the Baby-Friendly Hospital Initiative, which characterize hospital environments that promote breastfeeding (**Box 1**).[19,21–23] Baby-Friendly USA provides the baby-friendly designation to hospitals demonstrating that they undertake the Ten Steps.

Aligned with the Ten Steps, Healthy People 2020 set goals of reducing the proportion of breastfed infants who receive formula supplementation within the first 2 days of life from 24% to 14% and increasing the proportion of live births that occur in facilities providing the recommended care for breastfeeding mothers and their babies from 3% to 8%.[17] Yet the CDC recently reported that 95% of hospitals lack maternity care policies to fully support breastfeeding mothers and their infants.[24] (There is some debate surrounding exclusive breastfeeding and formula restriction in hospitals in response to the Joint Commission's inclusion of exclusive breastfeeding in its 2011 perinatal core measures set.[25] The investigators of a recent commentary in *Pediatrics* argued that providing small amounts of formula supplementation in the hospital may actually increase mothers' breastfeeding self-efficacy. They questioned whether entirely restricting formula and including exclusive breastfeeding as a quality indicator truly are warranted; their position prompted follow-up debate.[26–28])

A variety of policy-level interventions may promote baby-friendly hospitals and elements of the Ten Steps, from the micro level of a particular hospital undertaking the Ten Steps to national initiatives that promote regional or nationwide uptake of baby-friendly policies. In addition to recommending the creation and enforcement of specific policies at the hospital level, the Ten Steps speak of opportunities to train

---

Box 1
The ten steps to successful breastfeeding

1. Maintain a written breastfeeding policy that is routinely communicated to all health care staff.

2. Train all health care staff in skills necessary to implement this policy.

3. Inform all pregnant women about the benefits and management of breastfeeding.

4. Help mothers initiate breastfeeding within 1 hour of birth.

5. Show mothers how to breastfeed and how to maintain lactation, even if they are separated from their infants.

6. Give infants no food or drink other than breast milk, unless medically indicated.

7. Practice "rooming in," allowing mothers and infants to remain together 24 hours a day.

8. Encourage unrestricted breastfeeding.

9. Give no pacifiers or artificial nipples to breastfeeding infants.

10. Foster the establishment of breastfeeding support groups, and refer mothers to them on discharge from the hospital or clinic.

From World Health Organization. Evidence for the ten steps to successful breastfeeding. Geneva, Switzerland; World Health Organization, 1998; with permission.

health care staff in supporting breastfeeding and of establishing supports and connections after hospital discharge to provide linkage between the clinical and community environments. Specific policies at the organizational level may require these supports and training elements as well as specifically build them into individual accreditation requirements. In addition, health plans or government could play a role in policy change by offering enhanced financial incentives in the way of higher payment levels to hospitals that meet thresholds of exclusive breastfeeding or to facilities that achieve the baby-friendly designation, either directly or through incorporation of such practices into organizational accreditation processes.

Promoting breastfeeding in the community, including worksites and child care centers

Beyond the immediate postpartum, community and workplace environments may support mothers and infants in sustaining exclusive breastfeeding through the recommended 6 months and breastfeeding through 1 year of life. Regarding health policy and health insurance, the Department of Health and Human Services has adopted recommendations from the IOM requiring new health plans to cover costs of breastfeeding support, supplies (eg, breastfeeding equipment such as pumps), and counseling without cost sharing to mothers, beginning in August 2012.[29–31]

The work environment may support nursing mothers who return to work. When the Patient Protection and Affordable Care Act (ie, national health reform) was passed in 2010,[32] standards went into effect setting standards for worksites regarding breastfeeding. Specifically, the Affordable Care Act amended Section 7 of the Fair Labor Standards Act to require that worksites provide nursing mothers with sufficient break time and a clean private place that is not a bathroom to nurse or to express breast milk through the first year of a child's life.[33] In addition to worksites, child care facilities may support breastfeeding by providing places for women to nurse or to express breast milk, providing sufficient storage for breast milk, and training staff on supporting breastfeeding. These requirements may be reinforced through organizational policies and/or regulatory quality standards.

The IOM has recommended that "adults who work with infants and their families should promote and support exclusive breastfeeding for six months and continuation of breastfeeding in conjunction with complementary foods for one year or more."[6(Rec. 4-1)] This includes policies promoting baby-friendly initiatives; ensuring that public health staff, such as in the Women, Infants, and Children (WIC) program receive training in breastfeeding support; regulating how hospitals' promotional materials show first feeding and whether they may supply formula in newborn nurseries; and promoting supportive worksite policies. The Wisconsin Department of Health has developed the *Ten Steps to Breastfeeding-Friendly Childcare Centers Resource Kit*, a guide for centers to use in revising their own policies to support breastfeeding.[34] Regulatory bodies might include standards from this or similar guides in quality rankings.

Health plans again may take a role in policy change by providing sufficient reimbursement for continued breastfeeding counseling or by providing higher levels of reimbursement to pediatric practices that demonstrate improvement in breastfeeding support practices or outcomes, such as a meeting a certain threshold for breastfeeding or exclusive breastfeeding in their patient populations (accounting for case mix). Ideally, were health plans to implement such policies, they would partner with community agencies and organizations to support community-level programs and policies enabling mothers to sustain breastfeeding.[35]

At the local level, there are many opportunities to foster community environments supportive of breastfeeding. Local governments may strengthen and promote networks such as La Leche League and Nursing Mother's Councils via increased funding or public awareness campaigns or by providing space in municipal facilities for these groups to meet. These governments may enact, publicize, and enforce and monitor policies on how community facilities support breastfeeding (eg, incentives for restaurants that post breastfeeding-friendly signage). Additional policy opportunities include working with local health departments to expand programs that provide breastfeeding support in communities, such as the WIC Breastfeeding Peer Counseling program, Early Head Start, and home visitation programs.[5,6]

PROVIDING HEALTHY AFFORDABLE FOOD AND INFORMATION ABOUT FOOD IN COMMUNITY AND CHILD CARE SETTINGS

Children set patterns for eating in early childhood that carry through their lives. Yet, according to a 2011 report from the IOM, most young children do not eat nutritious diets.[6] Early childhood is an optimal period for providing children with a range of healthy foods because young children with early experiences eating a variety of healthy foods are more likely to continue to eat those foods subsequently.[36] Thus, the choices their caregivers have to improve nutrition choices in community settings and in the child care environment can set young children on a positive trajectory for healthy weight. A variety of environmental and policy factors related to healthy food may shape the food choices available to families and child care providers, which, in turn, may enable parents and caregivers to positively shape young children's eating environments by having the healthy choice be the easy choice in their environments.

Federal Food Assistance Programs and Food Access

Federal food assistance programs potentially affecting young children and their families include the Supplemental Nutrition Assistance Program (SNAP, more than one-quarter of US children will have enrolled in SNAP between birth and age 5 years), the Special Supplemental Nutrition Program for the WIC (serves more than 9 million women, infants, and children), the Child and Adult Care Food Program (CACFP, serves more than 3 million children), the WIC Farmers' Market Nutrition Program (serves more than 2 million WIC participants), and the Emergency Food Assistance Program.[37–40] Additional programs such as the School Breakfast Program, National School Lunch Program, and Summer Food Service Program focus on school-aged children.[6(pp4–15),37] The IOM recommends that government agencies promote access to healthy affordable foods by "maximizing participation in federal nutrition assistance programs and increasing access to healthy foods at the community level."[6(Rec.4-5)]

The neighborhood food environment, including both availability of healthy food in a family's environment and ease of access to those foods, influences a family's nutrition choices.[38] Supermarkets tend to provide the greatest variety of high-quality healthy food at the lowest cost, in contrast to convenience stores, which tend to offer more processed food and less fresh produce and at higher cost. Review of research demonstrates that better access to supermarkets is associated with healthier diet and possibly with lower rates of obesity.[39] Easy access to supermarkets may be particularly important for caregivers with young children. In those families, an errand to get food may be even more difficult when it entails one or more strollers, diaper bags, and/or highly active preschoolers in tow. Bringing access to these children and their families is thus even more important. According to the US Department of Agriculture's (USDA's) report on food deserts, 23.5 million people, including 6.5 million children, live in low-income areas more than 1 mile from a supermarket or larger grocery store.[5,40] Currently, the US Departments of the Treasury, Agriculture, and Health and Human

Services are collaborating to develop common evaluation measures of impacts of food deserts and of efforts to eliminate them.[41] These same 3 federal agencies comprise the Healthy Food Financing Initiative, which includes a variety of programs such as funding of private sector financing for healthy food options and promoting economic development in rural areas. The initiative aims to fund the creation of healthy food options and to work toward eliminating food deserts in underserved urban and rural communities nationwide.[42]

There are a variety of policy incentives and disincentives on multiple levels of government that may influence access to affordable healthy foods in communities. Indeed, there are actions community members themselves can take, working in partnerships with local governments. These members may, for example, work to bring supermarkets to underserved neighborhoods (eg, work to lower insurance premiums in neighborhoods where high premiums discourage chain supermarkets from opening a store), help convenience stores increase their supply of fresh produce, or ease permitting requirements to attract farmers' markets, farm stands, or mobile vendors into a community.[5]

Citizens and local governments also may create food policy councils for joint work on healthy food access. An area of policy in which they may work is land use and food planning urban policy to promote zoning and planning conducive to urban agriculture such as community gardens. The White House Task Force documented several examples of such policies: Vendors in Kansas City who sell healthy foods pay a reduced permit fee, New York City uses a combination of incentives and restrictions to get green produce carts in areas of the city with the least access to fresh fruits and vegetables, and Detroit and Cleveland have reclaimed acres of vacant land and lots for community gardens.[5(p53)]

Additional examples of food access policy change are on the level of the clinic/worksite setting, as we further describe in the section on dietary guidelines. Aligned with the IOM's recommendation, pediatric providers may encourage their hospital or worksite "to implement policies and practices consistent with the Dietary Guidelines, to promote healthy foods and beverages and reduce or eliminate the availability of calorie-dense, nutrient-poor foods."[6(Rec. 4-6)]

Food Marketing

Very young children are the target audience of significant and increasing food marketing,[43] and research has demonstrated that such marketing influences their preferences. For instance, young children may be more likely to choose food products featuring cartoon characters on the package.[44] National-level initiatives, both government-based, such as the 2006 Joint Task Force on Media and Childhood Obesity, and industry self-regulation attempts, such as the 2006 Children's Food and Beverage Advertising Initiative (CFBAI) of the Council of Better Business Bureaus, restricting marketing or even developing consensus-based nutrition standards have had challenges moving forward. The Joint Task Force was unable to agree on a uniform set of nutritional standards or on how media companies would be required to enforce advertising limits, and the Federal Trade Commission (FTC) released a report in 2008 recommending several enhancements to the standards set by the CFBAI (eg, originally, the standards applied only to certain forms of advertising; FTC criticized the quality and consistency of the nutritional standards).[5,45] The CFBAI did release a new agreement in July 2011 regarding regulating marketing and advertising directed at children.[46]

The FTC is limited in its ability to restrict food marketing to children because of free speech considerations. In 2011, the FTC created draft voluntary standards as required by Congress (the comment period for which closed in July), prompting mixed reactions from a variety of stakeholders from industry to public health. The Alliance for American Advertising opposed the standards, claiming that they would restrict advertising to adults in addition to children, would contain unnecessarily restrictive nutrition principles, were presented in the absence of an open process or supporting research evidence from the Working Group, would not pass a First Amendment analysis, and would eliminate thousands of jobs in their industry.[47] The Public Health Law Center strongly supported the standards and proposed revisions to further strengthen them, including providing uniform standards for what constitutes marketing or targeted to children and teenagers.[48]

Despite these challenges, the IOM continues to recommend that "the Federal Trade Commission, the U.S. Department of Agriculture, Centers for Disease Control and Prevention, and the Food and Drug Administration should continue their work to establish and monitor the implementation of uniform voluntary national nutrition and marketing standards for food and beverage products marketed to children."[6(Rec.5-3)] Separate from national-level regulatory efforts, local governments or worksites may establish policies to restrict food marketing directed at children. School systems, for example, may regulate commercial advertising from sugar-sweetened beverage companies.

Food Pricing

In addition to physical access to healthy food and food marketing, pricing of healthy food (both in the absolute and relative pricing of unhealthy foods) may drive families' purchasing choices. Research has demonstrated that families will purchase healthier foods when the prices of those foods are reduced, and they will decrease purchase of healthier foods as those prices increase.[49,50] According to the White House Task Force Report, the price of fruits and vegetables has increased nearly twice as fast as the price of carbonated beverages over the last 30 years.[5] Areas of policy influence on food pricing include agriculture policy, tax policy, and subsidy policy.

Agriculture policy

Regarding agriculture policy, nearly all agriculture subsidies to farmers are for 5 crops: soybeans, corn, rice, wheat, and cotton. Agriculture subsidies thus do not tend to promote lower prices for a range of crops that might, in turn, support a well-balanced diet for families. For the first time, the Food, Conservation, and Energy Act of 2008 (also known as the Farm Bill) did include $1.3 billion in new funding over 10 years for so-called specialty crops including fruits, vegetables, and nuts, which have higher production costs than the 5 most heavily subsidized crops,[51] and increased funding for programs that support local agriculture and healthy foods.[5]

In terms of food supply, the USDA's Economic Research Service has estimated the changes in agriculture that would be required to supply Americans to meet the 2010 Dietary Guidelines, and these changes are vast. USDA estimates that fruit production would have to increase by 117%, representing an additional 4.1 million acres; vegetable production would need to increase by 18% or 19.4 billion pounds per year; and farm milk production would have to increase approximately 108 billion pounds per year to meet potential demand for milk and milk products.[52]

In terms of agriculture policy, perhaps the most significant piece of Federal legislation is the Farm Bill. Set to expire in 2012, this legislation has potentially far-reaching implications for obesity prevention and public health efforts on the policy and environmental systems level because it includes provisions for nutrition, farm commodity support, conservation, crop insurance, livestock, and energy and forestry. The

Food, Conservation, and Energy Act of 2008 included $284 billion over 5 years and $604 billion over 10 years; 67% of those funds went toward nutrition provisions. Health-related initiatives in the 2008 bill included those related to distribution and access (eg, Farmers' Market Promotion Program), production practices, research (eg, a national study on food deserts[40]), education, and affordability and pricing. The anticipated reauthorization of this bill in 2012 thus represents a significant opportunity for public health coalition building around obesity prevention provisions, including those to benefit young children and their families.[51]

Tax policy: example of sugar-sweetened beverages
In addition to agriculture policy, tax policy relevant to food and beverage influences food pricing and may influence families' choices on food purchasing. The most current and hotly debated example is that of possible taxes on sugar-sweetened beverages. Nearly 60% of children aged 2 and 3 years drink at least one serving of 100% fruit juice in a day, and 46% drink sweetened beverages, including fruit-flavored drinks, soda, coffee, or tea.[53] The second largest source of energy in the diet of 2- and 3-year-old children is 100% fruit juice.[54] Researchers and policy advocates have proposed a penny-per-ounce tax on sugar-sweetened beverages. According to recently published modeling data from Yale's Rudd Center, a nationwide penny-per-ounce tax on sugar-sweetened beverages could bring in nearly $80 billion in revenue between 2010 and 2015, and this figure would increase to $118 billion if the tax included diet varieties of these beverages. In addition, they estimated that this tax could result in a 24% decrease in sugar-sweetened beverage consumption over this same period.[55]

Subsidy policy
An alternative policy approach to taxes on unhealthy food or beverages is subsidy policy to encourage families' purchasing and consumption of healthy food such as fresh fruits and vegetables. Some research has shown that subsidies do affect increased consumption of healthier foods. In one study, a 50% price reduction on fresh fruit and baby carrots in 2 secondary school cafeterias resulted in a 4-fold increase in fresh fruit sales and a 2-fold increase in baby carrot sales.[56] Emerging evidence suggests that programs such as the CACFP that subsidize nutritious meals in child care and other school settings may be associated with healthier weight, eg, with lower BMI.[37] Additional examples of subsidy programs are those such as Wholesome Wave's Double Value Coupon Program, which operates in 26 states and offers incentives for families to use their SNAP electronic benefit transfer cards to purchase fresh fruits and vegetables at farmers' markets.[57,58]

Dietary Guidelines

One area of environmental systems influence is the degree to which worksites, communities, and government programs disseminate and/or adopt nutritional standards and guidelines in their institutional policies. In 2010, the USDA and the Department of Health and Human Services released new Dietary Guidelines for Americans reflecting updated nutrition standards and thus providing up-to-date nutrition information for organizations or programs to use in policies they implement.[59] The reach of these programs (and therefore the policies guiding them) potentially is vast in terms of the number of children they serve. On the federal level alone, the SNAP (formerly Food Stamps) is one of several programs required to apply the Dietary Guidelines. One-half of all American children will participate in SNAP at some point during their childhood up to age 20 years, including 90% of African American children; more than a quarter of children will participate in SNAP between birth and age 5 years.[60]

Even outside of federal programs such as the SNAP, programs at the state, local, and even worksite level may adopt policies requiring that their programs adhere to federal dietary guidelines. A network of health care facilities, for example, may set a policy that its hospital cafeterias follow the Dietary Guidelines in its hospital cafeterias, eliminate fast food from its facilities, and also fund signage and other educational information for its patients on how to make healthier food choices. The 2010 Dietary Guidelines begin at age 2 years, and the IOM has recommended that future editions establish guidelines for children from birth to age 2 years.[6(Rec. 4-3)]

Access to Healthy Food in Child Care Centers

The Healthy, Hunger-Free Kids Act was enacted in December 2010 and represents landmark legislation particularly affecting school-aged children. In school-aged populations, the act included increasing access to universal free school meals, giving USDA authority to set nutritional standards for all foods regularly sold in schools during the school day and increasing funding to schools that meet updated nutritional standards. The act also contains important provisions affecting young children, including revisions to the CACFP and the WIC. Regarding CACFP, the act requires that nutrition standards must now comply with the new 2010 Dietary Guidelines; it enhances USDA training, providing technical assistance and educational materials available to child care providers in helping them to serve healthier food; authorizes research regarding implementation of healthy eating and wellness practices in child care settings, including barriers and facilitators to implementation; and expands eligibility and simplifies program requirements. Provisions related to the WIC include allowing WIC agencies to certify children for eligibility for 1 year rather than 6 months, promoting breastfeeding by expanding collection of WIC breastfeeding data and making funds available for purchase of breast pumps, and increasing WIC funding for infrastructure and research.[41,61,62]

PROMOTING PHYSICAL ACTIVITY IN CHILD CARE AND THE COMMUNITY

Physical activity represents another critical piece in the healthy weight equation, including fostering environments that are safe for and promoting of physical activity for young children and their families. National guidelines that advocate for increased physical activity as a strategy for obesity prevention include the 2010 Dietary Guidelines for Americans, The Surgeon General's Vision for a Healthy and Fit Nation, and the 2008 Physical Activity Guidelines for Americans (which start at age 6 years).[59,63,64] The IOM reported that many children younger than 5 years do not meet physical activity guidelines set by expert panels.[6] Further, this IOM panel recommended the following 3 goals for promoting physical activity in young children: (1) to increase young children's levels of physical activity, (2) to decrease their levels of sedentary behavior, and (3) to help adults adopt policies to accomplish the first 2 goals. The panel further recommended a variety of strategies to further these goals in the child care environment, which we overview in **Table 1**. These strategies included institutional-level and perhaps regulatory policies for providing indoor and outdoor play environments with adequate space per child and for promoting active time and limiting sitting or standing time in preschoolers and toddlers, as well as education-level policy changes to include curriculum content for early childhood providers on physical activity in young children.

Promoting Physical Activity in the Community

There are a variety of environmental and policy strategies to promote physical activity for young children in the community. One set of strategies relates to the community's

Table 1
Physical activity-related strategies to promote in the child care environment

Goal and Associated IOM Recommendation	Strategies in Child Care Settings
Increase physical activity in young children IOM Rec. 3-1: child care regulatory agencies should require child care providers and early childhood educators to provide infants, toddlers, and preschool children with opportunities to be physically active throughout the day	• Provide indoor and outdoor play environments at child care centers with adequate space per child and a variety of portable play equipment (note: centers currently vary in the degree to which their outdoor play spaces meet national physical activity and safety standards[65]) • Create environments that provide opportunities for children with disabilities to be physically active • Establish policies in child care centers promoting daily "tummy time" for infants younger than 6 y and opportunities for 15 min/h of physical activity for toddlers and preschoolers
Decrease sedentary behavior in young children IOM Rec. 3-3: child care regulatory agencies should require child care providers and early childhood educators to allow infants, toddlers, and preschoolers to move freely by limiting the use of equipment that restricts infants' movement and by implementing appropriate strategies to ensure that the amount of time toddlers and preschoolers spend sitting or standing still is limited	• Establish policies that limit sitting or standing activities for toddlers and preschoolers to a maximum of 30 min at a time • Establish policies for the use of strollers for toddlers and preschoolers only when necessary
Help adults increase young children's physical activity and decrease their levels of sedentary behavior IOM Rec. 3–4: Health and education professionals providing guidance to parents of young children and those working with young children should be trained in ways to increase children's physical activity and decrease their sedentary behavior, and in how to counsel parents about their children's physical activity	• Include content in undergraduate and graduate educational programs for early childhood professionals on increasing physical activity and decreasing sedentary behavior • Provide continuing education opportunities for providers on increasing physical activity and decreasing sedentary behavior in young children • Encourage child care regulatory agencies to establish policies fostering yearly consultation between centers and an early childhood experts on physical activity

Data from Committee on Obesity Prevention Policies for Young Children, Institute of Medicine. Early childhood obesity prevention policies. In: Birch LL, Parker L, Burns A, editors. Washington, DC: The National Academies Press; 2011. Available at: http://www.iom.edu/Reports/2011/Early-Childhood-Obesity-Prevention-Policies.aspx. Accessed July 21, 2011.

built environment, because the design of our communities may promote or inhibit physical activity. The built environment includes "spaces such as buildings and streets that are deliberately constructed as well as outdoor spaces that are altered in some way by human activity."[66(p1592)] Urban sprawl has been shown to be associated with obesity.[67] Conversely, communities that are more walkable and bikeable, with policies and funding for complete streets that promote safe transportation for pedestrians of all ages and abilities (including pedestrians pushing strollers or in wheelchairs), cyclists, public transportation, and cars,[68] may promote physical activity and therefore healthy weight. Neighborhood design and urban planning policies may increase incidental physical activity or the likelihood that a family will walk to the store or that their children will walk to school rather than ride in a car.[66] The IOM recommends that "the community and its built environment should promote physical activity for children from birth to age five"[6(Rec. 3-2)] in indoor and outdoor settings and for young children with a range of abilities.

In addition to the built environment, it is important to consider the social environment, that is, "how community members feel about their neighborhood, its safety, and their interest in participating in community-based physical activity."[5(p79)] For example, outdoor play environments such as community parks and playgrounds increase children's level of physical activity during unstructured time.[69] Children are more likely to use these facilities if they are easy and safe to access and if the sites, themselves, are safe and in good repair.[70] Across the country, there are disparities in access to safe places to play according to the socioeconomic position of the community and its residents.[66] Community members may work together with law enforcement, parks and recreation, and local governments to enhance safety and access to community facilities.

Another strategy for promoting physical activity for young children and families in the community is promoting the establishment of joint use agreements, which allow community members and programs to use schools' physical activity facilities during nonschool hours. According to the White House Task Force Report, as of 2010, 65% of schools allowed for joint use agreements.[5] The National Policy and Legal Analysis Network to Prevent Childhood Obesity offers a state-by-state analysis of state laws that affect joint use agreements that communities may apply in their efforts to implement these agreements.[71]

THE ROLE OF HEALTH CARE POLICY AND PEDIATRIC HEALTH CARE PROFESSIONALS
Role of Health Care Policy

Throughout this piece, we have considered a full range of policies that influence healthy weight, focusing on early childhood. We also have included a variety of examples of the roles for health care policy and health care professionals both inside and outside the clinic, including in clinical training (eg, staff education to support breast-feeding), the community environment (eg, partnering in the community to advance environmental changes), and clinical practice (eg, helping patients and families navigate community resources for obesity prevention). These examples are consistent with the recommendations of both a 2008 report by Simpson and colleagues[75] on the role of health policy in reversing childhood obesity and an article by Dietz and colleagues[35] regarding opportunities for health plans to engage in promoting environments and policies that support healthy weight.[72] An additional opportunity for health care sector involvement is in promoting BMI screening in the clinic and community.

BMI Screening

At the individual level, providing parents with information regarding their child's weight status via BMI may more effectively enable parents and caregivers to make healthy weight-promoting choices for their children. Research reviews have documented that parents whose children are at risk for or are overweight often misjudge their child's weight status (ie, not perceive that their child is at risk for or is overweight) and that parental involvement increases the effectiveness of obesity prevention.[73,74] Although BMI monitoring and clinical counseling programs (eg, the High Five for

Kids and LEAP 2 randomized trials) in isolation from other community efforts are not effective in reducing BMI,[75,76] at population levels, from schools to communities states, and nationally, current and updated BMI data will more effectively enable those communities to provide adequate services for obesity prevention and treatment of children and families. BMI screening can empower parents and caregivers with clear and actionable information and, when combined with community mobilization and environmental change, can help advance obesity prevention and treatment in their community. The AAP recommends that BMI assessment occur at each well-child visit starting at age 2 years.

Policy and environmental support for BMI screening may occur at a variety of levels. Pediatricians may work to create policies and systems within their clinics or hospitals to more effectively and easily assess and track BMI beginning with 2-year-old patients. Within communities, there are school-based initiatives to track BMI; these initiatives may be more relevant for children in kindergarten and beyond, although communities may work with child care centers to implement BMI screening initiatives for preschoolers. Community-level BMI screening may occur outside out of the school setting and also reach young children and their families; Shape Up Somerville in Somerville, MA, USA, is an example of a community that undertook a multipronged intervention with support from city leadership and saw reductions in children's BMI z scores.[77,78] Roughly 30 states have proposed or implemented statewide legislation for BMI assessment and tracking, as did Arkansas in its public schools.[79–81]

On the national level, the White House Task Force has set a goal for 100% of physicians to assess and track BMI in patients aged 2 years and more by 2012. The AAP has pledged 100% screening among its membership.[82] These efforts are supported by an Affordable Care Act provision at the health care policy level requiring that health plans cover screening for obesity without out-of-pocket costs to patients and families. Health plans additionally may set policies tying BMI assessment to payment. In a state system where there is more than one option for Medicaid managed care plans, the state may increase the proportion of previously unassigned new enrollees to be assigned to those plans that meet or exceed quality performance criteria such as the rate of BMI assessment.

BMI screening and monitoring is an example of overlap between measurement, quality improvement, and policy. A variety of stakeholders desire to improve quality of care and patient outcomes. Clinicians wish to identify children in need of counseling and follow-up, so their practices may begin to monitor BMI. Health plans wish to encourage monitoring, so they may build BMI monitoring into contracts and payment policies. Moving up a level, states want BMI data for monitoring population-level trends, so they may require BMI reporting, tracking, and monitoring and may facilitate entry into BMI registry systems. On the federal level, the Health Resources and Services Administration implemented a new data collection measure for all federally supported community health centers that tracks BMI assessment and counseling for pediatric patients.[41] Policies on BMI screening and monitoring thus may have far-reaching impacts, from improving health care quality to being used as assessment and monitoring tools for policy. The goal of all these efforts is, ultimately, improving information access, counseling, and care for patients and families.

NEXT STEPS: EVALUATING POLICY CHANGE AND PROMOTING HEALTH CARE PROFESSIONAL ADVOCACY
Evaluating and Monitoring Policy Change

A critical component regarding all the environmental and policy change strategies we have outlined is evaluation of both the implementation and effectiveness of those strategies as well as ongoing monitoring of policies once they are enacted. Once a bill is passed, there still must be ongoing advocacy for its effective implementation as well as monitoring and technical assistance to ensure that the intent of the original policy is fulfilled. In addition, there should be evaluation efforts to assess the implementation and effectiveness of policy. Although it is true that funding for evaluation research may be challenging, there are certain funding mechanisms to support research and evaluation, and state and federal programs may also require evaluation. The 2008 Farm Bill, for example, funded pilot projects such as the Healthy Incentives Pilot regarding use of SNAP cards at farmers' markets and also the evaluation of that project regarding whether fruit and vegetable use increased as a result of that program.[51] Ongoing monitoring as well as research on implementation, effectiveness, and return on investment are critical in understanding past policy change and setting policies in the future.

Role of health care professionals as advocates and resources for advocacy

Health care professionals themselves, including and perhaps especially pediatricians, have a unique and important role in promoting policy change and environments that support healthy weight. Pediatric health care professionals have daily exposure to the childhood obesity epidemic via the patients they treat, and they are trusted leaders in and resources for their communities.[83,84] Their scientific and clinical knowledge of the epidemic coupled with this trusted community role position health care professionals to participate in community-based advocacy outside their clinics.[85] Indeed, expert committees and professional organizations have called on health care professionals to collaborate with the public health community and to engage in community-based advocacy, and research has demonstrated that many clinicians are interested in advocacy.[86–91]

In response to this opportunity, the National Initiative for Children's Healthcare Quality, in partnership with the AAP, the California Medical Association Foundation, and the Robert Wood Johnson Center to Prevent Childhood Obesity created the Be Our Voice project with support from the Robert Wood Johnson Foundation. The project provides training and follow-up support to primary care providers to participate in community-based public health advocacy for childhood obesity prevention in their communities. Pediatric providers can visit www.nichq.org/advocacy for resources, including an advocacy training curriculum, examples of success stories from 8 Be Our Voice pilot communities, state fact sheets on policy issues affecting childhood obesity (eg, overall prevalence rates compared with other states and disparities by race/ethnicity, insurance status, and income level), and county-level fact sheets that compare healthy lifestyle indicators in one county to those of the entire state and its best-performing counties.

Additional resources are available to help guide providers in taking the first steps in advocacy and community engagement. At the national level, they include listservs from the AAP, Families USA, Voices for America's Children, and Zero to Three.[85] At the state level, state chapters of professional associations (eg, American Academy of Family Physicians) often lead advocacy efforts. On PreventObesity.net (www.preventobesity.net), people may connect with additional sources of data, individuals, or organizations in their area of advocacy interest.

SUMMARY

The earliest years of a child's life provide a key opportunity for supporting a developmental trajectory that will encourage healthy weight. Throughout this paper, we have highlighted a variety of policy strategies to promote environments that will support breastfeeding, foster access to healthy and affordable food and information about food, and promote physical activity. We have included policies on levels from the microinstitutional (eg, hospital/clinic) and community to more macro and public state and federal government levels and noted the importance of evaluating and monitoring the implementation and effectiveness of policies once they are passed. The health care sector and pediatric health care professionals have a unique and important role to play, both in implementing health care system policies (eg, via promoting BMI screening and counseling) and in advocating for policies that support healthy weight on multiple levels in the clinic and wider community.

ACKNOWLEDGMENTS

The authors thank Lisa Simpson for her assistance with the framing of this manuscript.

REFERENCES

1. Levi J, Segal LM, St Laurent R, et al. F as in Fat 2011. Trust for America's Health and the Robert Wood Johnson Foundation; 2011. Available at: http://www.rwjf.org/childhoodobesity/product.jsp?id=72575&cid=XEM_1095291. Accessed July 7, 2011.
2. Ogden CL, Carroll MD, Curtin LR, et al. Prevalence of high body mass index in us children and adolescents, 2007-2008. JAMA 2010;303(3):242–9.
3. Centers for Disease Control and Prevention. Communities Putting Prevention to Work. Available at: http://www.cdc.gov/CommunitiesPuttingPreventiontoWork/index.htm. Accessed August 3, 2011.
4. Robert Wood Johnson Foundation. Our strategy—childhood obesity. Available at: http://www.rwjf.org/childhoodobesity/strategy.jsp. Accessed September 8, 2010.
5. White House Task Force on Childhood Obesity. White House Task Force on Childhood Obesity Report to the President: Solving the Problem of Childhood Obesity Within a Generation. 2010. Available at: http://www.letsmove.gov/obesitytaskforce.php. Accessed June 2, 2010.
6. Committee on Obesity Prevention Policies for Young Children, Institute of Medicine. Early childhood obesity prevention policies. In: Birch LL, Parker L, Burns A, editors. Washington, DC: The National Academies Press; 2011. Available at: http://www.iom.edu/Reports/2011/Early-Childhood-Obesity-Prevention-Policies.aspx. Accessed July 21, 2011.
7. Laughlin L. Who's minding the kids? Child care arrangements: Spring 2005/Summer 2006. US Census Bureau; Available at: http://www.census.gov/population/www/socdemo/childcare.html. Accessed August 11, 2011. 2010. p. 26.
8. Kaphingst KM, Story M. Child care as an untapped setting for obesity prevention: state child care licensing regulations related to nutrition, physical activity, and media use for preschool-aged children in the United States. Prev Chronic Dis 2009;6(1). Available at: http://www.cdc.gov/pcd/issues/2009/jan/07_0240.htm. Accessed August 3, 2011.
9. Benjamin S, Cradock A, Walker E, et al. Obesity prevention in child care: a review of U.S. state regulations. BMC Public Health 2008;8(1):188.
10. Committee on Public Education. Children, adolescents, and television. Pediatrics 2001;107(2):423–6.
11. American Academy of Pediatrics, American Public Health Association, National Resource Center for Health and Safety in Child Care and Early Education. Caring for our children: national health and safety performance standards; guidelines for

early care and education programs. 3rd edition. 2011. Available at: http://nrckids. org/CFOC3/index.html. Accessed August 4, 2011.

12. Ip S, Raman G, Priscilla C, et al. Breastfeeding and maternal and infant health outcomes in developed countries. Rockville (MD): Agency for Healthcare Research and Quality; 2007. Available at: http://www.ahrq.gov/clinic/tp/brfouttp. htm. Accessed July 20, 2011.

13. Owen CG, Martin RM, Whincup PH, et al. Effect of infant feeding on the risk of obesity across the life course: a quantitative review of published evidence. Pediatrics 2005;115(5):1367–77.

14. Monasta L, Batty GD, Cattaneo A, et al. Early-life determinants of overweight and obesity: a review of systematic reviews. Obes Rev 2010;11(10):695–708.

15. CDC's Division of Nutrition, Physical Activity, and Obesity (DNPAO). Breastfeeding: Data: Report Card 2010. Available at: http://www.cdc.gov/breastfeeding/ data/reportcard.htm. Accessed July 20, 2011.

16. Taveras EM, Gillman MW, Kleinman K, et al. Racial/ethnic differences in early-life risk factors for childhood obesity. Pediatrics 2010;125(4):686–95.

17. U.S. Department of Health and Human Services. Healthy People 2020—maternal, infant, and child health objectives. Available at: http://www.healthypeople.gov/ 2020/topicsobjectives2020/objectiveslist.aspx?topicid=26. Accessed July 20, 2011.

18. Section on Breastfeeding. Breastfeeding and the use of human milk. Pediatrics 2005;115(2):496–506.

19. The World Health Organization. The World Health Organization's infant feeding recommendation. 2002. Available at: http://www.who.int/nutrition/topics/ infantfeeding_recommendation/en/index.html. Accessed July 20, 2011.

20. Committee on Health Care for Underserved Women. Committee on Obstetric Practice, ACOG. Breastfeeding: maternal and infant aspects. ACOG Clin Rev 2007;12(Suppl 1):1S–16S.

21. World Health Organization. Exclusive breastfeeding. Available at: http://www. who.int/nutrition/topics/exclusive_breastfeeding/en/. Accessed July 20, 2011.

22. World Health Organization, UNICEF. Protecting, promoting and supporting breastfeeding. Geneva, Switzerland: World Health Organization; 1989. Available at: http:// www.who.int/nutrition/publications/infantfeeding/9241561300/en/. Accessed July 27, 2011.

23. Baby-Friendly USA. The Ten Steps to Successful Breastfeeding. East Sandwich (MA): Baby-Friendly USA; Available at: http://www.babyfriendlyusa.org/eng/ docs/BFUSAreport.pdf. Accessed July 27, 2011.

24. Anon. CDC Vital signs—hospital support for breastfeeding. Available at: http:// www.cdc.gov/vitalsigns/Breastfeeding/index.html. Accessed August 3, 2011.

25. The Joint Commission. Specifications manual for Joint Commission National Quality Core Measures (v2011A). 2011. Available at: http://manual.jointcommission.org/ releases/TJC2011A/. Accessed July 20, 2011.

26. Flaherman VJ, Newman TB. Regulatory monitoring of feeding during the birth hospitalization. Pediatrics 2011;127(6):1177–9.

27. Perrine CG, Li R, Grummer-Strawn LM. The truth about exclusive breastfeeding during the hospital stay. Pediatrics 2011 [online letters]. Available at: http:// pediatrics.aappublications.org.ezp-prod1.hul.harvard.edu/content/127/6/1177/ reply#pediatrics_el_51546. Accessed August 14, 2011.

28. Labbok M, Marinelli KA. Support for exclusive breastfeeding (no formula supplements given) during hospital stay is associated with women achieving their exclusive breastfeeding intentions—will a joint commission indicator cause harm?

Pediatrics 2011 [online letters]. Available at: http://pediatrics.aappublications. org.ezp-prod1.hul.harvard.edu/content/127/6/1177/reply#pediatrics_el_51546. Accessed August 14, 2011.

29. Institute of Medicine (U.S.). Committee on Preventive Services for Women. Clinical preventive services for women: closing the gaps. Washington, DC: 2011. Available at: http://www.iom.edu/Reports/2011/Clinical-Preventive-Services-for-Women-Closing-the-Gaps.aspx. Accessed July 20, 2011.

30. Health Resources and Services Administration. Women's Preventive Services: required health plan coverage guidelines. 2011. Available at: http://www.hrsa. gov/womensguidelines/. Accessed August 4, 2011.

31. US Department of Health and Human Services. Affordable Care Act ensures women receive preventive services at no additional cost. 2011. Available at: http://www.hhs.gov/news/press/2011pres/08/20110801b.html. Accessed August 4, 2011.

32. Rep. Charles Rangel. H.R. 3590 [111th]. Patient Protection and Affordable Care Act. 2010. Available at: http://www.govtrack.us/congress/bill.xpd?bill=h111-3590. Accessed August 11, 2011.

33. Anon. Patient Protection and Affordable Care Act. Section 4207. Reasonable break time for nursing mothers. 2010. Available at: http://www.usbreastfeeding.org/ Portals/0/Workplace/HR3590-Sec4207-Nursing-Mothers.pdf. Accessed August 4, 2011.

34. Wisconsin Department of Health Services; Nutrition, Physical Activity and Obesity Program of the Division of Public Health. Ten steps to breastfeeding friendly child care centers resource kit. Wisconsin Department of Health Services; 2009. Available at: http://www.dhs.wisconsin.gov/health/physicalactivity/ pdf_files/BreastfeedingFriendlyChildCareCenters.pdf. Accessed August 14, 2011. p. 29.

35. Dietz W, Lee J, Wechsler H, et al. Health plans' role in preventing overweight in children and adolescents. Health Aff 2007;26(2):430–40.

36. Anzman SL, Rollins BY, Birch LL. Parental influence on children's early eating environments and obesity risk: implications for prevention. Int J Obes 2010; 34(7):1116–24.

37. Rank MR, Hirschl TA. Estimating the risk of food stamp use and impoverishment during childhood. Arch Pediatr Adolesc Med 2009;163(11):994–9.

38. Food and Nutrition Service, US Department of Agriculture. WIC fact sheet. Alexandria (VA): Food and Nutrition Service, US Department of Agriculture; 2011. Available at: http://www.fns.usda.gov/wic/wic-fact-sheet.pdf. Accessed August 18, 2011. p. 4.

39. Committee to Review Child and Adult Care Food Program Meal Requirements of the Institute of Medicine. Child and adult care food program: aligning dietary guidance for all. In: Murphy SP, Yaktine AL, Suitor CW, et al, editors. Washington, DC: National Academies Press; 2011. Available at: http://www.iom.edu/Reports/ 2010/Child-and-Adult-Care-Food-Program-Aligning-Dietary-Guidance-for-All.aspx? utm_medium=etmail&utm_source=Institute%20of%20Medicine&utm_campaign= 11.04.10+Report+-+Child+and+Adult+Care+Food+Program&utm_content= New%20Reports&utm_term=Non-profit. Accessed August 4, 2011.

40. Food and Nutrition Service, US Department of Agriculture. WIC farmers' market nutrition program fact sheet. 2011. Available at: http://www.fns.usda.gov/wic/ fmnp/fmnpfaqs.htm. Accessed August 18, 2011.

41. Kimbro RT, Rigby E. Federal food policy and childhood obesity: a solution or part of the problem? Health Aff 2010;29(3):411–8.

42. Mikkelsen L, Chehimi S. The links between the neighborhood food environment and childhood nutrition—RWJF. Oakland (CA): Prevention Institute for the Robert Wood Johnson Foundation; 2007. Available at: http://www.rwjf.org/programareas/resources/product.jsp?id=23551. Accessed August 8, 2011. p. 36.

43. Larson NI, Story MT, Nelson MC. Neighborhood environments: disparities in access to healthy foods in the U.S. Am J Prev Med 2009;36(1):74–81.e10.

44. Ver Ploeg M, Breneman V, Farrigan T, et al. Access to affordable and nutritious food—measuring and understanding food deserts and their consequences: report to Congress. USDA Economic Research Service; 2009. Available at: http://www.ers.usda.gov/publications/ap/ap036/. Accessed August 3, 2011. p. 160.

45. White House Task Force on Childhood Obesity. White House Task Force on childhood obesity: one year progress report. Washington, DC: White House; 2011. Available at: http://www.letsmove.gov/sites/letsmove.gov/files/Obesity_update_report.pdf. Accessed August 2, 2011. p. 6.

46. US Department of Health and Human Services, Office of Community Services. Healthy Food Financing Initiative. 2011. Available at: http://www.acf.hhs.gov/programs/ocs/ocs_food.html. Accessed August 15, 2011.

47. Harris JL, Schwartz MB, Brownell KD. Marketing foods to children and adolescents: licensed characters and other promotions on packaged foods in the supermarket. Public Health Nutr 2010;13(3):409–17.

48. Roberto CA, Baik J, Harris JL, et al. Influence of licensed characters on children's taste and snack preferences. Pediatrics 2010;126(1):88–93.

49. Federal Trade Commission. Marketing food to children and adolescents: a review of industry expenditures, activities, and self-regulation, a report to congress. Washington, DC: Federal Trade Commission; 2008. Available at: http://www.ftc.gov/os/2008/07/P064504foodmktingreport.pdf. Accessed August 18, 2011. p. 120.

50. Kolish ED. The children's food & beverage advertising initiative white paper on CFBAI's uniform nutrition criteria. Arlington (VA): Council of Better Business Bureaus; 2011. Available at: http://www.bbb.org/us/storage/16/documents/cfbai/White-Paper-on-CFBAI-Uniform-Nutrition-Criteria-July-2011.pdf. Accessed August 10, 2011. p. 41.

51. Alliance for American Advertising. Re: Interagency working group on food marketed to children: general comments and proposed marketing definitions. FTC Project No. P094513. 2011. Available at: http://www.aaaa.org/advocacy/gov/news/Documents/071511_comments_food.pdf. Accessed August 14, 2011.

52. Public Health Law Center. Interagency Working Group on Food Marketed to Children: proposed nutrition principles: FTC Project No. P094513. Interagency Working Group on Food Marketed to Children: general comments and proposed marketing definitions: FTC Project No. P094513. 2011. Available at: http://publichealthlawcenter.org/sites/default/files/resources/phlc-comments-iwg-nutritionstdsandmarketingdefs-2011.pdf. Accessed August 14, 2011.

53. Drewnowski A, Specter S. Poverty and obesity: the role of energy density and energy costs. Am J Clin Nutr 2004;79(1):6–16.

54. Drewnowski A, Darmon N. The economics of obesity: dietary energy density and energy cost. Am J Clin Nutr 2005;82(1):265S–73S.

55. Anon. Policy brief—the Farm Bill. Dallas (TX): American Heart Association; 2011. Available at: http://www.heart.org/idc/groups/heart-public/@wcm/@adv/documents/downloadable/ucm_429110.pdf. Accessed August 8, 2011. p. 15.

56. Buzby JC, Wells HF, Vocke G. Possible implications for U.S. agriculture from adoption of select dietary guidelines. USDA Economic Research Service; 2006. Available at: http://www.ers.usda.gov/Publications/ERR31/. Accessed August 8, 2011. p. 35.

57. Fox MK, Condon E, Briefel RR, et al. Food consumption patterns of young preschoolers: are they starting off on the right path? J Am Diet Assoc 2010; 110(12 Suppl 1):S52–9.

58. Reedy J, Krebs-Smith SM. Dietary sources of energy, solid fats, and added sugars among children and adolescents in the United States. J Am Diet Assoc 2010;110(10):1477–84.

59. Andreyeva T, Chaloupka FJ, Brownell KD. Estimating the potential of taxes on sugar-sweetened beverages to reduce consumption and generate revenue. Prev Med 2011;52(6):413–6. Available at: http://www.yaleruddcenter.org/resources/upload/docs/what/economics/SSBTaxesPotential_PM_4.11.pdf. Accessed August 8, 2011.

60. French SA. Pricing effects on food choices. J Nutr 2003;133(3):841S–3S.

61. Anon. Wholesome wave. Available at: http://wholesomewave.org/. Accessed August 9, 2011.

62. Ryan A. Vouchers double value of food stamps at Boston farmers' markets. Boston Globe. 2009. Available at: http://www.boston.com/news/local/breaking_news/2009/06/vouchers_double.html. Accessed August 9, 2011.

63. Office of Disease Prevention and Health Promotion, Department of Health and Human Services. Dietary Guidelines for Americans 2010. 2011. Available at: http://health.gov/dietaryguidelines/2010.asp. Accessed August 9, 2011.

64. Food Research & Action Center. Highlights: Healthy, Hunger Free Kids Act of 2010. Available at: http://frac.org/highlights-healthy-hunger-free-kids-act-of-2010/. Accessed August 9, 2011.

65. Senator Blanche Lincoln. S. 3307 [111th]: Healthy, Hunger-Free Kids Act of 2010. 2010. Available at: http://www.govtrack.us/congress/bill.xpd?bill=s111-3307. Accessed August 9, 2011.

66. U.S. Department of Health and Human Services, Office of Disease Prevention and Health Promotion. 2008 Physical Activity Guidelines for Americans: Contents. Washington, DC. 2008. Available at: http://www.health.gov/paguidelines/guidelines/default.aspx. Accessed August 10, 2011.

67. US Department of Health and Human Services. The surgeon general's vision for a healthy and fit nation. Rockville (MD): US Department of Health and Human Services, Office of the Surgeon General; 2010. Available at: http://www.surgeongeneral.gov/library/obesityvision/index.html. Accessed August 10, 2011. p. 21.

68. Cradock ALI, O'Donnell EM, Benjamin SE, et al. A review of state regulations to promote physical activity and safety on playgrounds in child care centers and family child care homes. J Phys Act Health 2010;7(Suppl 1): S108–19.

69. Committee on Environmental Health. The built environment: designing communities to promote physical activity in children. Pediatrics 2009;123(6):1591–8.

70. Zhao Z, Kaestner R. Effects of urban sprawl on obesity. National Bureau of Economic Research Working Paper Series; 2009. No. 15436. Available at: http://www.nber.org/papers/w15436. Accessed August 10, 2011.

71. National Complete Streets Coalition. Complete Streets. 2005. Available at: http://www.completestreets.org/. Accessed August 11, 2011.

72. Floriani V, Kennedy C. Promotion of physical activity in children. Curr Opin Pediatr 2008;20(1):90–5.

73. Grow HM, Saelens BE, Kerr J, et al. Where are youth active? Roles of proximity, active transport, and built environment. Med Sci Sports Exerc 2008;40(12): 2071–9.

74. NPLAN. Fifty-state scan of laws addressing community use of schools. 2010. Available at: http://www.nplanonline.org/nplan/products/community-use-charts. Accessed August 10, 2011.

75. Simpson L, Alendy C, Cooper J, et al. Childhood obesity: the role of health policy. Policy Sub-Committee of the Childhood Obesity Action Network, NICHQ; 2008. Available at: http://www.rwjf.org/childhoodobesity/product.jsp?id=35708. Accessed December 14, 2009.

76. Doolen J, Alpert PT, Miller SK. Parental disconnect between perceived and actual weight status of children: a metasynthesis of the current research [review]. J Am Acad Nurse Pract 2009;21(3):160–6.

77. Cislak A, Safron M, Pratt M, et al. Family-related predictors of body weight and weight-related behaviours among children and adolescents: a systematic umbrella review. Child: Care, Health and Development. Available at: http://onlinelibrary.wiley.com.ezp-prod1.hul.harvard.edu/doi/10.1111/j.1365-2214.2011.01285.x/abstract. Accessed August 18, 2011.

78. Taveras EM, Gortmaker SL, Hohman KH, et al. Randomized controlled trial to improve primary care to prevent and manage childhood obesity: the high five for kids study. Arch Pediatr Adolesc Med 2011;165(8):714–22.

79. Wake M, Baur LA, Gerner B, et al. Outcomes and costs of primary care surveillance and intervention for overweight or obese children: the LEAP 2 randomised controlled trial. BMJ 2009;339:b3308.

80. Economos CD, Curtatone JA. Shaping up Somerville: a community initiative in Massachusetts. Prev Med 2010;50(Suppl 1):S97–8.

81. Economos CD, Hyatt RR, Goldberg JP, et al. A community intervention reduces BMI z-score in children: shape up Somerville first year results. Obesity (Silver Spring) 2007;15(5):1325–36.

82. Thompson JW, Card-Higginson P. Arkansas' experience: statewide surveillance and parental information on the child obesity epidemic. Pediatrics 2009; 124(Suppl):S73–82.

83. Ryan KW, Card-Higginson P, McCarthy SG, et al. Arkansas fights fat: translating research into policy to combat childhood and adolescent obesity. Health Aff 2006;25(4):992–1004.

84. Longjohn M, Sheon AR, Card-Higginson P, et al. Learning from state surveillance of childhood obesity. Health Aff 2010;29(3):463–72.

85. American Academy of Pediatrics. Prepared remarks by Judith S. Palfrey, MD, FAAP, President, American Academy of Pediatrics: launch of First Lady of the United States Michelle Obama's "Let's Move!" campaign. 2010. Available at: http://www.aap.org/obesity/whitehouse/PalfreyObesityInitiativeRemarks.pdf. Accessed August 9, 2011.

86. Boyle M, Lawrence S, Schwarte L, et al. Health care providers' perceived role in changing environments to promote healthy eating and physical activity: baseline findings from health care providers participating in the healthy eating, active communities program. Pediatrics 2009;123(Suppl 5):S293–300.

87. Homer C, Barlow SE, Bolling CF, et al. The primary care pediatrician's role in obesity prevention, assessment, and management: voices of experience. Childhood Obesity 2011;7(3):169–76.

88. Armstrong SC, Best D, McPherson ME. Fighting childhood obesity: resources to help the community pediatrician curb this epidemic. Contemp Pediatr 2011; 28(2):40–51.

89. Committee on Nutrition, Krebs NF, Jacobson MS. Prevention of pediatric overweight and obesity. Pediatrics 2003;112(2):424–30.

90. Committee on Community Health Services, Rushton FE. The pediatrician's role in community pediatrics. Pediatrics 2005;115(4):1092–4.
91. Barlow SE, Expert committee. Expert committee recommendations regarding the prevention, assessment, and treatment of child and adolescent overweight and obesity: summary report. Pediatrics 2007;120(Suppl):S164–92.

Index

Note: Page numbers of article titles are in **boldface** type.

A

Academic performance, physical activity effects on, 1481–1485
Accelerometers, 1513–1514
Aceulfame, 1468–1469, 1474
Activity. *See* Physical activity.
Added sugars, **1455–1466**
    consumption of
        guidelines for, 1460–1461
        patterns for, 1457
        reduction of, 1461–1462, 1529
    definition of, 1455–1456
    examples of, 1456–1458
    health outcomes associated with, 1459–1460
    metabolism of, 1460
    obesity and, 1457, 1459–1460
    reasons for adding, 1455–1456
    statistics on, 1455
    versus artificial sweeteners, 1472
    versus naturally occurring sugars, 1456–1457
Addiction pathways, artificial sweetener effects on, 1474–1476
Adenovirus infections, obesity in, 1338
Adipocytokines, in NAFLD, 1382
Adiponectin
    in NAFLD, 1381–1382
    in weight control, 1336
Adiponutirin gene, in NAFLD, 1383
Adipose tissue, distribution of, 1357
Adiposity rebound, 1342
Adjustable gastric band, 1435
Advertising, of food products, 1497–1499
Advocacy, for policy change, 1534
Aerobic fitness, 1483
Agouti-related peptide, in weight control, 1336
Agricultural policy, 1528–1529
Albright hereditary osteodystrophy, 1338
American Academy of Pediatrics
    lipoprotein levels recommendations of, 1364
    obesity recommendations of, 1411–1412
    on artificial sweeteners, 1470–1471
    on screen viewing time, 1523
    television viewing limits of, 1486, 1501

Pediatr Clin N Am 58 (2011) 1543–1555
doi:10.1016/S0031-3955(11)00162-3
0031-3955/11/$ – see front matter © 2011 Elsevier Inc. All rights reserved.

pediatric.theclinics.com

M

N

Moving?

Make sure your subscription moves with you!

To notify us of your new address, find your **Clinics Account Number** (located on your mailing label above your name), and contact customer service at:

Email: journalscustomerservice-usa@elsevier.com

800-654-2452 (subscribers in the U.S. & Canada)
314-447-8871 (subscribers outside of the U.S. & Canada)

Fax number: 314-447-8029

Elsevier Health Sciences Division
Subscription Customer Service
3251 Riverport Lane
Maryland Heights, MO 63043